AF606490

INBORN ERRORS OF CALCIUM AND BONE METABOLISM

*Previous Symposia of the Society for the Study of Inborn Errors of Metabolism**

1. *Neurometabolic Disorders in Childhood. Ed. K. S. Holt and J. Milner 1963*
2. *Biochemical Approaches to Mental Handicap in Children. Ed. J. D. Allan and K. S. Holt 1964*
3. *Basic Concepts of Inborn Errors and Defects of Steroid Biosynthesis. Ed. K. S. Holt and D. N. Raine 1965*
4. *Some Recent Advances in Inborn Errors of Metabolism. Ed. K. S. Holt and V. P. Coffey 1966*
5. *Some Inherited Disorders of Brain and Muscle. Ed. J. D. Allan and D. N. Raine 1969*
6. *Enzymopenic Anaemias, Lysosomes and other papers. Ed. J. D. Allan, K. S. Holt, J. T. Ireland and R. J. Pollitt 1969*
7. *Errors of Phenylalanine Thyroxine and Testosterone Metabolism. Ed. W. Hamilton and F. P. Hudson 1970*
8. *Inherited Disorders of Sulphur Metabolism. Ed. N. A. J. Carson and D. N. Raine 1971*
9. *Organic Acidurias. Ed. J. Stern and C. Toothill 1972*
10. *Treatment of Inborn Errors of Metabolism. Ed. J. W. T. Seakins, R. A. Saunders and C. Toothill 1973*
11. *Inborn Errors of Hair, Skin and Connective Tissue. Ed. J. B. Holton and J. T. Ireland 1975*

The Society exists to promote exchanges of ideas between workers in different disciplines who are interested in any aspect of inborn metabolic disorders. Particulars of the Society can be obtained from the Editors of this Symposium.

*Symposia 1–10 published by E. & S. Livingstone

INBORN ERRORS OF CALCIUM AND BONE METABOLISM

MONOGRAPH BASED UPON
Proceedings of the Twelfth Symposium of
The Society for the Study of Inborn Errors of Metabolism

EDITED BY
H. Bickel
and
J. Stern

University Park Press
Baltimore

Published in USA and Canada by
University Park Press
Chamber of Commerce Building
Baltimore, Maryland, 21202

Published in UK by
MTP Press Ltd.
St. Leonards House
Lancaster, England

© 1976 MTP Press Ltd.

No part of this book may be reproduced in any form without permission from the publisher except for the quotation of brief passages for the purpose of review

Library of Congress Cataloging in Publication Data
Society for the Study of Inborn Errors of Metabolism.
Inborn errors of calcium and bone metabolism.

(Symposia of the Society for the Study of Inborn Errors of Metabolism; 12)
1. Bones—Diseases—Genetic aspects—Congresses.
2. Metabolism, Inborn errors of—Congresses.
I. Bickel, Horst. II. Stern, Jan. III. Title. IV. Series: Society for the Study of Inborn Errors of Metabolism. Symposia; 12.
RC930.S6 1976 · 616.7'1'042 76-6502
ISBN 0-8391-0853-2

Printed in Great Britain

Contents

Preface

For its 12th symposium the Society for the Study of Inborn Errors of Metabolism met in the ancient and illustrious university town of Heidelberg. The principal topic for discussion was 'Inborn Errors of Calcium and Bone Metabolism'—an apt choice in view of the important advances made in recent years in our understanding of bone disease. The pathways leading to the synthesis of 1,25-dihydroxycholecalciferol, the metabolically active form of vitamin D, have been elucidated, and sensitive and specific methods developed for the assay of parathyroid hormone. At the symposium, distinguished investigators from Europe and North America presented 18 papers which provide an up-to-date review of this important field, and besides contain much practical information not readily available elsewhere. In the third Milner Lecture Professor Charles Dent critically reviewed the rickets group of diseases from the unique perspective of the cases seen in his clinics over the past three decades.

A session of free communications, outside the main topic (nine papers) reflected on-going research by members of the Society, particularly in the field of aminoacidopathies, and included contributions on two recently discovered inborn errors of metabolism, α-aminoadipic aciduria and α-ketoadipic aciduria.

We are very grateful to Mr J. Milner for his generous support which made it possible to invite a number of eminent contributors. We are also greatly indebted to the City and University of Heidelberg for the warm welcome and hospitality to members of the Society, to the staff of the Kinderklinik, academic and non-academic for the smooth and efficient organisation of the meetings, and to Mrs J. Buck, Mrs S. Bones and the publishers for much appreciated help in the preparation of the manuscript.

Horst Bickel
Jan Stern

The following institutions and firms have contributed very kindly towards the cost of this meeting

Alete GmbH., München
Aponti GmbH., Köln
Bayer AG., Leverkusen
Behringwerke, Marburg
Boehringer Mannheim GmbH.
Braun B., Melsungen
CIBA Pharmazeutika, Wehr
Desitin-Werk C. Klinke GmbH., Hamburg
Dosch Karlheinz., Heidelberg
Engström GmbH., Darmstadt
Gödecke AG., Freiburg
Guttroff Friedr. GmbH., Reichholzheim
Heumann Ludwig & Co., Nürnberg
Hipp KG., Pfaffenhofen/llm
Hoechst Farbwerke AG., Frankfurt
Immuno GmbH., Heidelberg
Paul-Martini-Stiftung, Frankfurt
Milchwerke, Bielefeld
Milner Scientific, and Medical Research, Liverpool
Müller Karl, Heidelberg
Nutricia, Zoetermeer
Nestlé GmbH,. Frankfurt-Niederrad
Pfrimmer J. & Co., Erlangen
Rhein-Pharma GmbH., Heidelberg
Dr. Riese & Co., Rhöndorf
Sandoz AG., Nürnberg
Scientific Hospital Services, Liverpool
Springer Verlag, Heidelberg
Schering AG., Berlin
Schülke & Mayr GmbH., Hamburg
Upjohn GmbH., Heppenheim
Winthrop GmbH., Frankfurt

The editors wish to express the gratitude of all the members of the Society for the generous grants which have been received in support of this symposium from Mr J. Milner of Milner Scientific and Medical Research and to Scientific Hospital Services, Liverpool

Contributors and Active Participants

J. D. ALLAN
Paediatric Unit, West Park Hospital, Macclesfield, Cheshire, England.

K. BAERLOCHER
Kinderspital, Claudisstrasse, 9000 St Gallen, Switzerland.

SONIA BALSAN
Hôpital des Enfants Malades, 149 Rue de Sèvres, 75730 Paris Cedex 15, France.

K. BARTHOLOMÉ,
Universitäts-Kinderklinik, 6900 Heidelberg 1, Hofmeisterweg 1–9, West Germany.

G. F. BATSTONE
Division of Chemical Pathology, Southampton General Hospital, Southampton SO9 4XY, England.

N. R. BELTON
Department of Child Life and Health, University of Edinburgh, 17 Hatton Place, Edinburgh EH9 1UW, Scotland.

H. BICKEL
Universitäts-Kinderklinik, 6900 Heidelberg 1, Hofmeisterweg 1–9, West Germany.

U. BINSWANGER
Department of Medicine, University of Zürich, 8008 Zürich, Switzerland.

N. BLASKOVICS
Children's Hospital Los Angeles, 4650 Sunset Blvd., Los Angeles, California 90027, USA.

K. BLAU
Bernhard Baron Memorial Research Laboratories, Queen Charlotte's Maternity Hospital, Goldhawk Road, London W6 0XG, England.

W. BLOM
Sophia Children's Hospital, Gordelweg 160, Rotterdam, The Netherlands.

H. J. Bremer

Universitäts-Kinderklinik, Moorenstrasse 5, 4000 Düsseldorf 1, West Germany.

D. P. Brenton

Department of Human Metabolism, University College Hospital Medical School, University Street, London WC1E 6JJ, England.

J. BRODEHL

Medizinische Hochschule Hannover, Kinderklinik, 3 Hannover-Kleefeld, Karl-Wiechert-Allee 9, West Germany.

J. M. H. BUCKLER

Departments of Paediatrics and Child Health, University of Leeds, Leeds LS2 9NL, England.

N. R. M. BUIST

University of Oregon Medical School, Portland, Oregon 97225, USA.

F. CARNEVALE

Istituto Di Clinicia Pediatrica, Università Di Bari, 70124 Bari, Policlinica-Piazza Giulio Cesare, Italy.

NINA CARSON

Research Laboratory, Department of Child Health, Institute of Clinical Science, Grosvenor Road, Belfast BT12 6BJ, Northern Ireland.

C. O. CARTER

M.R.C. Clinical Genetics Unit, Institute of Child Health, 30 Guilford Street, London WC1N 1EH, England.

D. CARTON

Department of Pediatrics, Akademisch Ziekenhuis, De Pintelaan 135, 9000 Gent, Belgium.

BARBARA E. CLAYTON

Hospital for Sick Children, Great Ormond Street, London WC1N 3JH, England.

H. F. DELUCA

Department of Biochemistry, University of Wisconsin, Madison Wisconsin 53706, USA.

C. E. DENT

Department of Human Metabolism, University College Hospital Medical School, University Street, London WC1E 6JJ.

G. DI BITONTO

Istituto Di Clinica Pediatrica, Università Di Bari, 70124 Bari, Policlinico-Piazzo Giulio Cesare, Italy.

F. M. DIETRICH
Biological Research, Ciba-Geigy Ltd., R-1056.4.07, 4002 Basel, Switzerland.

J. F. DYMLING
Departments of Pathology and Endocrinology, Allmänna Sjukhuset, Malmö, Sweden.

R. S. ERSSER
Institute of Child Health, 30 Guilford Street, London WC1N 1EH, England.

ANGELA FAIRNEY
Department of Chemical Pathology, St Mary's Hospital Medical School, Praed Street, London W2 1NY, England.

A. FANCONI
Kinderklinik am Kantonspital, CH 8401 Winterthur, Switzerland.

J. A. FISCHER
Orthopädische Universitäts-Klinik Balgrist, Forchstrasse 346, CH 8008 Zürich, Switzerland.

M. H. FISCHER
Department of Pediatrics, University of Wisconsin Center for Health Sciences, Madison, Wisconsin 53706, USA.

D. FLYNN
Royal Free Hospital, Pond Street, London NW3 2QG, England.

B. FOWLER
Willink Clinical Genetics Unit, Pendlebury Children's Hospital, Pendlebury, Manchester M27 1HA, England.

R. GARABEDIAN
Hôpital des Enfants Malades, 149 Rue de Sèvres, 75730 Paris Cedex 15, France.

T. GERRITSEN
Room 613, Waisman Center, University of Wisconsin, 2605 Marsh Lane, Madison, Wisconsin 53706, USA.

R. GITZELMANN
Kinderspital, Steinwiesstrasse 75, CH 8032 Zürich, Switzerland.

F. H. GLORIEUX
DeBelle Laboratory for Biochemical Genetics McGill University—Montreal Children's Hospital Research Institute, 2300 Tupper Street, Montreal Qué. H3H 1P3, Canada.

D. GOMPERTZ

Department of Medicine, Royal Postgraduate Medical School, London, W12 0HS, England.

P. B. GREENBERG

Royal Melbourne Hospital, Parkville, Victoria, Australia 3050.

MARGARET I. GRIFFITH

Lea Castle Hospital, Welverly, Kidderminster, Worcester, England.

M. Th. Grimberg

Onze Lieve Vrouwe Gasthuis, Amsterdam, The Netherlands

F. HARRIS

Department of Child Health, Liverpool University, Alder Hey Hospital, Liverpool LI2 2AP, England.

CARMEL J. HILLYARD

Endocrine Unit, Royal Postgraduate Medical School, Ducane Road, London, W12 0HS, England.

M. F. HOLICK

Department of Biochemistry, University of Wisconsin, Madison, Wisconsin 53706, USA.

J. B. HOLTON

Biochemistry Department, Southmead Hospital, Westbury-on-Trym, Bristol BS10 5NB, England.

W. HUNZIKER

Orthopädische Universitäts-Klinik Balgrist, Forchstrasse 346, CH 8008 Zürich, Switzerland.

DOREEN JACKSON

Institute of Child Health, 30 Guilford Street, London WC1N 1EH, England.

H. P. KIND

Kinderspital, Steinwiesstrase 75, CH 8032 Zürich, Switzerland.

G. M. KOMROWER

Willink Clinical Genetics Unit, Pendlebury Children's Hospital, Pendlebury, Manchester M27 1HA, England.

O. LJUNGBERG

Departments of Pathology and Endrocrinology, Allmänna Sjukhuset, Malmö, Sweden.

INGRID LOMBECK

Universitäts-Kinderklinik, Moorenstrasse 5, 4000 Dusseldorf 1, West Germany.

P. LUTZ

Universitäts-Kinderklinik, 6900 Heidelberg 1, Hofmeisterweg 1–9, West Germany.

I. MACINTYRE

Endocrine Unit, Royal Postgraduate Medical School, Ducane Road, London W12 0HS, England.

O. MEHLS

Universitäts-Kinderklinik, 6900 Heidelberg 1, Hofmeisterweg 1–9, West Germany.

P. T. MOORE

St. James's Hospital, P.O. Box 580, Dublin 8, Ireland.

C. A. PENNOCK

Research Floor, Outpatients' Building, Bristol Royal Infirmary, Bristol BS2 8HW, England.

A. PRADER

Kinderspital, Steinwiesstrasse 75, CH 8032 Zürich, Switzerland.

Hildegard Przyrembel

Universitäts-Kinderklinik, 4000 Dusseldorf 1, Moorenstrasse 5, West Germany.

I. B. SARDHARWALLA

Willink Clinical Genetics Unit, Pendlebury Children's Hospital, Pendlebury, Manchester M27 1HA, England.

THERESA M. READE

DeBelle Laboratory for Biochemical Genetics McGill University—Montreal Children's Hospital Research Institute, 2300 Tupper Street, Montreal, Qué. H3H 1P3, Canada.

C. R. SCRIVER

DeBelle Laboratory for Biochemical Genetics McGill University—Montreal Children's Hospital Research Institute, 2300 Tupper Street, Montreal, Qué. H3H 1P3, Canada.

D. SCHEFFNER

Universitäts-Kinderklinik, 6900 Heidelberg 1, Hofmeisterweg 1–9, West Germany.

HILDEGARD SCHMIDT

Universitäts-Kinderklinik, 6900 Heidelberg 1, Hofmeisterweg 1–9, West Germany.

J. W. T. SEAKINS

Institute of Child Health, 30 Guilford Street, London WC1N 1EH, England.

A. C. SEWELL
Research Floor, Outpatients' Building, Bristol Royal Infirmary, Bristol BS2 8HW, England.

H. SHEPPARD
Department of Child Life and Health, University of Edinburgh, 17 Hatton Place, Edinburgh EH9 1UW, Scotland.

R. SMITH
Nuffield Department of Orthopaedic Surgery, Nuffield Orthopaedic Centre, Headington, Oxford OX3 7LD, England.

R. SORGNIARD
Hôpital des Enfants Malades, 149 Rue de Sèvres, 75730 Paris Cedex 15. France.

J. SPRANGER
Universitäts-Kinderklinik, 65 Mainz, West Germany.

T. C. B. STAMP
Royal National Orthopaedic Hospital, 234 Great Portland Street, London W1N 6AD, England.

S. W. STANBURY
Department of Medicine, The Royal Infirmary, Manchester M13 9WL, England.

R. STEENDIJK
Kinderklinik, Binnengasthuis, Amsterdam (C.), The Netherlands.

J. STERN
Queen Mary's Hospital for Children, Carshalton, Surrey SM5 4NR, England.

J. SYME
Department of Child Life and Health, University of Edinburgh, 17 Hatton Place, Edinburgh EH9 1UW, Scotland.

K. TADA
Department of Pediatrics, Osaka City University Medical School, Asahi-Machi, Abendo-Ku, Osaka, Japan.

W. TELLER
Universitäts-Kinderklinik, 79 Ulm 1/Donau, Prittwitzstrasse 43, West Germany.

H. S. TENENHOUSE
DeBelle Laboratory for Biochemical Genetics McGill University—Montreal Children's Hospital Research Institute, 2300 Tupper Street, Montreal, Qué. H3H 1P3, Canada.

C. TOOTHILL

Department of Paediatrics and Child Health, University of Leeds, Leeds LS2 9NL, England.

LINDA A. TYFIELD

Biochemistry Department, Southmead Hospital, Westbury on Trym, Britsol BS10 5NB, England.

N. S. UTTLEY

Department of Child Life and Health, University of Edinburgh, 17 Hatton Place, Edinburgh EH9 1UW, Scotland.

F. VECCHIO

Istituto di Clinica Pediatrica, Università di Bari, 70124 Bari, Policlinico-Piazza Guilio Cesare, Italy.

J. K. VISAKORPI

Teiskontie 37, 33520 Tampere 52, Finland.

S. K. WADMAN

Wilhelmina Kinderziekenhuis, Nieuwe Gracht 137, Utrecht, The Netherlands.

R. W. E. WATTS

M.R.C. Clinical Research Centre, Watford Road, Harrow, Middlesex HA1 3UJ, England.

U. WENDEL

Universitäts-Kinderklinik, Moorenstrasse 5, 4000 Düsseldorf 1, West Germany.

B. WINOKUR

Fieldhead Hospital, Wakefield, Yorkshire, England.

H. WOLF

Kinderklinik, Stadtkrankenhaus, 35 Kassel, Mönchberg Strasse 41–43 West Germany.

L. I. WOOLF

Kinsman Laboratory of Neurological Research, Department of Psychiatry, University of British Columbia, Vancouver 8 B.C., Canada.

I

Hormones derived from vitamin D : Their regulation and function

H. F. DeLuca

Introduction

During the past decade has come the remarkable discovery that vitamin D does not act directly on the target tissues of intestine and bone, but must be metabolically activated before it can carry out its important functions in mineral metabolism (Omdahl and DeLuca, 1973). In-depth investigation of these important phenomena has provided compelling evidence which shows that vitamin D is a prohormone giving rise to at least one and possibly more hormones. This hormone directs intestinal calcium and phosphorus absorption; the mobilisation of these mineral elements from previously formed bone and perhaps aids in the deposition of calcium and phosphate in the newly synthesised portions of bone. The endocrine system which uses vitamin D as its building block is located in the kidney and is regulated either directly or indirectly by serum calcium and serum phosphate concentrations. This system not only has great importance physiologically, but the application of the hormone(s) derived from vitamin D to bone disease in man is a very promising field of therapeutics. It will be the purpose of this communication to summarise the evidence which establishes the vitamin D endocrine system and to discuss possible medical applications of these findings.

Functions of vitamin D

It is well established that the primary function of vitamin D is to bring about normal mineralisation of bone (Omdahl and DeLuca, 1973; DeLuca, 1967). In the absence of any source of vitamin D, it is known that the disease rickets occurs in the young and osteomalacia in the adult; both diseases are characterised by a defect in the mineralisation process. It has been assumed that vitamin D must function in the mineralisation process *per se*, but so far evidence for this function is lacking. Although intellectually satisfying, the role for vitamin D or one of its active forms in this system remains to be established. It is known, however, that a deficiency of vitamin D results in a deficient supply of calcium and phosphate to the mineralisation sites (Shipley, *et al.*, 1925; Howland and Kramer, 1921). Thus in true deficiencies of vitamin D, serum calcium and/or phosphate concentrations fall below normal levels, which in turn results in a retardation of mineralisation. The essence of vitamin D function physiologically, therefore, is the elevation of plasma calcium and phosphate concentration to supersaturating levels. This is brought about by the stimulation of intestinal calcium absorption (Omdahl and DeLuca, 1973; Nicolaysen and Eeg-Larsen, 1953), intestinal phosphate absorption (Harrison and Harrison, 1961; Kowarski and Schachter, 1969; Wasserman and Taylor, 1973; Chen *et al.*, 1974) and a stimulation of the mobilisation of calcium and phosphate from previously formed bone mineral (Carlsson, 1952). The mobilisation of calcium from previously formed mineral requires the presence of parathyroid hormone (Harrison *et al.*, 1958; Rasmussen *et al.*, 1963). Both a form of vitamin D and the parathyroid hormone are required for this important physiologic process which plays a major role in the regulation of serum calcium concentration.

In the intestine, vitamin D activates an active calcium transport process in which metabolic energy is used to transfer calcium against an electro-chemical potential gradient (Omdahl and DeLuca, 1973). Vitamin D also activates independently a phosphate transport mechanism which has not been thoroughly studied at the present time.

At the kidney level it seems likely that vitamin D plays a role in renal tubular reabsorption of calcium (Gran, 1960; DeLuca *et al.*, 1974; Puschett *et al.*, 1972), but evidence to date suggests that it plays no role in renal tubular reabsorption of inorganic phosphorus.

In the case of all these functions, it is well known that there is a considerable lag between the time of vitamin D administration and the first appearance of a physiological response (Carlsson, 1952; DeLuca, 1969). This is illustrated in Figure 1.1, which shows that intestinal calcium transport does not respond immediately to an intravenous injection of vitamin D_3, but that a 10–12-hour period is required before the intestine responds. This is true for the bone calcium mobilisation system and for the intestinal phosphate transport system as well. Early

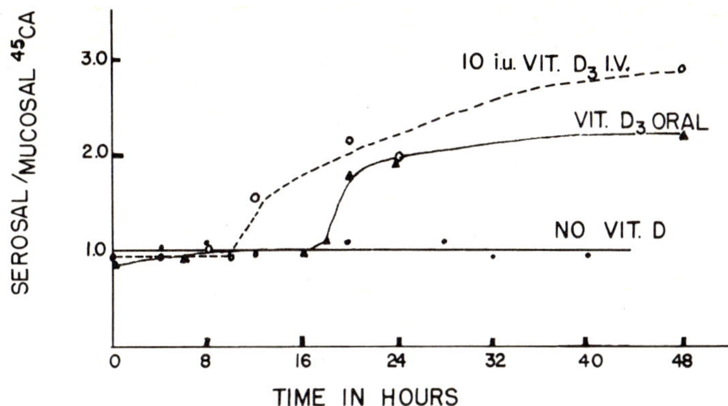

FIGURE 1.1 Time course of intestinal calcium transport response to a 0·25 μg dose of vitamin D_3 to rats.

work in our laboratory was directed at the biochemical reasons for this lag in vitamin D function. With radioactive vitamin D_3, which was successfully synthesised in our laboratory prior to 1966 (Neville and DeLuca, 1966), it was possible to demonstrate clearly that vitamin D disappears during the lag period and in its place appear polar metabolites (Lund and DeLuca, 1966). Following this demonstration and the demonstration that the polar metabolites possess biological activity, several important metabolites of the vitamin were isolated, identified and chemically synthesised (Blunt *et al.*, 1968; Blunt and DeLuca, 1969).

The path of functional vitamin D metabolism is shown in Figure 1.2. Vitamin D_3, which can be derived either from the skin by ultraviolet irradiation of the precursor 7-dehydrocholesterol, or from dietary sources, must largely go to the liver where it is hydroxylated on carbon-25 to form 25-hydroxyvitamin D_3 [25(OH)D_3] (Omdahl and DeLuca, 1973). This reaction is feed-back regulated by the liver level of 25(OH)D_3 in some unknown fashion (Bhattacharyya and DeLuca, 1974). The 25(OH)D_3 must then proceed to the kidney where it undergoes one of two different hydroxylations. If the animal is hypocalcaemic or hypophosphataemic, the 25(OH)D_3 is hydroxylated on carbon-1 to form 1,25-dihydroxyvitamin D_3 [1,25$(OH)_2D_3$] (Boyle *et al.*, 1972a; Tanaka and DeLuca, 1973). If on the other hand, the serum level of calcium and phosphorus are normal and the animal has been given a source of vitamin D, predominantly 24,25-dihydroxyvitamin D_3 [24,25$(OH)_2D_3$] is formed. To carry out the intestinal calcium transport function and the

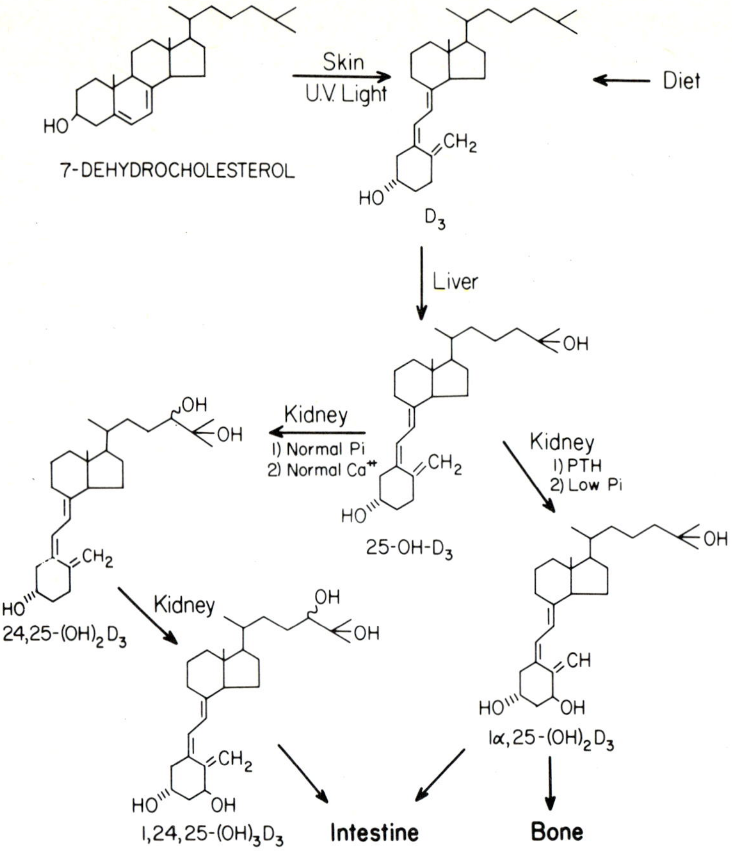

FIGURE 1.2 Functional metabolism of vitamin D_3.

bone calcium mobilisation function, the path must follow 25-hydroxylation followed by 1-hydroxylation.

The kidney as an endocrine organ for hormones derived from vitamin D

It is essential in this context to consider the evidence which established the kidney as an essential organ in the function of vitamin D. Following the identification of $25(OH)D_3$ in 1968, synthesis of this important metabolite was achieved which permitted the introduction of tritium into the side chain (Suda *et al.*, 1971) With the labelled metabolite it could be readily demonstrated that it is metabolised further before it can stimulate intestine and bone (DeLuca, 1970; Cousins, DeLuca *et al.*, 1970). Prior to the isolation and identification of 1,25$(OH)_2D_3$ came the discovery by Fraser and Kodicek (1970) establishing the kidney as the source of this metabolite. This important discovery was readily confirmed in our laboratory (Gray *et al.*, 1971). At the same time, however, we succeeded in isolating in pure form from the intestines of 1500 vitamin D-deficient chickens given radioactive vitamin D_3, the polar metabolite derived from 25$(OH)D_3$ (Holick *et al.*, 1971b). We were able to identify its structure as 1,25$(OH)_2D_3$ (Holick *et al.*, 1971b), and subsequently provide a chemical synthesis for it (Semmler *et al.*, 1972).

Thus it became clear that kidney tissue is the sole site of 1,25$(OH)_2D_3$ synthesis. Subsequent experiments on chick kidney preparations have revealed that the enzyme, 25$(OH)D_3$-1α-hydroxylase is exclusively a mitochondrial enzyme (Gray *et al.*, 1972), depends entirely on cytochrome P-450 (Ghazarian and DeLuca, 1974; Ghazarian *et al.*, 1974) and in all respects is a mixed-function oxidase (Ghazarian *et al.*, 1973). It has been successfully solubilised and is being studied in great detail biochemically.

The fact that the kidney is the exclusive site of synthesis made possible several experiments which demonstrate clearly that the kidney is an endocrine organ for the synthesis of the active form of vitamin D, which can in many respects be considered a hormone. Nephrectomised vitamin D-deficient animals do not respond to physiological doses of 25$(OH)D_3$ in terms of intestinal calcium transport or bone calcium mobilisation (Boyle *et al.*, 1972b; Holick *et al.*, 1972a). On the other hand, 1,25$(OH)_2D_3$ produces a clear response in intestine and bone in nephrectomised animals. Thus 1,25$(OH)_2D_3$ or a further metabolite is the metabolically active form of vitamin D in both intestine and bone. Further experiments revealed that 1,25$(OH)_2D_3$ is probably not metabolised further before it carries out these important functions (Frolik and DeLuca, 1971). Thus with the kidney as the sole source of 1,25$(OH)_2D_3$ one can visualise it as an endocrine organ producing a hormone which has its function in intestine and bone.

Regulation of the vitamin D endocrine system of kidney

Virtually all endocrine systems have some degree of feed-back regulation. The vitamin D dependent system of kidney is no exception. Following the work of Nicolaysen and his collaborators in 1937, it was recognised that animals fed a low calcium diet develop a high efficiency of intestinal calcium absorption, whereas those on high calcium diets have a low efficiency of intestinal calcium absorption (Nicolaysen *et al.*, 1953). Nicolaysen postulated the existence of an endogenous factor secreted by the skeleton which would direct the intestine to absorb calcium depending upon the skeletal needs. He further observed that the presence of vitamin D is required for this regulation to occur. We considered that $1,25(OH)_2D_3$ might well be the endogenous factor and dietary calcium might well regulate its synthesis. Examination of this question revealed that in fact animals maintained on a low calcium diet produce large amounts of $1,25(OH)_2D_3$, whereas those animals on a high calcium diet produce very little (Boyle *et al.*, 1971) When animals are made deficient in vitamin D this regulation does not occur. When the synthesis of $1,25(OH)_2D_3$ was turned off by high calcium diets, another metabolite was formed which was identified as $24,25(OH)_2D_3$ (Holick *et al.*, 1972b). These results, therefore, suggest very strongly that $1,25(OH)_2D_3$ may be the endogenous factor that

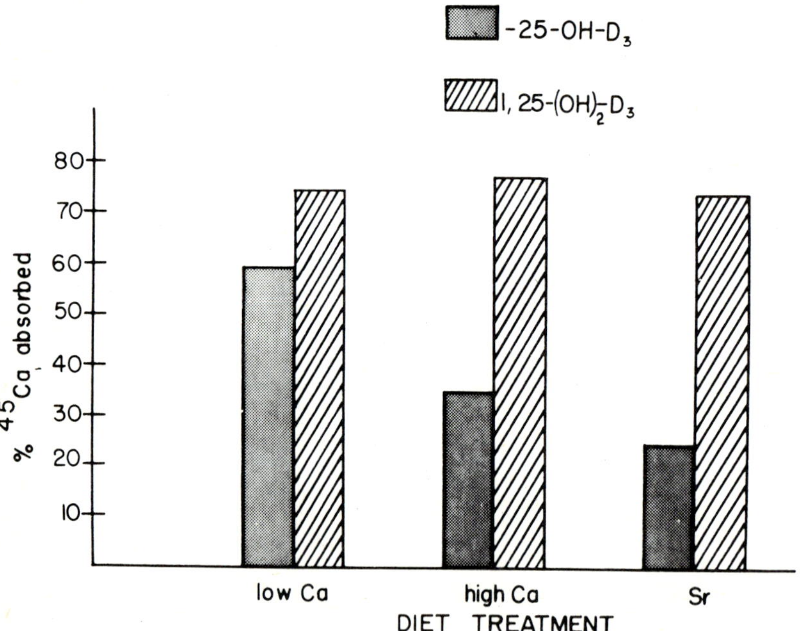

FIGURE 1.3 Failure of chicks given exogenous $1,25(OH)_2D_3$ to adapt to dietary calcium or strontium. Chicks were fed for 2 weeks on a low calcium, high calcium or strontium diet with either $25(OH)D_3$ or $1,25(OH)_2D_3$ supplement. Their intestinal calcium absorption rate was determined (Omdahl and DeLuca, 1973).

Nicolaysen had described. Proof of this was obtained when it could be shown that animals maintained on an exogenous source of $1,25(OH)_2D_3$ show high efficiencies of intestinal calcium absorption, independent of dietary calcium and strontium, whereas animals maintained on $25(OH)D_3$ show the expected adaptation (Omdahl and DeLuca, 1973) (Figure 1.3).

A major question, however, remained as to how the kidney was informed of either the skeletal need for calcium or dietary calcium level. The basis for this is shown in Figure 1.4 (Boyle *et al.*, 1972b). In both rats and chicks with intact parathyroid glands, there is a clear relationship between the synthesis of $1,25(OH)_2D_3$ and serum calcium concentration. At normal serum calcium levels, both $1,25(OH)_2D_3$ and

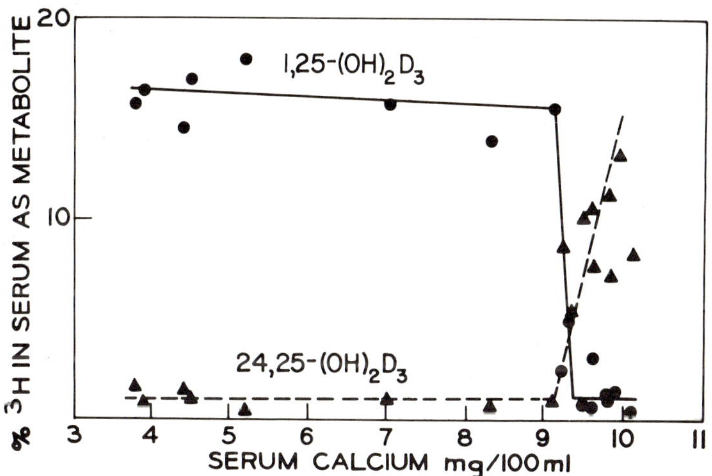

FIGURE 1.4 Relationship of serum calcium to the ability of rats to synthesise $1,25(OH)_2D_3$ or $24,25(OH)_2D_3$ (Boyle *et al.*, 1972a).

$24,25(OH)_2D_3$ are made. Under conditions of even slight hypocalcaemia the synthesis of $1,25(OH)_2D_3$ is turned on, whereas at normal to hypercalcaemia the synthesis of this hormone is shut down. Thus $1,25(OH)_2D_3$ is a hormone that mobilises calcium from both bone and intestine and its synthesis is regulated by the very product it seeks to affect, namely serum calcium concentration. Note that $24,25(OH)_2D_3$ whose function is unknown at the present time is synthesised whenever $1,25(OH)_2D_3$ synthesis is retarded.

The plot of serum calcium concentration versus $1,25(OH)_2D_3$ synthesis is very reminiscent of the parathyroid hormone secretion curve and suggests that the parathyroid hormone might well play a stimulatory role in the synthesis of 1,25$(OH)_2D_3$. We examined this question as shown in Figure 1.5 (Garabedian *et al.*, 1972). Animals fed a low calcium diet synthesise 1,25$(OH)_2D_3$ and no 24,25$(OH)_2D_3$. The initial double bar illustrates thyroparathyroidectomy. Following surgery the animals lose their ability to make 1,25$(OH)_2D_3$ and instead make 24,25$(OH)_2D_3$. The animals have completely lost their ability to make

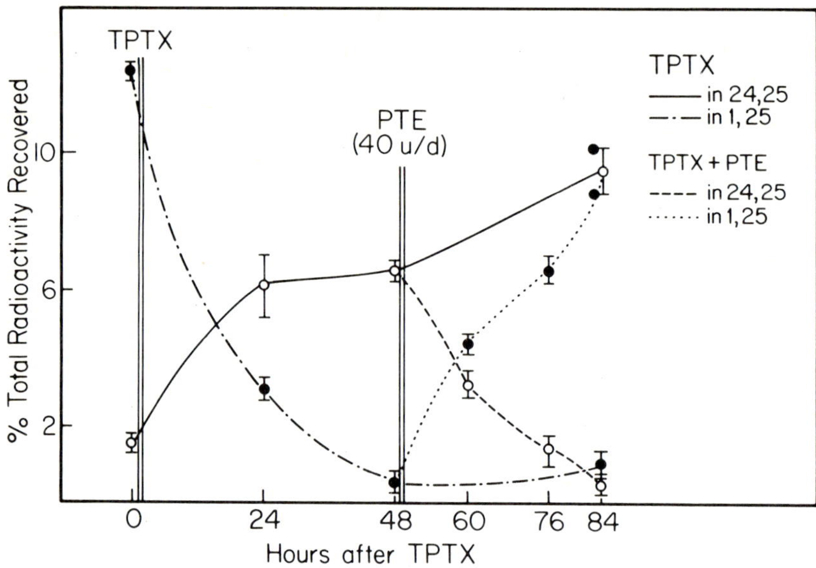

FIGURE 1.5 Role of parathyroid hormone in the regulation of vitamin D metabolism. Rats were fed a low calcium diet and thyroparathyroidectomised at the first double bar. Forty-eight hours later half the rats were given 10 units of parathyroid hormone every 6 hours (at second double bar). The *in vivo* synthesis of 1,25$(OH)_2D_3$ or 24,25$(OH)_2D_3$ was determined (Garabedian *et al.*, 1972).

1,25$(OH)_2D_3$ after 48 hours. At this stage restoration of 1,25$(OH)_2D_3$ synthesis is accomplished by administration of modest doses of parathyroid hormone (10 units/6 hours). This is accompanied by a shut down of 24,25$(OH)_2D_3$ synthesis. In experiments not shown here it could readily be demonstrated that the function of 1,25$(OH)_2D_3$ in intestine does not require the presence of parathyroid hormone whereas its function in bone requires that peptide hormone (Garabedian *et al.*, 1974). It could, therefore, be concluded that the function of parathyroid hormone in stimulating intestinal calcium transport is entirely mediated by its function in stimulating the synthesis of 1,25$(OH)_2D_3$.

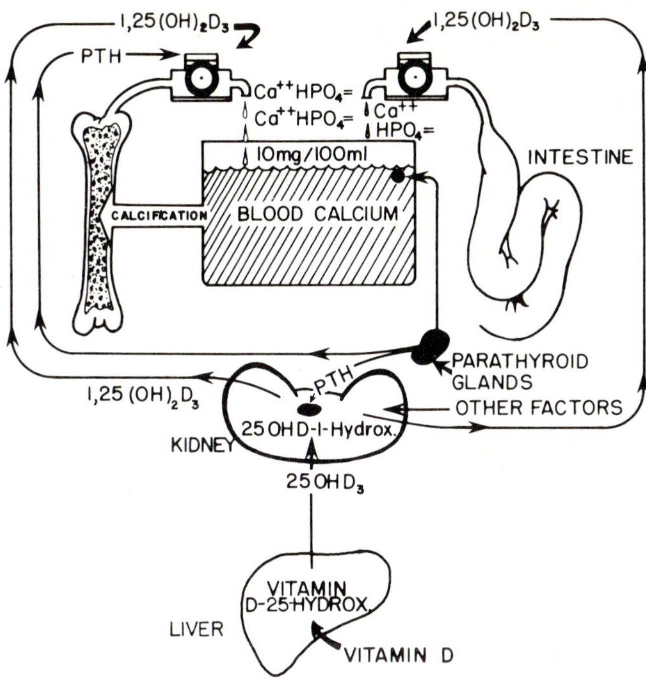

FIGURE 1.6 The role of the vitamin D endocrine system in calcium homeostasis.

A revision of the calcium homeostatic mechanism was, therefore, required (Figure 1.6). The sensing agent for serum calcium concentration is the parathyroid gland. Hypocalcaemia results in secretion of parathyroid hormone which acts directly on bone and which also acts on the kidney to stimulate synthesis of $1,25(OH)_2D_3$. The $1,25(OH)_2D_3$ proceeds to the intestine where it stimulates intestinal calcium transport without the parathyroid hormone and it proceeds to bone where, together with parathyroid hormone, mobilises calcium into the extracellular fluid. These two processes restore serum calcium to normal.

Role of vitamin D in phosphate metabolism

Vitamin D_3 has functions other than in the calcium homeostatic mechanism. Throughout the course of vitamin D investigation in recent years there has been an emphasis on its role in calcium metabolism with an ignorance of its role in phosphate metabolism. However, work from Harrison and Harrison (1961), Kowarski and Schachter (1969), and Wasserman and Taylor (1973) has suggested that vitamin D has an additional role in phosphate transport reactions. In the case of the rat it is known that the production of rickets requires not only a deficiency of vitamin D but also an accompanying deficiency of inorganic phosphate (McCollum *et al.*, 1922). The cure of the rachitic lesions in this species with some source of vitamin D is accompanied by a rise in serum phosphate concentration (McCollum *et al.*, 1922). During the course of

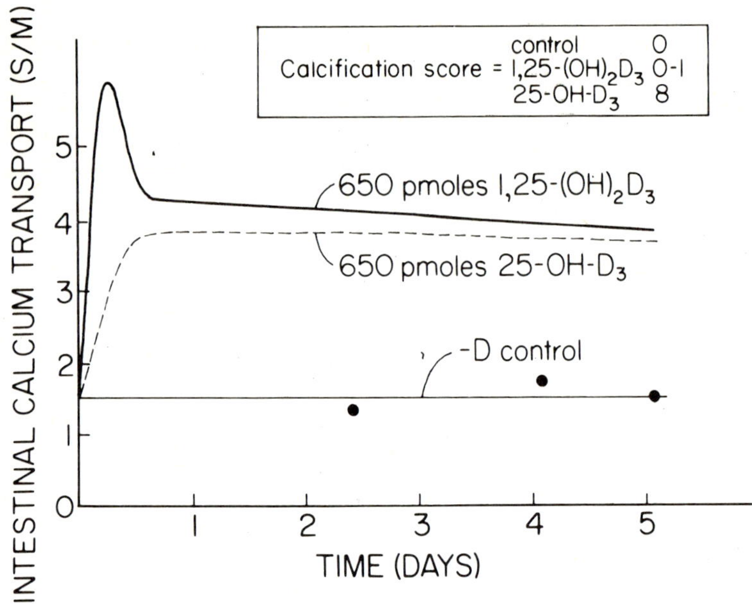

FIGURE 1.7 Intestinal calcium transport response of rachitic rats to a single 650 pmole dose of $25(OH)D_3$ or $1,25(OH)_2D_3$. Note the calcification score at the conclusion of the experiment (insert) (Tanaka and DeLuca, 1974).

our investigations of the effect of $1,25(OH)_2D_3$ in such animals we were surprised to learn that a single dose of $1,25(OH)_2D_3$ given intravenously resulted in the expected calcium transport response which was maintained over a period of 7 days as shown in Figure 1.7 (Tanaka and DeLuca, 1974). A similar dose of $25(OH)D_3$ did not produce the immediate response of $1,25(OH)_2D_3$ on intestinal calcium transport, but nevertheless the elevated intestinal calcium transport activity was maintained throughout the course of the study. Of great interest, however, was the fact that the single dose of $1,25(OH)_2D_3$ failed to mineralise the bone despite the fact that it produced very high intestinal calcium transport activity whereas $25(OH)D_3$ produced marked mineralisation of bone although its effect on calcium transport was similar to that produced by $1{,}25(OH)_2D_3$ (Figure 1.7). It, therefore, became clear that the mineralisation of bone under these circumstances was not related to intestinal calcium transport response and that some other factor was involved. That factor is shown in Figure 1.8, which illustrates that serum inorganic phosphate concentration is probably responsible.

The $25(OH)D_3$ dosage resulted in a sustained elevation of serum inorganic phosphate whereas the $1{,}25(OH)_2D_3$ produced an initial response which decreased to deficiency levels within 2–3 days. The administration of small amounts of $1{,}25(OH)_2D_3$ each day during the course of the experiment produced a sustained elevation of serum inorganic phosphate and resulted in marked mineralisation of bone. It is, therefore, clear that $1{,}25(OH)_2D_3$ is responsible for the elevation of serum inorganic phosphate by activating a system (or systems) which is independent of the intestinal calcium transport system. A recent series of experiments not shown here has demonstrated that the source of phosphorus in this case is bone and that there is, therefore, a phosphate mobilisation system in bone responsive to $1{,}25(OH)_2D_3$.

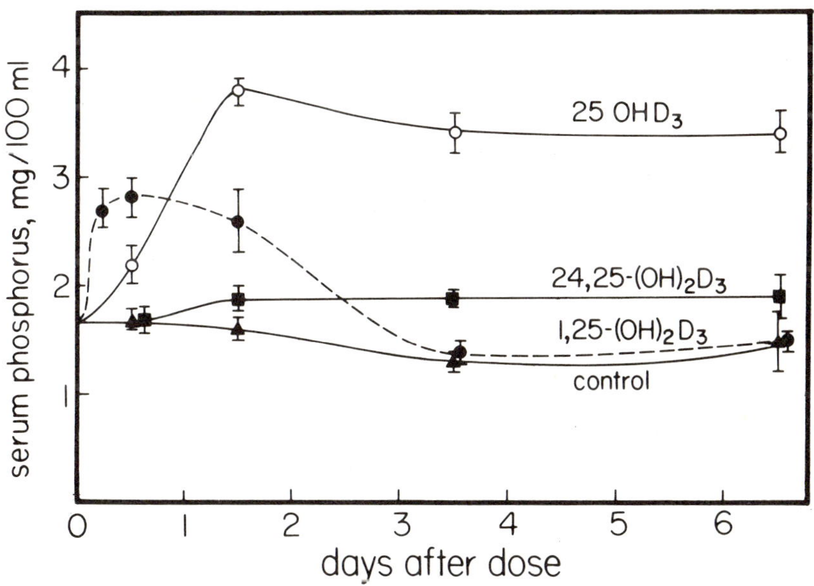

FIGURE 1.8 Serum inorganic phosphorus response of rachitic rats on a low phosphorus diet to Vitamin D metabolites.

Intestinal phosphate transport in the jejunum is also vitamin D dependent and not related to calcium transport. This system also shows a marked response to 1,25$(OH)_2D_3$ and 25$(OH)D_3$ but not 24,25$(OH)_2D_3$ (Chen *et al.*, 1974). Under these circumstances 24,25$(OH)_2D_3$ is hydroxylated on carbon-1 to form 1,24,25-trihydroxyvitamin D_3 [1,24,25$(OH)_3D_3$] (Holick *et al.*, 1973a), which stimulates the intestine to absorb calcium but appears not to stimulate the phosphate transport system of intestine. Of great interest is that nephrectomy prevents intestinal phosphate transport response to physiological doses of 25$(OH)D_3$ but that it does not prevent the response to the 1,25$(OH)_2D_3$ compound, again illustrating that 1,25$(OH)_2D_3$ is probably the metabolically active form in this system as well.

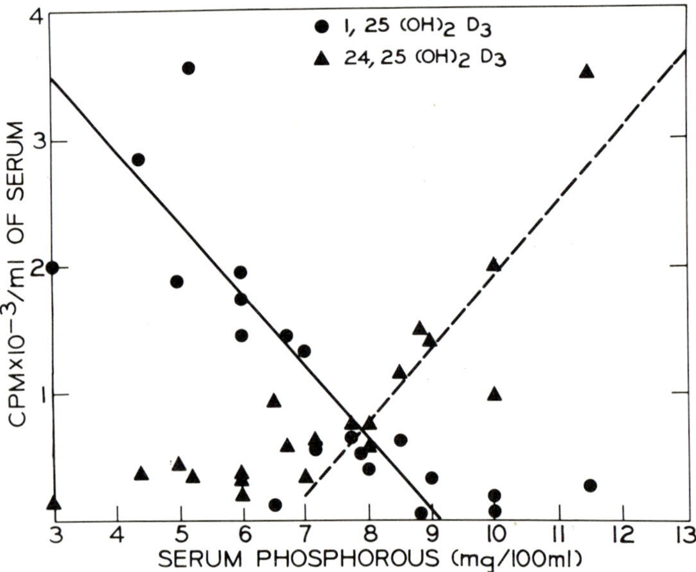

FIGURE 1.9 Relationship of serum inorganic phosphorus level add to serum levels of 1,25$(OH)_2D_3$ or 24,25$(OH)_2D_3$ in thyroparathyroidectomised rats (Tanaka and DeLuca, 1974).

Regulations of 1,25$(OH)_2D_3$ synthesis by serum inorganic phosphate

In view of the fact that 1,25$(OH)_2D_3$ is a hormone which has a function in stimulating phosphate transport reactions, it is reasonable to suspect that its synthesis may be regulated by serum inorganic phosphorus concentration (Tanaka and DeLuca, 1973). This can be demonstrated in thyroparathyroidectomised animals where the serum inorganic phosphate concentration can then be regulated without interference with the parathyroid hormone regulating system. In such animals it is clear that there is a relationship between synthesis of $1,25(OH)_2D_3$ and serum inorganic phosphate concentration as shown in Figure 1.9. It may, therefore, be concluded that $1,25(OH)_2D_3$ is not only a calcium mobilising hormone but a phosphate mobilising hormone and its synthesis is regulated both by serum calcium concentration through the parathyroid hormone system and by serum inorganic phosphorus concentration.

Specific correction of hypocalcaemia or hypophosphataemia by stimulation of $1,25(OH)_2D_3$ synthesis

It might be reasonable to suspect that $1,25(OH)_2D_3$, a hormone with dual functions in calcium and phosphate metabolism, might suffer a lack of specificity in its response to either a hypophosphataemic stimulus or a hypocalcaemic stimulus. By considering the sequence of events following such stimuli, this can be considerably clarified. Parathyroid hormone which is secreted in response to hypocalcaemic stimulus not only triggers $1,25(OH)_2D_3$ synthesis but also causes a phosphate diuresis (Figure 1.10). Although $1,25(OH)_2D_3$ mobilises both calcium

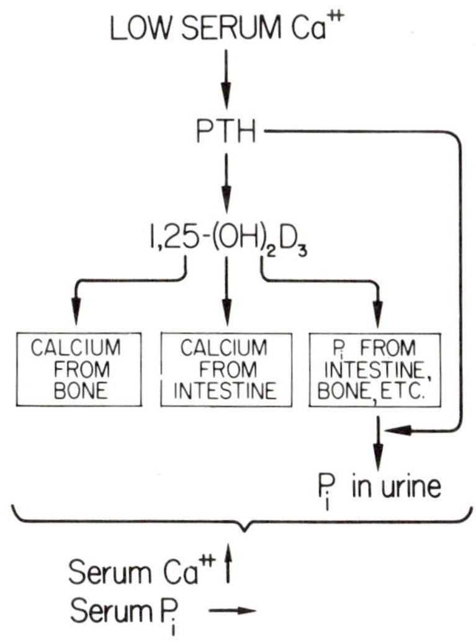

FIGURE 1.10 Sequence of events following hypocalcaemic stimulation of $1,25(OH)_2D_3$ synthesis.

and phosphate, the phosphate which is mobilised in response to $1,25(OH)_2D_3$ is lost by parathyroid induced phosphate diuresis resulting in the net elevation of serum calcium concentration and little change in serum phosphate in response to $1,25(OH)_2D_3$. On the other hand, hypophosphataemic stimulus of $1,25(OH)_2D_3$ synthesis is not accompanied by secretion of parathyroid hormone (Figure 1.11). In this circumstance, mobilisation of calcium from bone does not occur because of the absence of parathyroid hormone. Furthermore, parathyroid hormone does not cause a phosphate diuresis. The overall net effect is to elevate serum phosphorus concentration with little effect on calcium concentration. Thus the specific correction of the original stimulus is dictated by whether parathyroid hormone is secreted or not. It is,

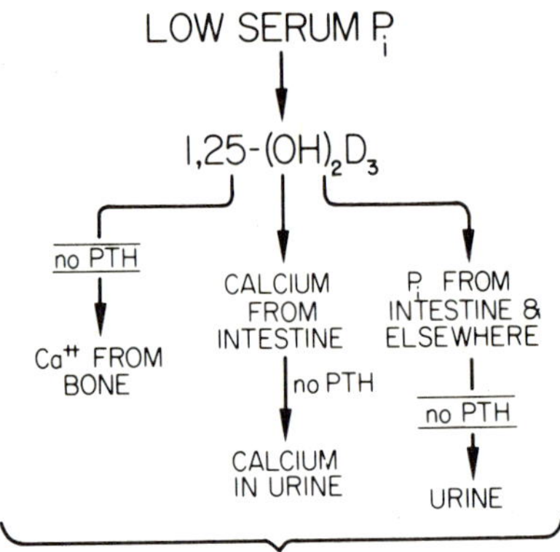

FIGURE 1.11 Sequence of events following a hypophosphataemic stimulation of $1.25(OH)_2D_3$ synthesis.

therefore, evident that $1,25(OH)_2D_3$ hormone can function both as a phosphate mobilisation hormone and as a calcium mobilising hormone in a rather specific manner physiologically.

1,24,25-trihydroxyvitamin D_3

The puzzling synthesis of $24,25(OH)_2D_3$ in large amounts in normal man and animals and its presence as an alternate metabolite to the $1,25(OH)_2D_3$ has raised a number of questions regarding its function (Omdahl and DeLuca, 1973). In the rat, radioactive $24,25(OH)_2D_3$

survived for sufficient periods of time to exclude the idea that it might be an excretory product. The fact that its synthesis is regulated and that it is the most abundant dihydroxy metabolite in normal man and animals suggests that it probably plays an important physiological role. Attempts in our laboratory to study this have led to the conclusion that $24,25(OH)_2D_3$ is converted to the $1,24,25(OH)_3D_3$. This substance, which may be another hormone derived from vitamin D, has marked intestinal calcium transport activity and possesses no activity in the mobilisation of calcium from bone and in phosphate transport reactions (Holick *et al.*, 1973a; Boyle *et al.*, 1973).

Vitamin D as a prohormone

It is evident that vitamin D either from the diet or from skin must be metabolised to $25(OH)D_3$ in the liver and subsequently in the kidney (Figure 1.2). In the kidney two options are available. When an emergency situation exists such as hypocalcaemia or hypophosphataemia, $1,25(OH)_2D_3$ is synthesised. This hormone proceeds to the intestine and bone where it mobilises calcium and phosphate. On the other hand, if normal calcium and normal phosphorus is present in the serum, $24,25(OH)_2D_3$ is made in large amounts. It is possible that this substance proceeds further to the $1,24,25(OH)_3D_3$, which may be a maintenance hormone whose sole responsibility may be to stimulate intestinal calcium absorption. Whether this is actually the case remains to be established. Nevertheless, this system illustrates the endocrine nature of the vitamin D system and furthermore shows that there are many possibilities for defects in vitamin D metabolism which may ultimately result in bone disease.

Vitamins and metabolism in disease

It is readily apparent that renal disease is often associated with marked osteomalacia and/or osteitis fibrosa (Slatopolsky *et al.*, 1972). It is now clear that an important component of this disease is a failure to synthesise $1,25(OH)_2D_3$. Furthermore, it is also clear that hypoparathyroid patients probably lack the ability to produce $1,25(OH)_2D_3$ in response to the hypocalcaemic stimulus (S. W Stanbury, these proceedings). These defects in vitamin D metabolism have already been exploited with the demonstration that $1,25(OH)_2D_3$ at 1 microgram/day is markedly effective in correcting the calcium metabolism defects in renal osteodystrophy and hypoparathyroidism.

Of great interest to this conference is the demonstration of the existence of a specific metabolic block in vitamin D metabolism, resulting in a well-known disease. This disease was originally discovered by Prader and associates and is termed vitamin D dependency disease, Prader's syndrome, or pseudo vitamin D deficiency disease. In this autosomal recessive disease, children develop severe rickets even with normal amounts of vitamin D. This can be completely corrected by the

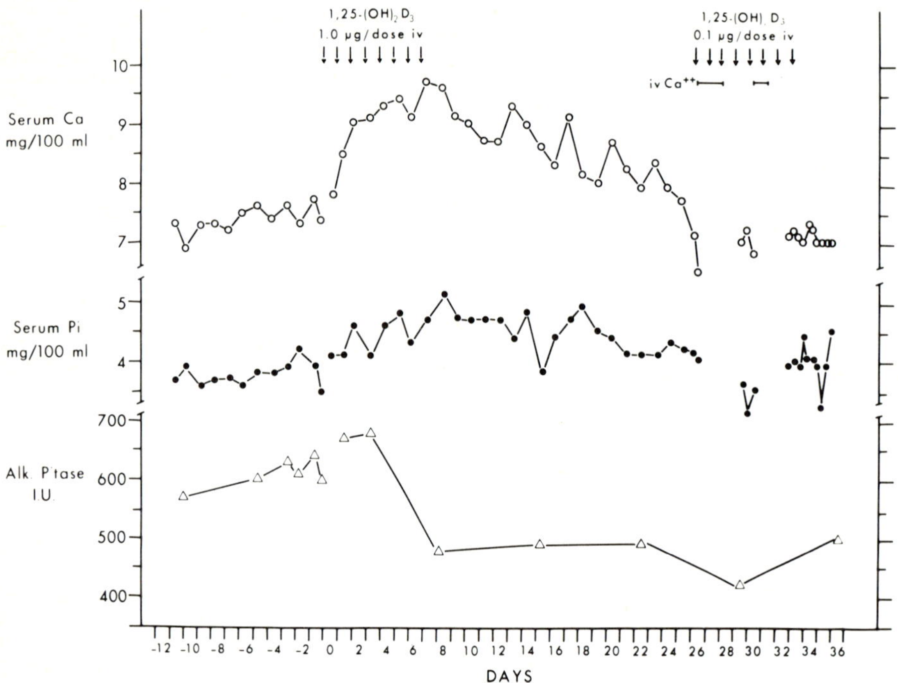

FIGURE 1.12 Response of serum parameters of a vitamin D dependency disease patient to physiological doses of $1,25(OH)_2D_3$ (Fraser *et al.*, 1973).

administration of large amounts of vitamin D (in the order of 50 000–150 000 units/day). When $25(OH)D_3$ became available the question of whether a metabolic block existed in the 25-hydroxylation stage appeared. Administration of this substance is very effective in correcting these lesions but pharmacological amounts are required of the order of 10 000–25 000 units/day. Of great interest, however, is the response of these patients to $1,25(OH)_2D_3$. In work carried out with Dr Donald

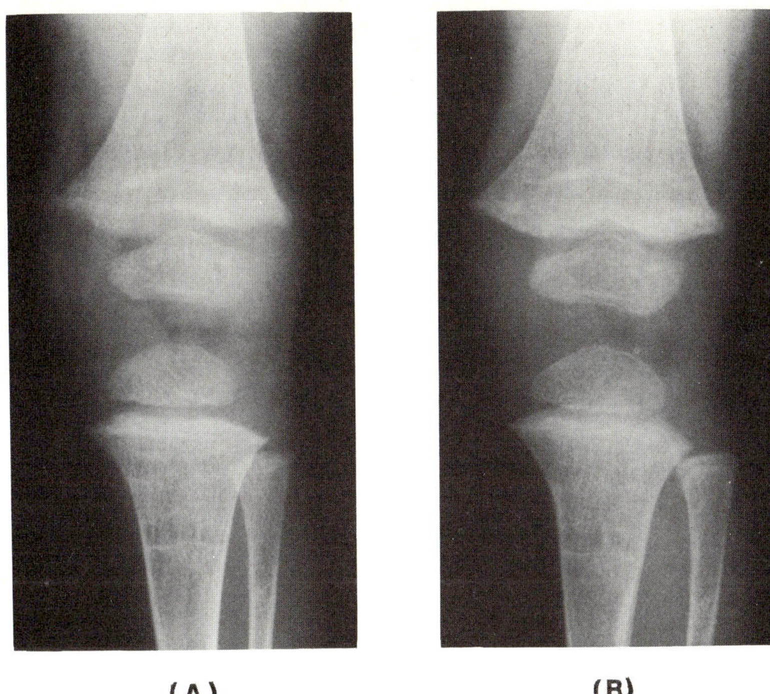

FIGURE 1.13 Radiographic healing in response to $1,25(OH)_2D_3$ of a vitamin D dependency rachitic patient. The patient received 1·0 μg/day of $1\alpha,25(OH)_2D_3$ on zero to 7th day. X-rays were taken on zero day (A) and on the 19th day (B).

Fraser in Toronto (Fraser *et al.*, 1973), it is clear that the patients respond remarkably to $1,25(OH)_2D_3$ as shown in Figure 1.12. One microgram per day produced a large serum calcium response. In addition, even after 7 days' treatment with 1 microgram $1,25(OH)_2D_3$/day, bone mineralisation can be ascertained on X-rays shown in Figure 1.13. By inference, therefore, this disease may represent a metabolic block in which 1α-hydroxylase enzyme may require large amounts of substrate before it can catalyse significant amounts of 1-hydroxylation.

1α-hydroxyvitamin D_3

During the course of chemical synthesis of $1,25(OH)_2D_3$ (Semmler *et al.*, 1972), 1α-hydroxyvitamin D_3 ($1\alpha(OH)D_3$) was synthesised (Holick *et al.*, 1973b). It possessed marked biological activity very similar to $1,25(OH)_2D_3$. This activity has been estimated in rats to be about 3–5 times that of vitamin D_3 (Holick *et al.*, 1975) whereas $1,25(OH)_2D_3$

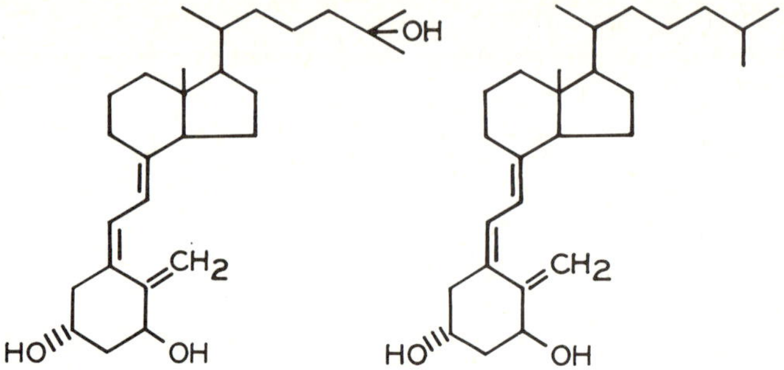

FIGURE 1.14 Structure of $1\alpha,25(OH)_2D_3$ and $1\alpha(OH)D_3$.

given parenterally is approximately 10 times more active than vitamin D_3 (Tanaka *et al.*, 1973). This substance, whose structure is shown in Figure 1.14 (II) is inexpensive to synthesise, is fully effective when given orally, and is apparently less likely to cause hypercalcaemia than is $1,25(OH)_2D_3$. It is likely that this substance may become the therapeutic compound of choice for patients who have difficulty with the 1-hydroxylation stage of vitamin D metabolism. The availability of the compound together with $25(OH)D_3$ could provide the physician with the necessary forms of vitamin D to correct the specific defect in vitamin D metabolism which may be encountered in metabolic bone disease.

Summary

Although only one genetic metabolic block has been observed in vitamin D metabolism, many bone diseases may be in part related to defects in vitamin D metabolism. With the understanding that vitamin D is a prohormone, the nature of the hormone, its function, its regulation and with its availability or its anglogues, the physician may be armed with new important agents to treat metabolic bone disease.

Acknowledgement

Some of the original research reported here was supported by a grant from the National Institutes of Health No. AM–15512 and the Harry Steenbock Professorship Fund.

REFERENCES

BHATTACHARYYA, M. H., and DELUCA, H. F. (1974) The regulation of calciferol 25-hydroxylase in the chick. *Biochem. Biophys. Res. Commun.*, **59**, 734

BLUNT, J. W., DELUCA, H. F. and SCHNOES, H. K. (1968) 25-Hydroxycholecalciferol. A biologically active metabolite of vitamin D. *Biochemistry*, **7**, 3317

BLUNT, J. W., and DELUCA, H. F. (1969). The synthesis of 25-hydroxycholecalciferol. A biologically active metabolite of vitamin D_3. *Biochemictry*, **8**, 671

BOYLE, I. T., GRAY, R. W., and DELUCA, H. F. (1971). Regulation by calcium of *in vivo* synthesis of 1,25-dihydroxycholecalciferol and 21,25-dihydroxycholecalciferol. *Proc. Natl. Acad. Sci. USA*, **68**, 2131

BOYLE, I. T., GRAY, R. W., OMDAHL, J. L. and DELUCA, H. F. (1972a). Calcium control of the *in vivo* biosynthesis of 1,25-dihydroxyvitamin D_3: Nicolaysen's endogenous factor. In S. Taylor (ed.), *Endocrinology 1971*, p. 468. (London : Wm. Heinemann Medical Books)

BOYLE, I. T., MIRAVET, L., GRAY, R. W., HOLICK, M. F. and DELUCA, H. F. (1972b). The response of intestinal calcium transport to 25-hydroxy and 1,25-dihydroxyvitamin D in nephrectomized rats. *Endocrinology*, **90**, 605

BOYLE, I. T., OMDAHL, J. L., GRAY, R. W. and DELUCA, H. F. (1973). The biological activity and metabolism of 24,25-dihydroxyvitamin D_3. *J. Biol. Chem.*, **248**, 4174

CARLSSON, A. (1952). Tracer experiments on the effect of vitamin D on the skeletal metabolism of calcium and phosphorus. *Acta Physiol. Scand.*, **26**, 212

CHEN, T. C., CASTILLO, L., KORYCKA-DAHL, M. and DELUCA, H. F. (1974). Role of vitamin D metabolism in phosphate transport of rat intestine. *J. Nutr.*, **104**, 1056

COUSINS, R. J., DELUCA, H. F., SUDA, T., CHEN, T. and TANAKA, Y. (1970). Metabolism and subcellular location of 25-hydroxycholecalciferol in intestinal mucosa. *Biochemistry*, **9**, 1453

DELUCA, H. F. (1967). Mechanism of action and metabolic fate of vitamin D. *Vit. and Horm.*, **25**, 315

DELUCA, H. F. (1969). Recent advances in the metabolism and function of vitamin D. *Fed. Proc.*, **28**, 1678

DELUCA, H. F. (1970). Metabolism and function of vitamin D. In H. F. DeLuca and J. W. Suttie (eds.), *The Fat-Soluble Vitamins*, p. 3. (Madison : University of Wisconsin Press)

DELUCA, H. F., TANAKA, Y. and CASTILLO, L. (1974). Interrelationships between vitamin D and phosphate metabolism. Presented at the 5th Parathyroid Conference, Oxford

FRASER, D. R. and KODICEK, E. (1970). Unique biosynthesis by kidney of a biologically active vitamin D metabolite. *Nature*, **228**, 764

FRASER, D., KOOH, S. W., KIND, H. P., HOLICK, M. F., TANAKA, Y. and DELUCA, H. F. (1973). Pathogenesis of hereditary vitamin D dependent rickets: an inborn error of vitamin D metabolism involving defective conversion of 25-hydroxyvitamin D to 1α,25-dihydroxyvitamin D. *N. Engl. J. Med.*, **289**, 817

FROLIK, C. A. and DELUCA, H. F. (1971). 1,25-Dihydroxycholecalciferol: the metabolite of vitamin D responsible for increased intestinal calcium transport. *Arch. Biochem. Biophys.*, **147**, 143

GARABEDIAN, M., HOLICK, M. F., DELUCA, H. F. and BOYLE, I. T. (1972). Control of 25-hydroxycholecalciferol metabolism by the parathyroid glands. *Proc. Natl. Acad. Sci. USA*, **69**, 1673

GARABEDIAN, M., TANAKA, Y., HOLICK, M. F. and DELUCA, H. F. (1974). Response of intestinal calcium transport and bone calcium mobilization to 1,25-dihydroxyvitamin D_3 in thyroparathyroidactomized rats. *Endocrinology*, **94**, 1022

GHAZARIAN, J. G. and DELUCA, H. F. (1974). 25-Hydroxycholecalciferol 1-hydroxylase: a specific requirement for NADPH and a hemoprotein component in chick kidney mitochondria. *Arch. Biochem. Biophys.*, **160**, 63

GHAZARIAN, J. G., SCHNOES, H. K. and DELUCA, H. F. (1973). Mechanism of 25-hydroxycholecalciferol 1α-hydroxylation. Incorporation of oxygen-18 into the 1α position of 25-hydroxycholecalciferol. *Biochemistry*, **12**, 2555

GHAZARIAN, J. E., JEFCOATE, C. R., KNUTSON, J. C., ORME-JOHNSON, W. H. and DELUCA, H. F. (1974), Mitochondrial cytochrome P450 : a component of chick kidney 25-hydroxycholecalciferol-1α-hydroxylase. *J. Bio. Chem.*, **249**, 3026

GRAN, F. C. (1960). The retention of parenterally injected calcium in rachitic dogs. *Acta Physiol. Scand.*, **50**, 132

GRAY, R., BOYLE, I. and DELUCA, H. F. (1971). Vitamin D metabolism: the role of kidney tissue. *Science*, **172**, 1232

GRAY, R. W., OMDAHL J. L., GHAZARIAN, J. G. and DELUCA, H. F. (1972). 25-Hydroxycholecalciferol 1-hydroxylase: subsellular location and properties. *J. Biol. Chem.*, **247**, 7528

HARRISON, H. E. and HARRISON, H. C. (1961). Intestinal transport of phosphate: action of vitamin D, calcium, and potassium. *Am. J. Physiol.*, **201**, 1007

HARRISON, H. C., HARRISON, H. E. and PARK, E. A. (1958). Vitamin D and citrate metabolism. Effect of vitamin D in rats fed diets adequate in both calcium and phosphorous. *Am. J. Physiol.*, **192**, 432

HOLICK, M. F., SCHNOES, H. K., DELUCA, H. F., SUDA, T. and COUSINS, R. J. (1971). Isolation and identification of 1,25-dihydroxycholecalciferol. A metabolite of vitamin D active in intestine. *Biochemistry*, **10**, 2799

HOLICK, M. F., GARABEDIAN, M. and DELUCA, H. F. (1972a). 1,25-Dihydroxycholecalciferol: metabolite of vitamin D_3 active on bone in anephric rats. *Science*, **176**, 1146

HOLICK, M. F., SCHNOES, H. K., DELUCA, H. F., GRAY, R. W., BOYLE, I. T. and SUDA, T. (1972b). Isolation and identification of 24,25-dihydroxycholecalciferol: a metabolite of vitamin D_3 made in the kidney. *Biochemistry*, **11**, 4251

HOLICK, M. F., KLEINER-BOSSALLER, A., SCHNOES, H. K., KASTEN, P. M., BOYLE, I. T. and DELUCA, H. F. (1973a). 1,24,25-Trihydroxyvitamin D_3: a metabolite of vitamin D_3 effective on intestine. *J. Biol. Chem.*, **248**, 6691

HOLICK, M. F., SEMMLER, E. J., SCHNOES, H. K. and DELUCA, H. F. (1973b) 1α-Hydroxy derivative of vitamin D_3: a highly potent analog of 1α, 25-dihydroxyvitamin D_3. *Science*, **180**, 190

HOLICK, M. F., GARABEDIAN, M., SCHNOES, H. K. and DELUCA, H. F. (1975). Relationship of 25-hydroxyvitamin D_3 side chain structure to biological activity. *J. Biol. Chem.*, **250**, 226

HOWLAND, J. and KRAMER, B. (1921). Calcium and phosphorus in the serum in relation to rickets. *Am. J. Dis. Child.*, **22**, 105

KOWARSKI, S. and SCHACHTER, D. (1969). Effects of vitamin D on phosphate transport and incorporation into mucosal constituents of rat intestinal mucosa. *J. Biol. Chem.*, **244**, 211

LUND, J. and DELUCA, H. F. (1966). Biologically active metabolite of vitamin D_3 from liver, and blood serum. *J. Lipid Res.*, **7**, 739

MCCOLLUM, E. V., SIMMONDS, N., SHIPLEY, P. G. and PARK, E. A. (1922). Studies on experimental rickets. XV. The effect of starvation on the healing of rickets. *Bull. Johns Hopkins Hosp.*, **22**, 31

NEVILLE, P. F., and DELUCA, H. F. (1966). The synthesis of [1,2-^{3}H] vitamin D_3 and the tissue localisation of a 0.25 μg (10 IU) dose per rat. *Biochemistry*, **5**, 2201

NICOLAYSEN, R. and EEG-LARSEN, N. (1953). The biochemistry and physiology of vitamin D. *Vit. and Horm.*, **11**, 29

NICOLAYSEN, R., EEG-LARSEN, N, and MALM, O. J. (1953). Physiology of calcium metabolism. *Physiol. Rev.*, **33**, 424

OMDAHL, J. L. and DELUCA, H. F. (1973). Regulation of vitamin D metabolism and function. *Physiol. Rev.*, **53**, 327

PUSCHETT, J. B., FERNANDEX, P. C., BOYLE, I. T., GRAY, R. W., OMDAHL, J. L. and DELUCA, H. F. (1972). The acute renal tubular effects of 1,25-dihydroxycholecalciferol. *Proc. Soc. Exp. Biol. Med.*, **141**, 379

RASMUSSEN, H., DELUCA, H., ARNAUD, C., HAWKER, C. and VON STEDINGK, M. (1963). The relationship between vitamin D and parathyroid hormone. *J. Clin. Invest.*, **42**, 1940

SEMMLER, E. J., HOLICK, M. F., SCHNOES, H. K. and DELUCA, H. F. (1972). The synthesis of 1α,25-dihydroxycholecalciferol—a metabolically active form of vitamin D_3. *Tetrahedron Lett.* **40**, 4147

SHIPLEY, P. G., KRAMER, B. and HOWLAND, J. (1925). Calcification of rachitic bone *in vitro*. *Am. J. Dis. Child.*, **30**, 37

SLATOPOLSKY, E., RUTHERFORD, W. E., HOFFSTEN, P. E., ELKAN, I. O., BUTCHER, H. R. and BRICKER, N. S. (1972). Non-suppressible secondary hyperparathyroidism in chronic progressive renal disease. *Kidney Int.*, **1**, 38

SUDA, T., DELUCA, H. F. and HALLICK, R. B. (1971). Synthesis of [26,27-^{3}H]-hydroxycholecalciferol. *Anal. Biochem.*, **43**, 139

TANAKA, Y. and DELUCA, H. F. (1973). The control of 25-hydroxyvitamin D metabolism by inorganic phosphorus. *Arch. Biochem. Biophys.*, **154**, 566

TANAKA, Y. and DELUCA, H. F. (1974). Role of 1,25-dihydroxyvitamin D_3 in maintaining serum phosphorus and curing rickets. *Proc. Natl. Acad. Sci. USA*, **71**, 1040

TANAKA, Y., FRANK, H. and DELUCA, H. F. (1973). Biological activity of 1,25-dihydroxyvitamin D_3 in the rat. *Endocrinology*, **92**, 417

WASSERMAN, R. H. and TAYLOR, A. N. (1973). Intestinal absorption of phosphate in the chick: effect of vitamin D_3 and other parameters. *J. Nutr.*, **103**, 586

2

Intestinal absorption of calcium and phosphorus in adult man in health and disease

S. W. Stanbury

Some 8 years ago, realising that I would never be able to acquire sufficient data of my own from healthy individuals to act as controls for metabolic balance studies in disease, I began to collate such information from the published nutritional literature. This collection was made, from careful studies by reputable nutritionists, with the principal aim of establishing the pattern of calcium balance in the healthy adult; to this end, it was possible to extract a total of 549 balance periods from 309 subjects (Stanbury, 1968). Parallel studies of phosphorus metabolism were less well represented but observations in 130 healthy individuals produced 275 metabolic balance periods (Stanbury, 1971); and a similar independent collection was made of the pattern of magnesium metabolism in the adult (King and Stanbury, 1970).

These data will be used for comparison with selective studies of the intestinal net absorption of calcium and phosphorus in disease, which will be almost exclusively personal observations. Certain points must be made quite clear. Firstly, the collected control data were from adults of both sexes between the ages of 17 and 77 years; children are not represented. Secondly, one is concerned only with absolute data, the mass of calcium or phosphorus in the diet or the faeces, or the net mass absorbed The data to be discussed will be presented in the simplest possible form as the relationship between the two independently measured variables, the dietary intake and the faecal output. It is fully appreciated that the external balance, or the measurement of intestinal net absorption, provides an incomplete account of events in the intestine. Much has been made of the need to take into account also the digestive juice calcium and its absorption and contribution to the faecal output. But the methods used to study the fate of digestive juice calcium are far from foolproof and it is probably true to say that studies involving its measurement have added nothing basically important to the concepts derived from the simple external balance.

In the case of calcium, the collected metabolic data confirm the observation, made 20 years ago by Brine and Johnson (1955), that the relationship between the dietary and faecal calcium is curvilinear and not linear as often assumed (Figure 2.1). There can be little doubt that this curvilinearity has a functional significance; the relationship may

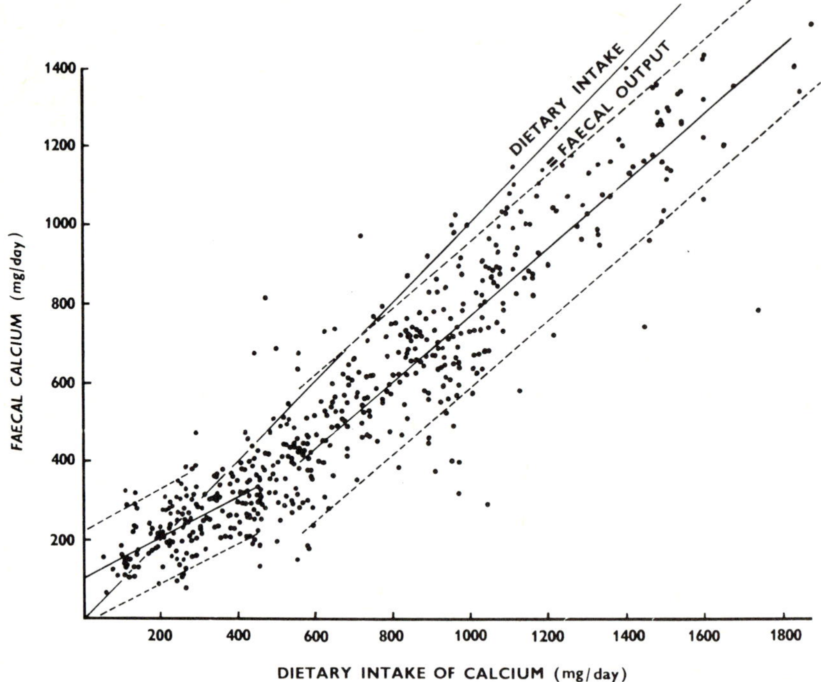

FIGURE 2.1 The relationship between dietary and faecal calcium in healthy adults. Data from 549 balance periods in 309 subjects. Separate regressions, with 95% confidence limits (interrupted lines), are inserted for intakes less than 450 mg/day and from 550 mg/day upwards.

represent the effects of a relatively small saturable component of active calcium transport plus an unsaturable component of passive permeation or exchange diffusion (Wassermann, 1968). But it is not considered justifiable to extrapolate from this simple relationship and the data have been used only to provide a 'normal standard'—an approximated curvilinear regression with confidence limits (Figure 2.1)—for comparison with the state of affairs in disease (Stanbury, 1968). Above an intake of about 450 mg/day the faecal calcium is statistically less than the dietary calcium in virtually all subjects; beyond this level, up to an intake of about 1·8 g/day, there is a progressive but small increase in net absorption.

In the case of phosphorus, within a range of intake between 0·5 and 2·0 g/day, the dietary and faecal phosphorus are related linearly (Figure 2.2; Stanbury, 1971). The faecal phosphorus is equivalent to about one-third of the dietary phosphorus. Net absorption of phosphorus is more complete than of calcium and it increases progressively with intake.

These control data from healthy individuals were collected originally for comparison with the metabolic state in chronic renal failure and in

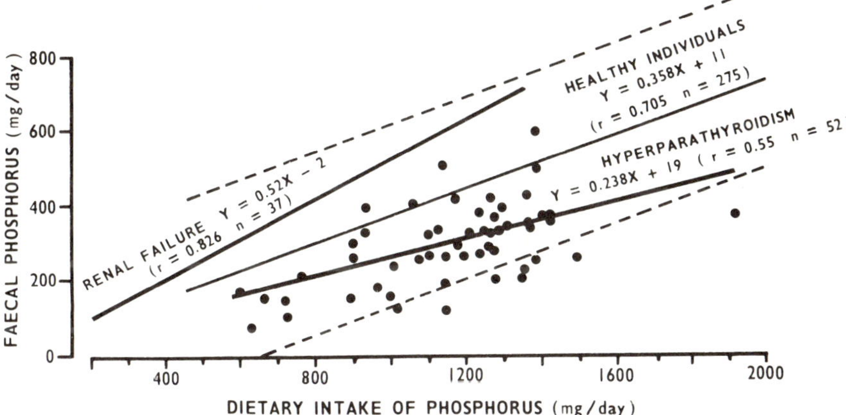

FIGURE 2.2 The relationship between dietary and faecal phosphorus in healthy adults and patients with renal failure and with primary hyperparathyroidism. Modified from Stanbury (1971). Individual data are shown from 52 cases of primary hyperparathyroidism.

primary hyperparathyroidism. Personal studies of more than 30 patients with CHRONIC RENAL FAILURE showed that the dietary and faecal calcium were statistically equivalent, implying that the net absorption of calcium in uraemia was effectively nil (Stanbury, 1968; 1973). This observation, together with many other biological observations on the state of the bone, etc., led to the conclusion that the uraemic state was one of apparent vitamin D deficiency (Stanbury and Lumb, 1962; Lumb *et al.*, 1971). In ultimate confirmation of this, following the classical observation of Fraser and Kodicek (1970) on the role of the kidney in synthesising $1,25(OH)_2D_3$, it was shown that patients with chronic renal failure produced little or none of this metabolite of vitamin D (Mawer *et al.*, 1973).

Since one was dealing with an apparent absolute deficiency of 1,25-dihydroxycholecalciferol, it was of interest to examine also intestinal net absorption of phosphorus in chronic renal failure. In simple vitamin D deficiency in man, or in osteomalacia complicating intestinal malabsorption, the faecal phosphorus is above the normal regression on intake —in the upper half of the normal range or outside it (Figure 2.8). The same is true of chronic renal failure (Stanbury, 1971) but, in both situations, it was evident that phosphorus absorption increased with intake as in healthy individuals (Figures 2.2 and 2.8).

This phenomenon—a net absorption less than normal at a particular level of intake, associated with a proportionate increase of absorption with increased intake—indicates that there are two components in the intestinal absorption of phosphorus. This was further emphasised by the pattern of absorptive response to treatment with vitamin D. In the original metabolic studies of Stanbury and Lumb (1962), it was shown that the treatment of renal osteodystrophy with effective doses of vitamin D produced equimolar increments in the intestinal net absorption of calcium and phosphorus. At first sight, this suggested that the effect of vitamin D on the absorption of phosphorus was dependent on the influence of the vitamin on calcium absorption; and further that there was perhaps some obligatory linkage between the calcium and phosphorus absorption mediated by vitamin D. Two observations made the latter unlikely. In some patients with a high rate of calcium absorption induced by vitamin D, the accompanying absorption of phosphorus was much less than equimolar. Secondly, in patients receiving a low intake of phosphorus, vitamin D may promote calcium absorption without accompanying increase of phosphorus absorption (Stanbury, 1971). A third observation, on which it has been difficult to acquire additional data, is that in some of the studies of Stanbury and Lumb (1962) treatment with vitamin D increased net absorption of phosphorus without increasing calcium absorption.

This enhancement of phosphorus absorption by vitamin D is, of course, not a phenomenon seen only in renal osteodystrophy. In simple vitamin D deficiency, the initial incremental absorption of calcium and phosphorus is equimolar; but, when calcium absorption exceeds 10–12 mmol/day, the incremental P : Ca molar ratio falls progressively (Figure 2.3). This fall off is probably simply due to reduced availability

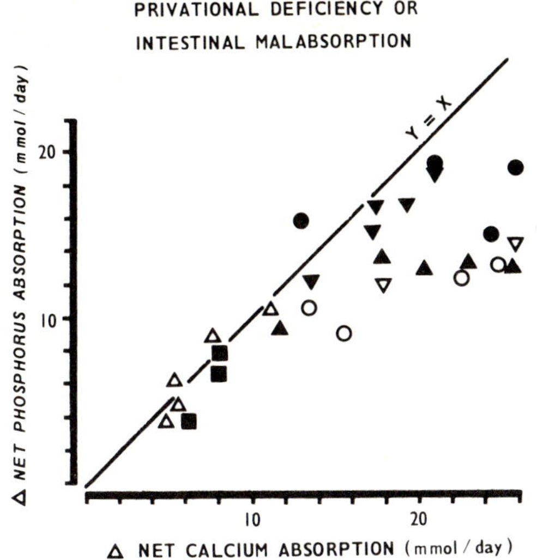

FIGURE 2.3 The incremental intestinal net absorption of calcium and of phosphorus produced by treatment with vitamin D in six patients with osteomalacia due to vitamin D deficiency (cf. Figure 2.10).

of phosphorus within the intestinal lumen; and, as is shown later, the provision of additional dietary phosphorus during the action of vitamin D can produce incremental P : Ca molar ratios of 2 : 1 or greater (Figure 2.10).

Irrespective of their precise interpretation, the data so far demonstrated provide empirical patterns of intestinal absorptive function with which to compare diseases purportively associated with hyper- or hypo-absorption.

It is generally accepted that PRIMARY HYPERPARATHYROIDISM is associated with intestinal hyperabsorption of calcium, although the published firm data on which this belief is based have been very scanty. Starting with metabolic balance studies on 50 patients of our own, we have examined net calcium absorption in a total collection of 95 patients with this disease and shown that the net absorption of calcium is statistically greater than normal at all levels of dietary intake (Stanbury, 1973). The regression of faecal on dietary calcium in primary hyperparathyroidism falls on the lower 95% confidence limit of normal and 50% of the data fall below the lower confidence limit shown in Figure 2.1. This immediately suggests the involvement of vitamin D, or of 1,25-dihydroxyvitamin D (1,25$(OH)_2D_3$) in the production of this phenomenon of hyperabsorption. Compatible with this, one finds that the intestinal net absorption of phosphorus also tends to be statistically increased in primary hyperparathyroidism (Figure 2.2). Even more impressive indirect evidence for an involvement of vitamin D in this phenomenon, is that such hyperabsorption is no longer present when primary hyperparathyroidism is complicated by advanced secondary renal disease. Intestinal net absorption may then be nil as in advanced primary renal failure, where we know the synthesis of $1,25(OH_2)D_3$ is also effectively nil (Mawer *et al.*, 1973).

Since it has been claimed that parathyroid hormone may actually inhibit the synthesis of $1,25(OH)_2D_3$ (Galante *et al.*, 1972), evidence from inference is not sufficient to establish this point. In a group of otherwise normal individuals with varying degrees of vitamin D insufficiency, we have shown that the increment in serum $1,25(OH)_2D_3$ produced from an intravenous pulse of radioactive cholecalciferol is related inversely to the serum calcium; none of this metabolite was formed when the serum calcium exceeded 9·6 mg/100 ml. Hypercalcaemic patients with primary hyperparathyroidism and intact renal function all produced significant amounts of $1,25(OH)_2D_3$: and, whereas formation of this metabolite in the controls was significantly correlated with the serum concentration of immunoreactive parathyroid hormone, there was no such correlation in primary hyperparathyroidism (Stanbury *et al.*, 1975; Mawer *et al.*, 1975).

It seems probable that a continued and apparently inappropriate secretion of $1,25(OH)_2D_3$ in response to increased circulating parathyroid hormone, is an essential component in the hyperabsorption of calcium in primary hyperparathyroidism. For a variety of reasons, however, we are not yet convinced that $1,25(OH)_2D_3$ itself *directly* regulates or determines this hyperabsorption. Firstly, although intestinal absorption of calcium is unequivocally increased, estimates of the concentrations of $1,25(OH)_2D_3$ in the serum in primary hyperparathyroidism (Mawer *et al.*, 1975) give values no higher than those assayed in the serum of healthy vitamin D replete individuals (Hill *et al.*, 1974). Secondly, hyperabsorption of calcium may persist after the autonomous hyperparathyroidism has been eliminated by parathyroidectomy (Figure 2.4).

A continued high rate of calcium absorption after parathyroidectomy is especially likely to be seen when the primary hyperparathyroidism has been complicated by florid bone disease, and we are still attracted by the concept of a regulatory influence on the intestine that originates in

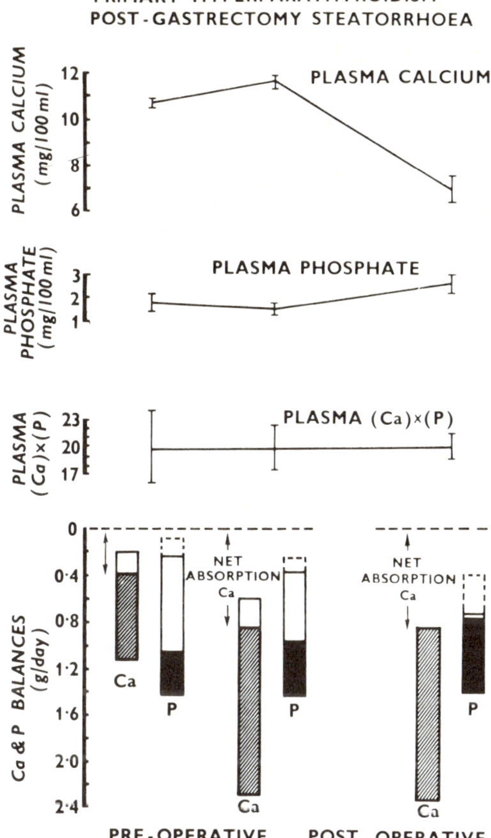

FIGURE 2.4 Effects of parathyroidectomy in a patient with primary hyperparathyroidism and hyperparathyroid bone disease. Metabolic data charted in conventional manner. Faecal calcium, cross-hatched; faecal phosphorus, black; urinary calcium and phosphorus, white. The interrupted lines on the P columns indicate theoretical P balance. Note that the net calcium absorption of *c.* 800 mg/day remained unchanged after successful parathyroidectomy.

bone—Nicolaysen's 'endogenous factor'. Experimental studies on RETARDED AND ACCELERATED GROWTH in the rat and chick, made by Adams in this laboratory (Adams *et al.*, 1975b; Adams *et al.*, 1975a) indicate that the relative rate of growth is an important determinant of calcium absorption—and incomplete observations suggest that calcium absorption in this experimental situation may vary independently of the concentration of $1,25(OH)_2D_3$ in the intestinal mucosa. We have no direct observations on the effects of induced alterations in growth rate on calcium absorption in man but a particular personal clinical experience may be relevant. In Figure 2.5 are shown the results of metabolic balance studies in three adolescents with coeliac disease, each of whom had presented clinically with rickets. Each patient was shown to have jejunal villous atrophy and, at the time of the metabolic studies, each was eating gluten-containing bread but all showed intestinal hyperabsorption of calcium. No completely satisfactory explanation for this phenomenon can be offered but it is known that each patient had grown rapidly—by as much as 15 cm—during the immediately preceeding months. The phenomenon may be analogous to the increased calcium absorption that accompanies the 'catch-up' growth of young animals on re-feeding after a period of calorie deprivation (Adams *et al.*, 1975 a, b).

It might be questioned also whether the impaired intestinal absorption of calcium sometimes reported in FAMILIAL X-LINKED HYPOPHOSPHATAEMIC RICKETS may be a consequence of the retarded growth rate in affected children rather than an attribute of the disease itself. This potential influence of growth is irrelevant in the adult and one might better assess calcium absorption in this syndrome by studying affected

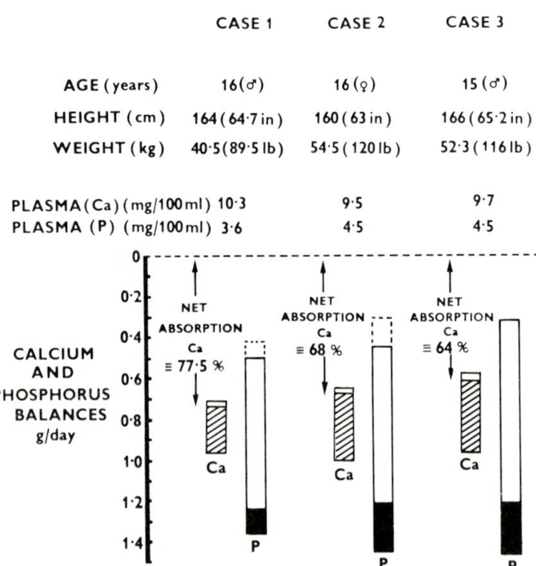

FIGURE 2.5 Calcium and phosphorus balances in three adolescents with gluten enteropathy, presenting with rickets following a period of rapid growth.

adults rather than children. The relationship between the dietary and faecal calcium in 11 such adults studied personally and in three cases of Nagant and Krane (1967) is shown in Figure 2.6. All the data are within the confidence limits of the regression for healthy adults; and they contrast with the data from eight adults with simple vitamin D deficiency which lie along the line of equivalence (Figure 2.6). Taking this further, calcium absorption has been examined in six hypophosphataemic adults with calcium intakes as high as 3·5 g/day (Figure 2.7): each point in this diagram represents metabolic collections over a period of 16 to 32 days. Net calcium absorption increased with intake in all patients;

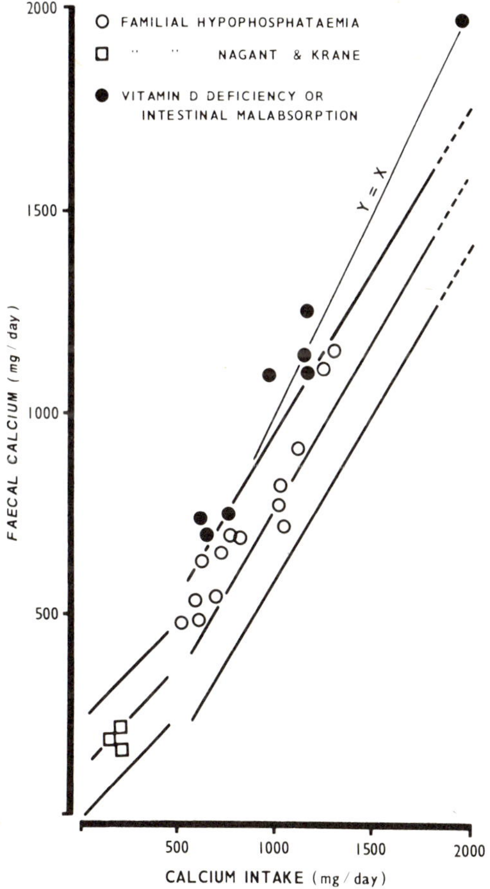

FIGURE 2.6 The relationship between the dietary and faecal calcium in adults with osteomalacia due to familial x-linked hypophosphataemia, contrasted with eight cases of untreated vitamin D deficiency osteomalacia. Data are superimposed upon the regression and confidence limits for healthy adults, taken from Figure 2.1.

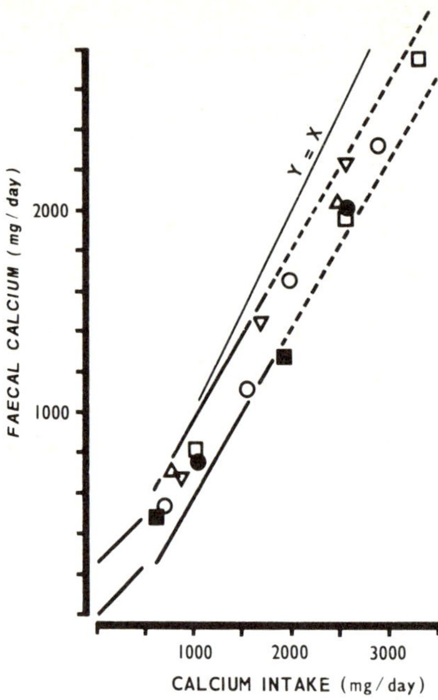

FIGURE 2.7 Effects of a high oral intake of calcium in adults with familial hypophosphataemic osteomalacia. The confidence limits from Figure 2.1 are extended between intake levels of 1·8 and 3·5 g/day; interrupted lines.

no adequate control data from healthy individuals are available at this range of intake but all the data from the patients fall within the extrapolation of the 'normal range'. There is little convincing evidence for a primary disturbance of calcium absorption, and even less reason to seek a primary disturbance of vitamin D metabolism, in this syndrome.

There is, however, a contemporary—and probably also unwarranted—tendency to assume that there is a primary disorder of the intestinal absorption of phosphorus in this syndrome. If there is a genetically determined defect of phosphate transport in the renal tubule it would be intellectually more tidy if the defect were also shared with the intestinal epithelium. Some, accepting that the faecal calcium may be high but believing the mechanisms of calcium transport to be intact, have attributed the supposedly high faecal calcium to a failure of phosphorus absorption—which is nonsense. And, although Short *et al.* (1973) appear to have demonstrated two components in the uptake of phosphate by human intestinal epithelium in vitro, the data on which they claim to show a defect in familial hypophosphataemia are as yet extremely scanty and cannot be accepted without reservations unless confirmed by further studies.

The relationship between the dietary and faecal phosphorus in 19 cases of familial hypophosphataemia is shown in Figure 2.8. The data are distributed evenly within the 'normal range'; there was no difference in the distribution of data from affected males and females; and the pattern is very different from vitamin D deficiency, in which it is accepted that phosphate absorption is impaired. There was thus no

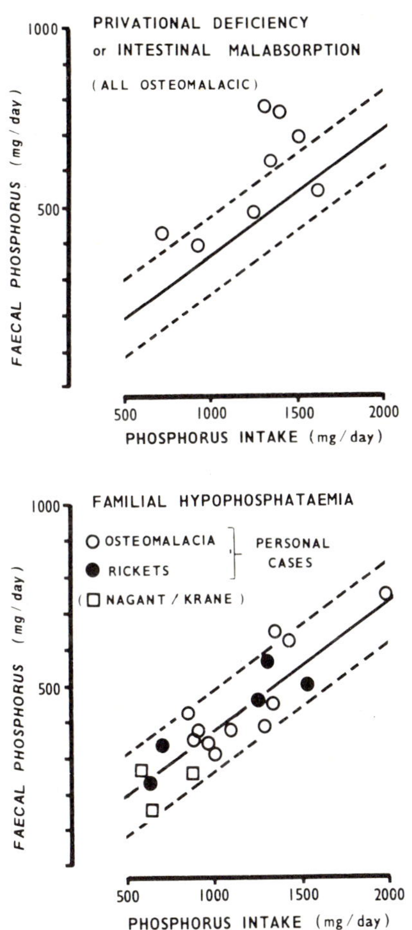

FIGURE 2.8 The relationship between the dietary and faecal phosphorus in 19 cases of familial hypophosphataemia (below) and eight cases of osteomalacia due to vitamin D deficiency (above). Data are superimposed upon the regression and confidence limits for healthy adults, taken from Figure 2.2.

suggestion of an impaired absorption of phosphorus when the patients were eating normal diets. Further evidence for a normal absorptive capacity is provided in six adults who received supplementary phosphate to increase the daily intake to levels approaching 4 g (Figure 2.9). Again normal control data are lacking at this level of intake; but, above intakes of about 2·5 g/day, most data fall well below an extrapolation of the normal range. That is, the faecal phosphorus at this level of intake

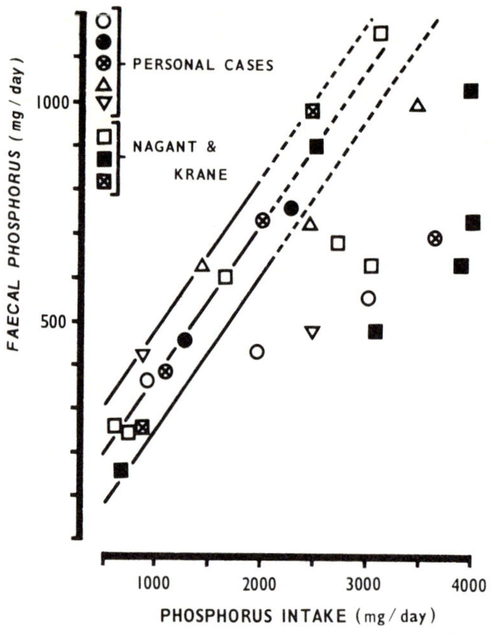

FIGURE 2.9 The relationship between dietary and faecal phosphorus in patients with familial hypophosphataemia receiving high doses of supplementary phosphorus. The confidence limits of Figure 2.2 are extrapolated (interrupted lines) to intakes between 2 and 4 g/day.

was lower—not higher—than might be expected from the behaviour of normal individuals. Rather than impaired absorption, it might even be questioned whether these adults have an intestinal epithelium excessively permeable to phosphate!

The vitamin D dependent component of phosphorus absorption in this syndrome also appears to be indistinguishable from normal (Figure 2.10). As already shown in simple vitamin D deficiency (Figure 2.3) and in renal osteodystrophy, the initial incremental absorption of calcium and phosphorus in response to vitamin D is on

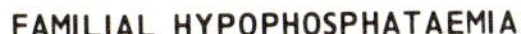

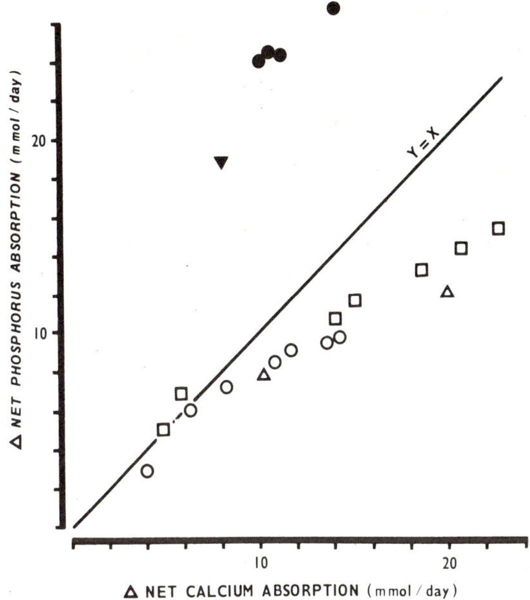

FIGURE 2.10 The incremental net absorption of calcium and of phosphorus in four adults with X-linked hypophosphotaemia during treatment with pharmacological doses of ergocalciferol (cf. Figure 2.3). Note the fall in the ratio △ : P△Ca when calcium absorption increased by more than 10 mmol/day. Case ▼ was receiving supplementary phosphorus before starting treatment with vitamin D; case ○ received supplementary P (●) when the P : Ca ratio began to diminish; in both cases the P : Ca ratio exceeded 2 : 1 (see text).

an equimolar basis: and, when the incremental absorption of calcium exceeds 10–12 mmol/day, the incremental P : Ca molar ratio falls as in simple vitamin D deficiency treated with vitamin D. But, if additional oral phosphorus is provided when the ratio has fallen, the P : Ca ratio may exceed 2 : 1 (Figure 2.10). Similarly, if the patient has been treated with large amounts of supplementary phosphorus before receiving vitamin D, the *incremental* absorption of phosphorus and calcium may be in ratio exceeding 2 : 1 (Figure 2.10). This is further evidence for the suggestion made earlier that the increase of phosphorus absorption produced by vitamin D may be due to the vitamin itself and not to an obligatory concomitant absorption of calcium. Parenthetically, the moderate increase in faecal phosphorus produced by massive supplements of phosphorus in X-linked hypophosphataemia does not cause an increase in faecal calcium (unpublished observations).

These data on X-linked hypophosphataemic osteomalacia have been examined in some detail to make the point that hypotheses must be repeatedly checked against native data. As we interpret the observations, they provide no evidence for impaired calcium absorption in X-linked hypophosphataemia; and they demonstrate that the two components we identify in the intestinal absorption of phosphorus are apparently intact. This in no way challenges the importance of renal phosphaturia in this syndrome, nor the analysis of the nature of this renal leak by Scriver and his colleagues (Glorieux and Scriver, 1972). But it does emphasise the dangers of extrapolating without data. Also, it is perhaps unfortunate that most interest has been directed at affected children with this syndrome. As I commonly encounter the syndrome in the adult, it is extremely difficult to believe that it is due to phosphorus deficiency. In such adults, one has a densely osteosclerotic skeleton with excess endosteal, cortical and periosteal bone; ossification occurring in tendons, ligaments and joint capsules in company with a failure of mineralisation of bone. A syndrome simulating skeletal fluorosis and atypical ankylosing spondylitis; and, in respect of these changes, affecting male and females with equal severity. If all this is due to phosphorus deficiency, we have much to learn about the functions of phosphorus in the supporting tissues. One has frequently wondered if a primary abnormality of the bone cells might not cause the renal phosphaturia, rather than the latter being responsible for the observed bony changes!

Having strayed into what is generally regarded as paediatric territory, I shall compound my trespass by making my last example an internist's look at IDIOPATHIC HYPERCALCAEMIA. We had the opportunity to make observations on a case of the severe type of infantile hypercalcaemia, who was one of the first patients to be treated successfully by deprivation of calcium by Professor Capon at Liverpool. At the age of 16 years, she was still hypercalcaemic and the creatinine clearance was also low at 16 ml/min. Despite this advanced renal impairment, she had an intestinal net absorption of calcium equivalent to 40% of an intake of 700 mg/day. We have made many observations in patients of this age with a comparable degree of renal impairment due to primary renal disease; none has shown a net absorption of this magnitude. Compatible with the conventional view that intestinal hyperabsorption contributes to the hypercalcaemia, the serum calcium diminished immediately when the intake of calcium was reduced to 140 mg/day. But, despite sustained negative calcium balance, hypercalcaemia was fairly rapidly re-established

—indicating that factors other than intestinal hyperabsorption were contributing to the elevation of the serum calcium. At about this time, Rasmussen (1969) mentioned having encountered evidence of hyperparathyroidism and benefit from parathyroidectomy in two children with idiopathic hypercalcaemia; and he kindly provided more details of this experience. In our patient, Dr Eric Reiss found the concentration of immunoreactive parathyroid hormone in the plasma to be ten times the highest value encountered in normal individuals; and no significant change in immunoreactive hormone concentration occurred when we varied the serum calcium experimentally between 8 and 16 mg/100ml. Thus we had a state of hyperparathyroidism that was apparently almost completely autonomous; and, after serious consideration and debate, we undertook sub-total parathyroidectomy. The serum calcium fell to within the normal range and, in a balance study carried out afterwards, there appeared to be a reduced intestinal net absorption of calcium. But, during ensuing months, hypercalcaemia became re-established and at 6 months it was again possible to demonstrate intestinal hyperabsorption and the same pattern of response to calcium deprivation.

This may appear to have been an interesting but perhaps misguided therapeutic adventure. There are, however, some additional points of theoretical interest. Firstly, despite the advanced renal insufficiency and a moderate degree of hyperphosphataemia, there was hyperabsorption of phosphorus as well as calcium. In other words, the pattern of intestinal absorption suggests an intestine under the influence of vitamin D. But, with the patient's degree of renal insufficiency, previous experience would lead one to expect a failure of the synthesis of the metabolite of vitamin D acting on the intestine (Mawer *et al.*, 1973). In fact, studies with doubly-labelled radioactive cholecalciferol in this patient showed no evidence of the formation of $1,25(OH)_2D_3$.

This vitamin D-like effect in the intestine, in the apparent absence of the formation of $1,25(OH)_2D_3$ is reminiscent of the action of the polyene antibiotic, filipin. Filipin alters the permeability of cellular membranes and, in the vitamin D deficient chick, it has been shown capable of increasing the intestinal transport of calcium in vitro in a manner similar to that produced by correction of the vitamin D deficiency (Adams *et al.*, 1970). If the intestinal mucosa in infantile hypercalcaemia were congenitally abnormal—conceivably, with an increased permeability to calcium at the brush border or with the activation of some other biochemical component of the calcium transport mechanism—this might explain some features of the syndrome. And if this hypothetical abnormality of cellular membranes were shared by other tissues concerned with the translocation of calcium—such as by the cells of parathyroid glands—one wonders if this might in some way underlie the paradoxical development of hyperparathyroidism in a state of alimentary hypercalcaemia.

This is, of course, unbridled speculation deliberately intended as provocation! But it may be recalled that in SARCOIDOSIS, in which intestinal hyperabsorption of calcium contributes to the development of hypercalcaemia, there is an apparently high incidence of 'primary' hyperparathyroidism. As first pointed out by Jackson and Dancaster (1959), the intestinal hyperabsorption in sarcoidosis involves phosphorus as well as calcium (Figure 2.11), so there are some analogies with in-

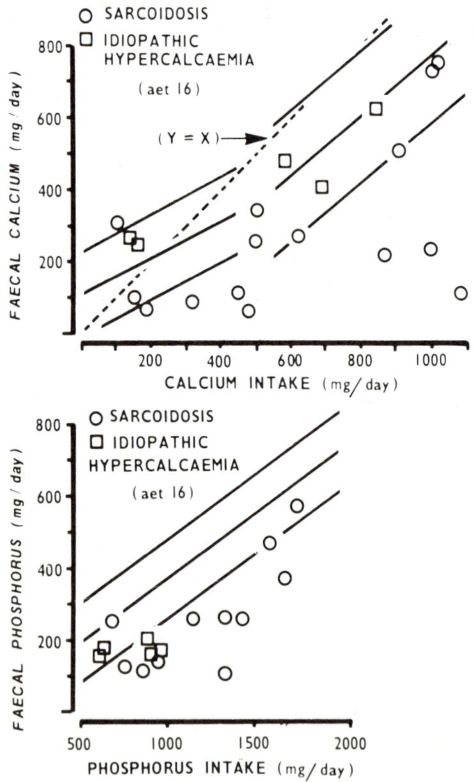

FIGURE 2.11 The relationship between dietary and faecal calcium (above) and dietary and faecal phosphorus (below) in sarcoidosis and a surviving case of infantile hypercalcaemia. Appropriate regressions, etc. taken from Figures 1 and 2. Data for sarcoidosis from Jackson and Dancaster (1959).

fantile hypercalcaemia. It would be unwise to take the analogy further. I am unaware of any studies of the formation of $1,25(OH)_2D_3$ in hypercalcaemic sarcoidosis; and, according to Reiss, hypercalcaemia in sarcoidosis is invariably associated with absence of immunoreactive parathyroid hormone from the blood (personal communication).

None the less, the intestinal hyperabsorption in infantile hypercalcaemia and in sarcoidosis—which it is suggested tentatively may occur independently of $1,25(OH)_2D_3$—is suppressed by treatment with CORTISONE. Whereas the intestinal hyperabsorption in primary hyperparathyroidism, in which we have produced evidence for an involvement of $1,25(OH_2)D_3$ is not so influenced by adrenal glucorticoids. In the rat, we and others have shown that these adrenal steroids may produce impairment of the intestinal transport of calcium, despite the presence of normal concentrations of $1,25(OH)_2D_3$ in the intestinal mucosa (Lukert *et al.*, 1973; Favus *et al.*, 1973). These clinical and experimental phenomena, together with the effects on calcium absorption of retarded and accelerated growth, suggest to us that there could be many as yet unidentified factors influencing or controlling calcium absorption. Although DeLuca's hypothesis that $1,25(OH)_2D_3$ directly controls the intestinal absorption of calcium is attractive, we would prefer to leave open the option that its function may be permissive and that other factors determine the quantitative extent of absorption.

Acknowledgements

Many of the researches reported were supported by grants from the Medical Research Council. The author is also grateful to his many colleagues who shared in obtaining the original data described.

REFERENCES

ADAMS, P. H., FYANS, P., HILL, L. F., LUMB, G. A., MAWER, E. B. and TAYLOR, C. M. (1975a). Interrelationship of growth, calcium absorption and vitamin D metabolism. In R. V. Talmadge, M. Owen and J. A. Parsons (eds.), *Calcium-regulating Hormones*. (Amsterdam: Excerpta Medica)

ADAMS, P. H., HILL, L. F., WAIN, D. and TAYLOR, C. M. (1975b). The effects of undernutrition and its relief on intestinal calcium transport in the rat. *Calcif. Tissue Res.*, **16**, 293

ADAMS, T. H., WONG, R. G. and NORMAN, A. W. (1970). Studies on the mechanism of action of calciferol, II. Effects of the polyene antiobiotic, filipin, on vitamin D mediated calcium transport. *J. Biol. Chem.*, **245**, 4432

BRINE, C. L. and JOHNSTONE, F. A. (1955). Endogenous calcium in the feces of adult man and the amount of calcium absorbed from food. *Am. J. Clin. Nutr.*, **3**, 418

FAVUS, M. J., KIMBERG, D. V., MILLAR, G. N. and GERSHON, E. (1973). Effects of cortisone administration on the metabolism and localisation of 25-hydroxycholecalciferol in the rat. *J. Clin. Invest.*, **49**, 1288

FRASER, D. R. and KODICEK, E. (1970). Unique biosynthesis by kidney of a biologically active vitamin D metabolite. *Nature*, **228**, 764

GALANTE, L., COLSTON, K., MACAULEY, S. and MACINTYRE, I. (1972). Effect of parathyroid extract on vitamin-D metabolism. *Lancet*, **i**, 985

GLORIEUX, F. and SCRIVER, C. R. (1972). Loss of a parathyroid-sensitive component of phosphate transport in x-linked hypophosphatemia. *Science*, **175**, 997

HILL, L. E., TAYLOR, C. M. and MAWER, E. B. (1974). Bioassay of 1,25-dihydroxy-cholecalciferol. Proceedings of the Medical Research Society. *Clin. Sci. Mol. Med.*, **47**, 14

JACKSON, W. P. U. and DANCASTER, C. (1959). A consideration of the hypercalciuria in sarcoidosis, idiopathic hypercalciuria, and that produced by vitamin D. A new suggestion regarding calcium metabolism. *J. Clin. Endocrinol.*, **19**, 658

KING, R. G. and STANBURY, S. W. (1970). Magnesium metabolism in primary hyper-parathyroidism. *Clin. Sci.*, **39**, 281

LUKERT, B. P., STANBURY, S. W. and MAWER, E. B. (1973). Vitamin D and intestinal transport of calcium: effects of prednisolone. *Endocrinology*, **93**, 202

LUMB, G. A., MAWER, E. B. and STANBURY, S. W. (1971). The apparent vitamin D resistance of chronic renal failure: a study of the physiology of vitamin D in man. *Am. J. Med.*, **50**, 421

MAWER, E. B., BACKHOUSE, J., HILL, L. F., LUMB, G. A., DE SILVA, P., TAYLOR, C. M. and STANBURY, S. W. (1975). Parathyroid function and vitamin D metabolism in man. *Clin. Sci. Mol. Med.*, **48**, 349

MAWER, E. B., BACKHOUSE, J., TAYLOR, C. M., LUMB, G. A. and STANBURY, S. W. (1973). Failure of formation of 1,25-dihydroxycholecalciferol in chronic renal insufficiency. *Lancet*, **i**, 626

NAGANT, C. and KRANE, S. M. (1967). The treatment of adult phosphate diabetes and Fanconi syndrome with neutral sodium phosphate. *Am. J. Med.*, **43**, 508

RASMUSSEN, H. (1969). Differentiation of parathyroid hyperplasia from adenoma. *N. Engl. J. Med.*, **280**, 1416

SHORT, E. M., BINDER, H. J. and ROSENBERG, L. E. (1973). Familial hypophosphatemic rickets: defective transport of inorganic phosphate by intestinal mucosa. *Science*, **179**, 700

STANBURY, S. W. (1968). The intestinal absorption of calcium in normal adults, primary hyperparathyroidism and renal failure. In G. M. Berlyne (ed.), *Nutrition in Renal Disease*, p. 118. (Edinburgh : E. & S. Livingstone)

STANBURY, S. W. (1971). The phosphate ion in chronic renal failure. In D. J. Hioco (ed.), *Phosphate et Metabolisme Phosphocalcique*, p. 187. (Paris : Sandoz Editions)

STANBURY, S. W. (1973). Parathyroid hormone and the intestinal absorption of calcium. In *Metabolism of Water and Electrolytes*, Siena, Italy

STANBURY, S. W. and LUMB, G. A. (1962). Metabolic studies of renal osteodystrophy. I. Calcium, phosphorus and nitrogen metabolism in rickets, osteomalacia and hyperparathyroidism complicating chronic uremia and in the osteomalacia of the adult Fanconi syndrome. *Medicine (Baltimore)*, **41**, 1

STANBURY, S. W., MAWER, E. B., HILL, L. F., TAYLOR, C. M., DE SILVA, P. and LUMB, G. A. (1975). Vitamin D metabolism in adult man in health and in disease. In R. V. Talmadge, M. Owen and J. A. Parsons (eds.), *Calcium-regulating Hormones*. (Amsterdam: Excerpta Medica)

WASSERMAN, R. H. (1968). Calcium transport by the intestine: a model and comment on vitamin D action. *Calcif. Tissue Res.*, **2**, 301

3

Human parathyroid hormone: Immunochemical studies and determination of circulating hormone in patients with primary hyperparathyroidism and renal insufficiency

F. M. Dietrich, U. Binswanger, W. Hunziker and J. A. Fischer

Introduction

Methods of precisely and reproducibly quantitating parathyroid hormone (PTH) and calcium levels in human peripheral serum, are a prerequisite to both the diagnosis and the elucidation of the pathogenesis of the various forms of hypo- and hyperparathyroidism. Until recently, immunoreactive PTH (iPTH) in man was estimated by means of a heterologous radioimmunoassay systems (Berson and Yalow, 1966; Reiss and Canterbury, 1968; Lequin *et al.*, 1970; Arnaud *et al.*, 1971b; Potts *et al.*, 1971; Roof *et al.*, 1973; Blair *et al.*, 1973; Conaway and Anast, 1974). In all these studies, human iPTH was estimated by competitive displacement of radioiodinated bovine PTH (bPTH) from antibodies raised to the bovine or porcine hormone. The validity of this is, however, questionable for two reasons. Firstly, parathyroid hormones originating from different species are structurally different and exhibit varying degrees of immunological cross-reactivity to human PTH (hPTH). Secondly, and more seriously, circulating iPTH is known to consist of several PTH peptides, which not only differ in their biological properties, but are also heterogeneous with regard to their reactivity with antisera to PTH (cf. Arnaud *et al.*, 1974). In order to estimate absolute concentrations of PTH in normal and pathological conditions, we have been trying to establish homologous immunoassay systems. To this end, we first studied the quantitative and qualitative properties of antibodies raised against the synthetic amino-terminal fragment of hPTH comprising the aminoacid residues 1–34 (Fischer *et al.*, 1974a). More recently, we characterised antibodies to a human glandular extract and to the synthetic amino-terminal hPTH fragments 1–12 and 1–34 (Fischer *et al.*, 1974b). We showed that some of these antibodies are useful for quantitating iPTH levels in the sera of patients with primary hyperparathyroidism, as well as in sera of control subjects. In this communication, we present additional immunological data on these new assay systems and report on their usefulness for the quantitation of circulating PTH in patients suffering from primary hyperparathyroidism and renal insufficiency. The materials and methods used in the present study are identical with those fully described in one of our previous publications (Fischer *et al.*, 1974b).

Chemistry and immunoheterogeneity of human parathyroid hormone

PTH was isolated from parathyroid tumours and the sequence of its 34 amino-terminal amino acids was determined by Brewer *et al.* (1972). Further chemical and conformational properties of PTH were summarised in a recent publication by Brewer *et al.* (1974). As shown in Figure 3.1, the structure of hPTH-(1–34) differs from that of the bovine peptide in five amino acid residues. Human PTH-(1–34) was synthesised by Rittel and co-workers (Andreatta *et al.*, 1973). An alternative structure for this amino-terminal peptide, which differs in three amino acids, was proposed by Potts' group (Niall *et al.*, 1974) who additionally determined residues 35–37. Very recently, further structural features of hPTH became known, such as the 44–69 sequence (Keutmann *et al.* 1975).

Biosynthetic precursors of hPTH having molecular weights of about 12 000 were isolated by Habener *et al.* (1972) and by Chu *et al.* (1973). Jacobs *et al.* (1974) determined the sequence of six additional amino acids at the amino-end of hPTH-(1–84) and found it to be identical with the structure of bPTH (Hamilton *et al.*, 1974). Most recently, Hamilton *et al.* (1975) presented evidence of the existence of additional amino acid residues at the carboxy-terminal end of bPTH-(1–84). Human parathyroid hormone species greater in size than hPTH-(1–84) were demonstrated by gel filtration in the sera of patients with primary hyperparathyroidism (Benson *et al.*, 1974; Fischer *et al.*, 1974b) and in culture medium of parathyroid tumour explants (Arnaud *et al.*, 1971a; Martin *et al.*, 1973).

Immune heterogeneity of circulating hPTH was first suggested by Berson and Yalow (1968) and subsequently demonstrated to be a

	1				5					10					15		
hPTH	Ser	Val	Ser	Glu	Ile	Gln	Leu	Met	His	Asn	Leu	Gly	Lys	His	Leu	Asn	Ser
bPTH	Ala	Val	Ser	Glu	Ile	Gln	Phe	Met	His	Asn	Leu	Gly	Lys	His	Leu	Ser	Ser

			20					25					30				34
hPTH	Met	Glu	Arg	Val	Gln	Trp	Leu	Arg	Lys	Lys	Lys	Gln	Leu	Val	His	Asn	Phe - R
bPTH	Met	Glu	Arg	Val	Gln	Trp	Leu	Arg	Lys	Lys	Leu	Gln	Asp	Val	His	Asn	Phe - R

FIGURE 3.1 NH_2-terminal amino acid sequence (residues 1–34) of human and bovine PTH (Brewer *et al.*, 1974).

property of glandular and serum PTH by Arnaud *et al.* (1970). The concept of the presence of more than one molecular weight species of PTH was later confirmed by gel filtration of the incubation media obtained from parathyroid tumour explants maintained under tissue culture conditions (Sherwood *et al.*, 1970; Arnaud *et al.*, 1971a). Habener *et al.* (1971) demonstrated that the major species of iPTH in the venous parathyroid effluent consisted of glandular hPTH-(1–84) with a molecular weight of 9500, whereas the major component of circulating iPTH was a fragment having a molecular weight of 7000. Various authors furnished evidence that this fragment is generated from the hormone comprising 84 amino acid residues by deletion of an amino-terminal peptide sequence (Segre *et al.*, 1972; Silverman and Yalow, 1973; Arnaud *et al.*, 1974; Segre *et al.*, 1974). Immunoreactive PTH exhibiting chromatographic properties compatible with the notion that it consists of various molecular weight peptide species is also demonstrable with our new assay systems in sera from patients suffering from primary hyperparathyroidism (Fischer *et al.*, 1974b) and from renal insufficiency (unpublished observations). A representative finding is shown by the chromatograms reproduced in Figure 3.2, obtained upon analysis of serum PTH by gel filtration and by two immunoassay systems. In immunoassay system (a) consisting of [^{131}I]bPTH-(1–84)), antibodies to a trichloroacetic acid extract of human parathyroid tumours (hPTH-TCA) and a Sephadex G-100-purified extractive PTH (hPTH-(1–84) G–100) as standard, iPTH was eluted as a single peak between hPTH-(1–84) and hPTH-(1–34), thus corresponding to the 7000 dalton species reported in the literature. Gel filtration and immunochemical analysis of iPTH in which a totally homologous hPTH-(1–34) assay was employed (system b, see legend to Figure 3.2), revealed three elution peaks: the first was eluted between the void volume and hPTH-(1–84), the second coeluted with hPTH-(1–84) and the third was located between the markers hPTH-(1–34) and [^{131}I]hPTH-(1 –12). As is the case with sera from patients with primary hyperparathyroidism, a large molecular weight component represented only a minor fraction of iPTH in sera of patients with renal insufficiency, whereas patients with ectopic hyperparathyroidism seemed to have a considerable amount of an iPTH species with a molecular weight greater than 9500 in their circulation (Benson *et al.*, 1974). The quantity of iPTH corresponding to peptides having a molecular weight of approximately 9500 daltons was also very small in the sera of patients with renal insufficiency. A large part of the iPTH consisted of molecular species ranging in size from approximately the tetratriacontapeptide to the dodecapeptide. The finding of small molecular weight fragments is reminiscent of the results reported by Canterbury and Reiss (1972), who detected iPTH

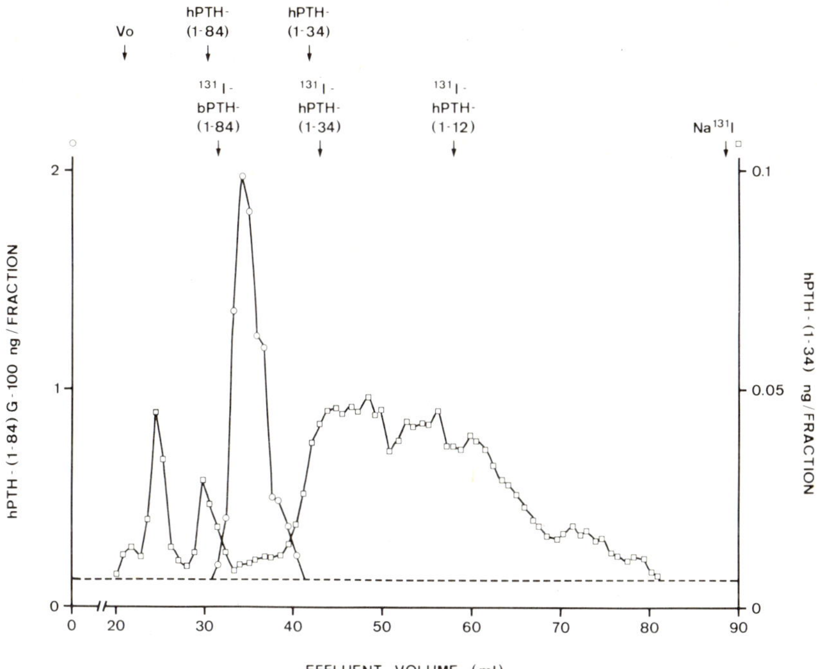

FIGURE 3.2 Characterisation of immunoreactive PTH (iPTH) from a patient with primary hyperparathyroidism. [^{131}I]bPTH-(1–84), [^{131}I]hPTH-(1–34), [^{131}I]hPTH-(1–12) and Na^{131}I were added as markers to a 1 ml sample of serum. The void volume (Vo) and the elution volumes of hPTH-(1–84) and -(1–34) are indicated by arrows (top row). Gel filtration: Bio-Gel P-10, 1 × 100 cm column, 0·2 M ammonium acetate pH 4·7 and human serum albumin (2·5 mg/ml) as eluant, 1·5 ml/hour flow rate, 0·75 ml fractions. iPTH was analysed by means of two radioimmunoassay systems: (a) [^{131}I]bPTH-(1–84), anti-hPTH-(TCA) (goat 3, day 253, 1:1500) and hPTH-(1–84)G-100 as standard (○); (b) [^{131}I]hPTH-(1–34), anti-hPTH-(1–34) (Goat 11, day 116, 1:200 000) and hPTH-(1–34) as standard (□). The broken line indicates the sensitivity limits of the radioimmunoassays.

fragments with molecular weights of 4500 to 5000 daltons in hyperparathyroid sera. These peptides were recognised by antibodies specific for determinants located in the amino-terminal half of hPTH-(1–84) (Goldsmith *et al.*, 1974; Silverman and Yalow, 1973; Canterbury *et al.*, 1973; Arnaud *et al.*, 1974).

Immunochemical analysis of antibodies employed to assay PTH in human sera

Various qualitative properties of goat anti-hPTH-(TCA) and anti-hPTH-(1–34) are demonstrated in Figure 3.3. As judged by inhibition

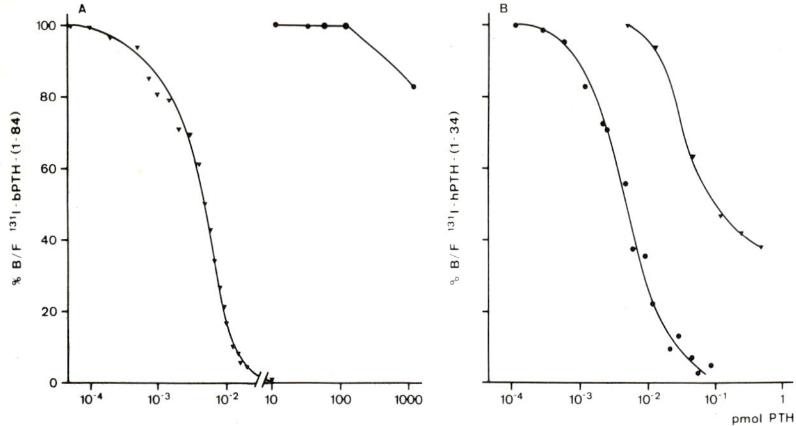

FIGURE 3.3 Qualitative properties of antibodies to extracted hPTH-(TCA) and synthetic hPTH-(1–34) employed in the radioimmunological determination of iPTH in human serum (the source of the antisera is specified in the legend of Figure 3.2). (A) inhibition of specific binding of [^{131}I]bPTH-(1–84) to anti-hPTH-(TCA); (B) inhibition of specific binding of [^{131}I]hPTH-(1–34) to anti-hPTH-(1–34). Inhibitors: hPTH-(1–84)G-100 (▼), hPTH-(1–34) (●); Ordinate: per cent initial ratio of antibody-bound and free ligand (B/F) without inhibitor added.

patterns obtained with hPTH-(1–84) G-100 and hPTH-(1–34), the antibody raised against the full-length extracted hPTH-(TCA) is directed to COOH-terminal parts of the hPTH-(1–84) molecule. Whether or not the amino-terminal-specific antibody raised to the amino-acid sequence 1–34 has also some cross-reactivity with carboxy-terminal parts of hPTH-(1–84) remains to be shown. The substantiation of this possibility depends on the availability of synthetic carboxy-terminal fragments. Figure 3.4 demonstrates qualitative properties of antibodies to hPTH-(TCA) obtained from a different goat. As compared with a serum sample taken 117 days after the first immunisation, there was, however, a considerable increase in reactivity against the amino-terminal sequence of hPTH-(1–84) in the antiserum obtained on day 306 (Figure 3.4, bottom panels). Interestingly enough, antisera of this particular goat taken at various times showed only a

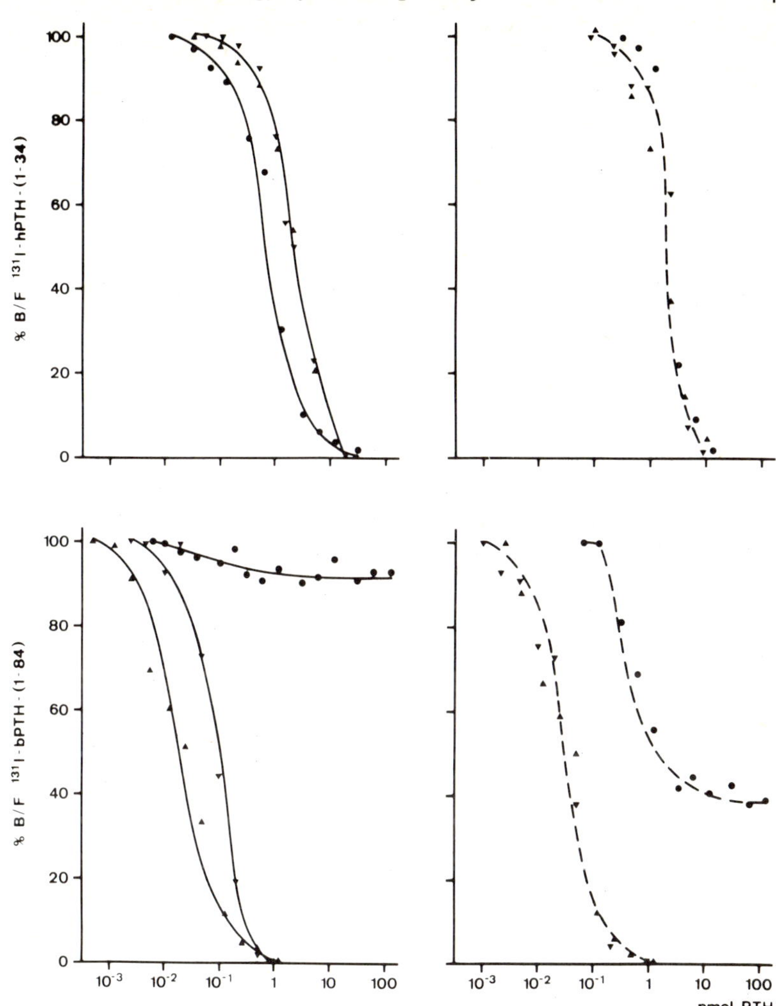

FIGURE 3.4 Qualitative properties of antibodies to extracted hPTH-(TCA). Inhibition of specific binding of [131I]hPTH-(1–34) (upper panels) and of [131I]bPTH-(1–84) (lower panels) to anti-hPTH-(TCA) obtained from goat 1 on day 117 (———) and on day 306 (– – – –). Inhibitors: hPTH-(1–34) (●), pPTH-(1–84)G-100 (▼), bPTH-(1–84) (▲); Ordinate: per cent initial B/F (without inhibitor added).

slight, marginal degree of discrimination between hPTH-(1–84) and bPTH-(1–84), or none at all. This is in contrast to the findings made with different antibodies, which clearly discriminated between the full-length human and bovine hormones when tested with [131I] hPTH-(1–34) as ligand (Fischer *et al.*, 1974b).

The intensity and quality of the immune response to synthetic

TABLE 3.1 *The immune response to synthetic hPTH-(1–34)*

Goat	Antigen*	Day of blood sampling: 26		56		91		116	
	μg		pg		pg		pg		pg
10	35	8·0†	168‡	10†	76‡	2·5†	110‡	15†	41‡
12	35	25	92	15	81	5·0	71	22	36
13	35	1·5	713	4·0	84	2·0	144	5·9	41
11	280	60	129	40	69	12	95	45	32
14	280	3·0	212	3·0	113	1·2	153	13·5	33
15	280	7·0	346	5·0	101	2·0	149	15	38

* Injected on days 0 and 112.
† Dilution-50 (× 10^3) [serum dilution giving 50% binding of [^{131}I]hPTH-(1–34)].
‡ Inhibition dose-50 [amount of hPTH-(1–34) required for a 50% reduction of specific binding of [^{131}I]hPTH-(1–34) to anti-hPTH-(1–34) serum].

hPTH-(1–34) are shown in Table 3.1. High titre antisera were already obtained after a single injection of either 35 μg or 280 μg of peptide incorporated in aluminium hydroxide and complete Freund's adjuvant. After reinjection on day 112, the ID_{50}-values ranged from 32 to 41 pg, indicating that every animal yielded a potent antiserum with high-affinity antibodies. As demonstrated previously (Fischer *et al.*, 1974a and 1974b), these antisera are directed to antigenic sites located in several parts of hPTH-(1–34), including both the carboxy-terminal and amino-terminal regions of the tetratriacontapeptide.

Applicability of radioimmunological methods for the quantitation of circulating parathyroid hormone in clinical medicine

The clinical usefulness of a PTH assay may be assessed first of all by its effectiveness in revealing differences in serum PTH levels in primary hyperparathyroidism and in health. Secondly, it is essential that it should be specific and adequately sensitive. With a single exception (Reiss and Canterbury, 1968), the first criterion was only partially met by the heterologous radioimmunoassay systems reported in the literature. There was always a certain number of hyperparathyroid patients showing serum levels of PTH overlapping those found in the circulation of control subjects. When the antibodies used in the assay system were directed preferentially to the amino-terminal, the overlap was more pronounced than with antibodies exhibiting specificity for antigenic determinants located in the carboxy-terminal part of PTH-(1–84) (Silverman and Yalow, 1973; Arnaud *et al.*, 1974). A similar finding was made in our laboratories in experiments with the homologous radioimmunoassay systems.

In addition, our results confirmed those obtained by Arnaud *et al.* (1971a), who found that the elevation of serum calcium (total and ionised) paralleled the elevation of PTH levels, suggesting that the

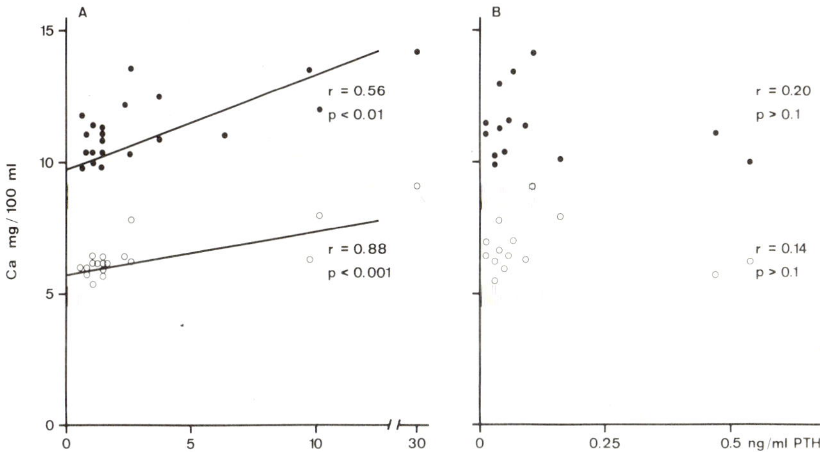

FIGURE 3.5 Correlation between immunoreactive PTH and calcium levels in peripheral sera from patients with primary hyperparathyroidism: A: immunoassay system (a); B: immunoassay system (b) (see legend to Figure 3.2). Ordinate: EGTA-titratable calcium (●) and ionised calcium (O) (Orion calcium specific electrode, Model 99–20). Normal ranges are indicated by shaded areas.

carboxy-specific assay system was biologically valid. This point is made by the data presented in Figure 3.5. There was a statistically significant linear correlation between the calcium and PTH levels when the latter were determined by immunoassay systems (a) (Figure 3.5, Panel A), whereas no correlation was detectable when immunoassay system (b) was used (Figure 3.5, Panel B). As is shown in Figure 3.6A, the immunoassay system (a) also revealed clear-cut differences in the PTH levels in patients with chronic renal insufficiency who were kept on haemodialysis and in control subjects. Again, system (b) employing amino-terminal specific antibodies revealed no such differences (Figure

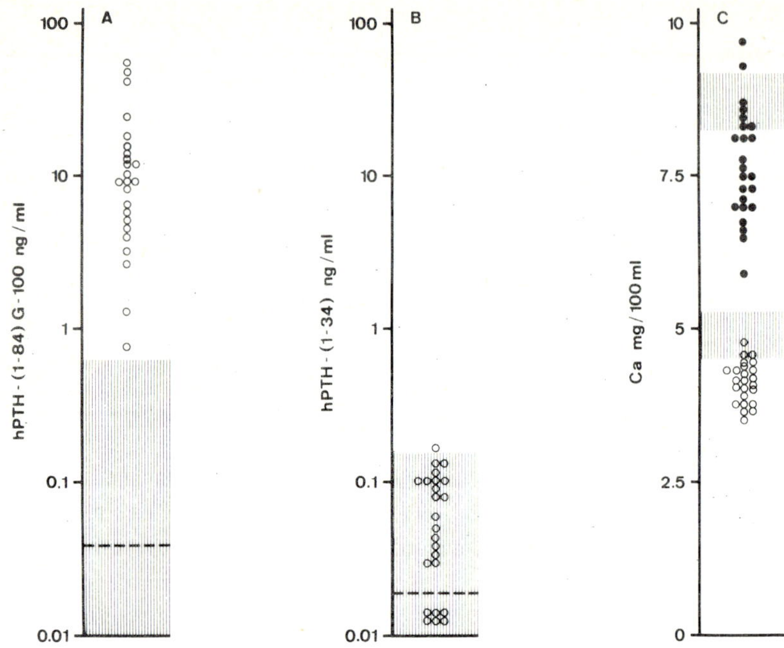

FIGURE 3.6 Immunoreactive PTH and calcium in peripheral serum from patients suffering from chronic renal insufficiency and maintained on haemodialysis. A: immunoassay system (a); B: immunoassay system (b) (see legend to Figure 3.2); C: EGTA-titratable calcium (●) and ionised calcium (O). Normal ranges are indicated by shaded areas.

3.6B). As can be seen in Figure 3.6C, ionised calcium was not elevated in the sera of patients with chronic renal insufficiency; in most cases, it was below the normal range. Elevated PTH levels may be explained by slower metabolic turnover of carboxy-terminal fragments as compared to full-length PTH. Indeed, this seems to be the case in primary hyperparathyroidism (Silverman and Yalow, 1973) and in renal insufficiency (Goldsmith *et al.*, 1973). Alternatively, the postulated suppression of PTH secretion by vitamin D or its biologically active metabolites, which is thought to be effective under normal conditions, may not function in cases of renal insufficiency (Fischer *et al.*, 1973).

Summary and conclusions

The present study provides additional immunological data on newly elaborated PTH assay systems, denoted

(a) [^{131}I]bPTH-(1–84), anti-hPTH-(TCA) and hPTH-(1–84) G-100 as standard, and
(b) [^{131}I]hPTH-(1–34), anti-hPTH-(1–34) and hPTH-(1–34) as standard.

With system (a), mainly carboxy-terminal fragments of hPTH-(1–84) having a molecular weight of approximately 7000 daltons were detected, whereas system (b) detected several molecular species of iPTH. System (a) proved sensitive enough to detect differences in PTH levels in pathological conditions (primary hyperparathyroidism and renal insufficiency) and in health, whereas system (b) did not. The elevated PTH levels determined with system (a) in the sera of patients with primary hyperparathyroidism paralleled calcium concentrations, whereas in the sera of patients suffering from chronic renal insufficiency they were associated with normal or subnormal calcium levels. An increase in PTH and calcium is characteristic of primary and ectopic hyperparathyroidism, whereas increased PTH associated with normal and subnormal calcium is diagnostic for secondary hyperparathyroidism (vitamin D deficiency, renal insufficiency and pseudohypoparathyroidism).

REFERENCES

ANDREATTA, R. H., HARTMANN, A., JOEHL, A., KAMBER, B., MAIER, R., RINIKER, B., RITTEL, W. and SIEBER, P. (1973). Synthese der Sequenz 1–34 von menschlichem Parathormon. *Helv. Chim. Acta*, **56**, 40

ARNAUD, C. D., TSAO, H. S. and OLDHAM, S. B. (1970). Native human parathyroid hormone: an immunochemical investigation. *Proc. Natl. Acad. Sci. USA*, **67**, 415

ARNAUD, C. D., SIZEMORE, G. W., OLDHAM, S. B., FISCHER, J. A., TSAO, H. S. and LITTLEDIKE, E. T. (1971a). Human parathyroid hormone: glandular and secreted molecular species. *Am. J. Med.*, **50**, 630

ARNAUD, C. D., TSAO, H. S. and LITTLEDIKE, T. (1971b). Radioimmunoassay of human parathyroid hormone in serum. *J. Clin. Invest.*, **50**, 21

ARNAUD, C. D., GOLDSMITH, R. S., BORDIER, P. J. and SIZEMORE, G. W. (1974). Influence of immunoheterogeneity of circulating parathyroid hormone on results of radioimmunoassays of serum in man. *Am. J. Med.*, **56**, 785

BENSON, R. C. Jr., RIGGS, B. L., PICKARD, B. M. and ARNAUD, C. D. (1974). Immunoreactive forms of circulating parathyroid hormone in primary and ectopic hyperparathyroidism. *J. Clin. Invest.*, **54**, 175

BERSON, S. A. and YALOW, R. S. (1966). Parathyroid hormone in plasma in adenomatous hyperparathyroidism, uremia, and bronchogenic carcinoma. *Science*, **154**, 907

BERSON, S. A. and YALOW, R. S. (1968). Immunochemical heterogeneity of parathyroid hormone in plasma. *J. Clin. Endocrinol. Metab.*, **28**, 1037

BLAIR, A. J. Jr., HAWKER, C. D. and UTIGER, R. D. (1973). Ectopic hyperparathyroidism in a patient with metastatic hypernephroma. *Metabolism*, **22**, 147

BREWER, H. B. Jr., FAIRWELL, T., RONAN, R., SIZEMORE, G. W. and ARNAUD, C. D. (1972). Human parathyroid hormone: amino-acid sequence of the amino-terminal residues 1–34. *Proc. Natl. Acad. Sci. USA*, **69**, 3585

BREWER, H. B. Jr., FAIRWELL, T., RITTEL, W., LITTLEDIKE, T. and ARNAUD, C. D. (1974). Recent studies on the chemistry of human, bovine and porcine parathyroid hormones. *Am. J. Med.*, **56**, 759

CANTERBURY, J. M. and REISS, E. (1972). Multiple immunoreactive molecular forms of parathyroid hormone in human serum. *Proc. Soc. Exp. Biol. Med.*, **140**, 1393

CANTERBURY, J. M., LEVEY, G. S. and REISS, E. (1973). Activation of renal cortical adenylate cyclase by circulating immunoreactive parathyroid hormone fragments. *J. Clin. Invest.*, **52**, 524

CHU, L. L. H., MACGREGOR, R. R., LIU, P. I., HAMILTON, J. W. and COHN, D. V. (1973). Biosynthesis of proparathyroid hormone and parathyroid hormone by human parathyroid glands. *J. Clin. Invest.*, **52**, 3089

CONAWAY, H. H. and ANAST, C. S. (1974). Double-antibody radioimmunoassay for parathyroid hormone. *J. Lab. Clin. Med.*, **83**, 129

FISCHER, J. A., BINSWANGER, U., FANCONI, A., ILLIG, R., BAERLOCHER, K. and PRADER, A. (1973). Serum parathyroid hormone concentrations in vitamin D deficiency rickets of infancy: effects of intravenous calcium and vitamin D. *Horm. Metab. Res.*, **5**, 381

FISCHER, J. A., BINSWANGER, U., RITTEL, W. and DIETRICH, F. M. (1974a). Human parathyroid hormone: immunological characterisation of antibodies against the synthetic amino-terminal fragment 1–34, and their use in the determination of immunoreactive hormone in human serum. In S. Taylor (ed.), *Endocrinology* 1973, p. 229. (London : Heinemann)

FISCHER, J. A., BINSWANGER, U. and DIETRICH, F. M. (1974b). Human parathyroid hormone: immunological characterisation of antibodies against a glandular extract and the synthetic amino-terminal fragment 1–12 and 1–34 and their use in the determination of immunoreactive hormone in human sera. *J. Clin. Invest.*, **54**, 1382

GOLDSMITH, R. S., FURSZYFER, J., JOHNSON, W. J., FOURNIER, A. E., SIZEMORE, G. W. and ARNAUD, C. D. (1973). Etiology of hyperparathyroidism and bone disease during chronic hemodialysis. III. Evaluation of parathyroid suppressibility. *J. Clin. Invest.*, **52**, 173

HABENER, J. F., POWELL, D., MURRAY, T. M., MAYER, G. P. and POTTS, J. T. Jr. (1971). Parathyroid hormone: secretion and metabolism in vivo. *Proc. Natl. Acad. Sci. USA*, **68**, 2986

HABENER, J. F., KEMPER, B., POTTS, J. T. Jr. and RICH, A. (1972). Proparathyroid hormone: biosynthesis by human parathyroid adenomas. *Science*, **178**, 630

HAMILTON, J. W., NIALL, H. D., JACOBS, J. W., KEUTMANN, H. T., POTTS, J. T. Jr. and COHN, D. V. (1974). The N-terminal amino-acid sequence of bovine proparathyroid hormone. *Proc. Natl. Acad. Sci. USA*, **71**, 653

HAMILTON, J. W., HUANG, D. W. Y., CHU, L. L. H., MACGREGOR, R. R. and COHN, D. V. (1975). Chemical and biological properties of proparathyroid hormone. In R. V. Talmadge, M. Owen, and J. A. Parsons (eds.), *Calcium-regulating Hormones*, p. 40. (Amsterdam: Excerpta Medica).

JACOBS, J. W., KEMPER, B., NIALL, H. D., HABENER, J. F. and POTTS, J. T. Jr. (1974). Structural analysis of human proparathyroid hormone by a new microsequencing approach. *Nature*, **249**, 155

KEUTMANN, H. T., BARLING, P. M., HENDY, G. N., SEGRE, G. V., NIALL, H. D., AURBACH, G. D., POTTS, J. T. Jr. and O'RIORDAN, J. L. H. (1974). Isolation of human parathyroid hormone. *Biochemistry*, **13**, 1646

LEQUIN, R. M., HACKENG, W. H. L. and SCHOPMAN, W. (1970). A radioimmunoassay for parathyroid hormone in man. II. Measurement of parathyroid hormone concentrations in human plasma by means of a radioimmunoassay for bovine hormone. *Acta Endocrinol.*, **63**, 655

MARTIN, T. J., GREENBERG, P. B. and MICHELANGELI, V. (1973). Synthesis of human parathyroid hormone by cultured cells: evidence for relase of prohormone by some adenomata. *Clin. Sci.*, **44**, 1

NIALL, H. D., SAUER, R. T., JACOBS, J. W., KEUTMANN, H. T., SEGRE, G. V., O'RIORDAN, J. L. H., AURBACH, G. D. and POTTS, J. T. Jr. (1974). The amino-acid sequence of the amino-terminal 37 residues of human parathyroid hormone. *Proc. Natl. Acad. Sci. USA*, **71**, 384

NIALL, H. D., JACOBS, J. W., BARLING, P. M., HENDY, G. N., O' RIORDAN, J. L. H. and POTTS, J. T., Jr. (1975). A reinvestigation of the amino-terminal sequence of parathyroid hormone and analysis of the residues 44-69. In R. V. Talmadge, M. Owen and J. A. Parsons (eds.), *Calcium-regulating Hormones*, p. 9. (Amsterdam: Excerpta Medica)

POTTS, J. T. Jr., MURRAY, T. M., PEACOCK, M., NIALL, H. D., TREGEAR, G. W.,

KEUTMANN, H. T., POWELL, D. and DEFTOS, L. J. (1971). Parathyroid hormone sequence, synthesis, immunoassay studies. *Am. J. Med.*, **50**, 639

REISS, E. and CANTERBURY, J. M. (1968). A radioimmunoassay for parathyroid hormone in man. *Proc. Soc. Exp. Biol. Med.*, **128**, 501

ROOF, B. S., GORDAN, G. S., GOLDMAN, L. and PIEL, C. F. (1973). Berson and Yalow's radioimmunoassay for parathyroid hormone: a clinical progress report. *Mt. Sinai J. Med., N.Y.*, **40**, 433

SEGRE, G. V., HABENER, J. F., POWELL, D., TREGEAR, G. W. and POTTS, J. T. Jr. (1972). Parathyroid hormone in human plasma: immunochemical characterisation and biological implication. *J. Clin. Invest.*, **51**, 3163

SEGRE, G. V., NIALL, H. D., HABENER, J. F. and POTTS, J. T. Jr. (1974). Metabolism of parathyroid hormone, physiologic and clinical significance. *Am. J. Med.*, **57**, 774

SHERWOOD, L. M., RODMAN, J. S. and LUNDBERG, W. B. (1970). Evidence for a precursor to circulating parathyroid hormone. *Proc. Nat. Acad. Sci. USA*, **67**, 1631

SILVERMAN, R. and YALOW, R. W. (1973). Heterogeneity of parathyroid hormone: clinical and physiologic implications. *J. Clin. Invest.*, **52**, 1958

4

Parathyroid hormone in hereditary diseases of mineral metabolism

A. Fanconi and J. A. Fischer

The recent development of a reliable radioimmunoassay for the determination of parathyroid hormone (PTH) levels in human sera is of great importance for clinical research. In this report we present results obtained in children with hereditary disorders of mineral metabolism: pseudovitamin D deficiency, familial hypophosphataemic vitamin D resistant rickets and pseudohypoparathyroidism. Some of the data have recently been published (Fischer *et al.*, 1973; Fanconi *et al.*, 1974), others are unpublished.

Methods

Circulating PTH was estimated radioimmunologically (Arnaud *et al.*, 1971a; Fischer *et al.*, 1974) by a heterologous system with ^{131}I labelled bovine PTH-(1–84), anti-porcine PTH, and a standard obtained from a tissue culture medium of parathyroid tumour explants *in vitro*.* Since the human PTH-(1–34) (Brewer *et al.*, 1972; Andreatta *et al.*, 1973) is not recognised in this system, the antibodies used are presumably directed to the carboxy-terminal half of the human PTH-(1–84). On gel filtration of hyperparathyroid sera, immunoreactive PTH fragments with an apparent molecular weight of about 7000 are primarily recognised. The upper limit of normal immunoreactive PTH (iPTH) levels in control children older than 6 months and in adults amounts to 40 ng/ml. Undetectable values are found in less than 5% of adult control subjects (Fischer *et al.*, 1973; Fischer *et al.*, 1974).

Serum calcium concentrations were determined either by automatic EGTA titration (normal range for adults 8·3–9·7 mg/100ml), or, in the case of pseudovitamin D deficiency, by atomic absorption spectrophotometry (normal range 8·9–10·2 mg/100 ml).

* The antiserum (GP1M) and the tissue culture standard were kindly provided by Dr C. D. Arnaud, Rochester, Minn.

Pseudovitamin D deficiency rickets (vitamin D dependency)

Clinical, pathogenetical and therapeutical aspects of this disease are reported in detail by Prader and Kind in this symposium (p. 115). Our iPTH results concern two siblings, a girl of 8 years and her 6-year-old sister. The initial iPTH determinations were performed when both patients developed a relapse of their disease during a therapeutic trial with dihydrotachysterol in small amounts (30 μg/day) which proved to be ineffective. During that time, the serum calcium in the older girl

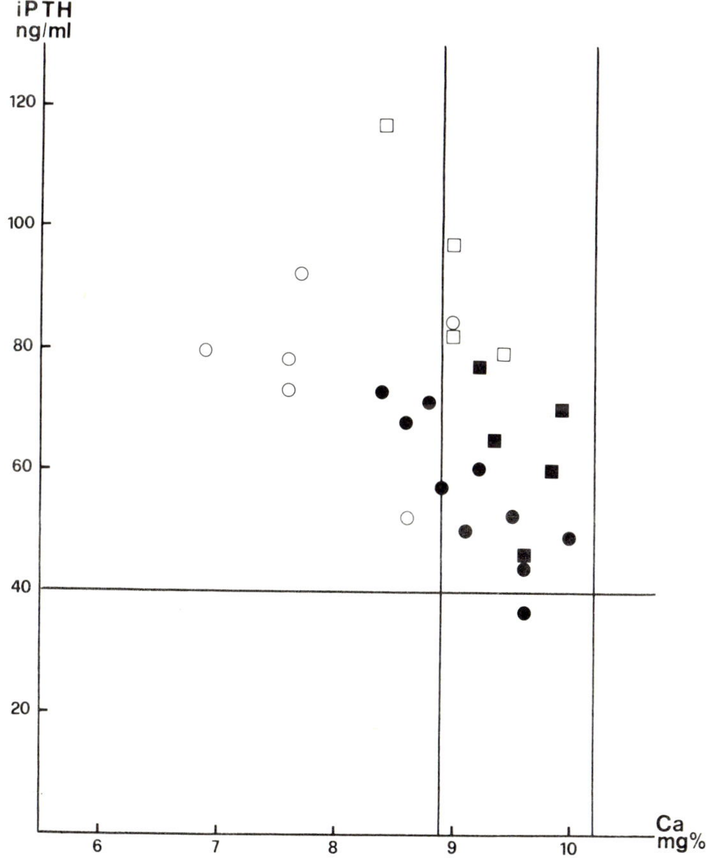

FIGURE 4.1 iPTH and serum calcium in pseudovitamin D deficiency rickets. Measurements in two siblings (□ and ○). Open symbols: No treatment or inefficient treatment. Closed symbols: effective treatment with 1-25-dihydroxycholecalciferol or 1α-hydroxycholecalciferol. The solid lines indicate the normal limits.

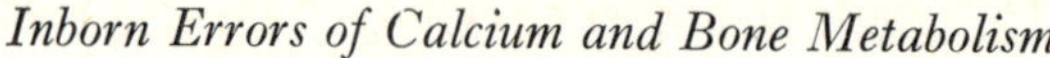

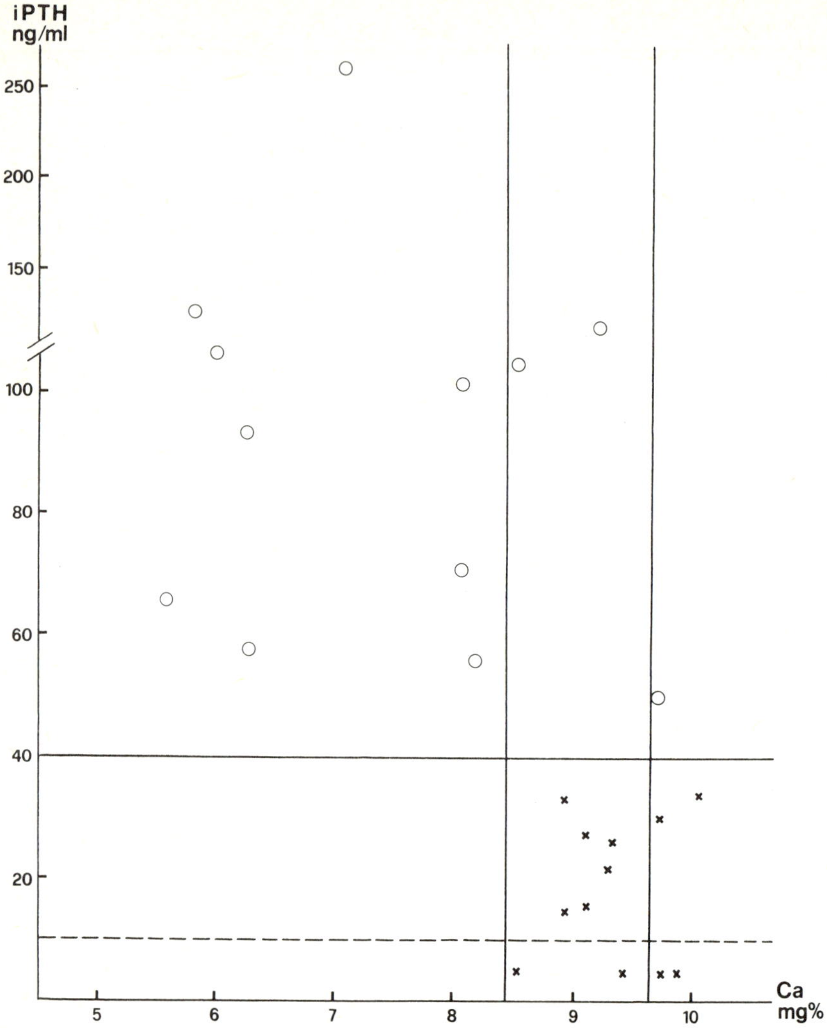

FIGURE 4.2 iPTH and serum calcium in vitamin D deficiency rickets. ○, 12 patients with rickets; ×, 12 control children. The solid lines indicate the normal limits, the broken line the sensitivity limit of the iPTH assay.

decreased from 9·6 to 7·6 mg/100 ml, and in the younger one from 9·9 to 8·4 mg/100 ml. The alkaline phosphatase was highly elevated, and radiological signs of rickets reappeared in both patients. iPTH increased to 92 ng/ml in the older and to 117 ng/ml in the younger sister.

The patients were subjected to a therapeutical trial with small amounts of 1,25-dihydroxycholecalciferol (1 μg/day) in one case, and 1αhydroxycholecalciferol (2 μg/day) in the other case, just enough to induce remineralisation. The changes in the iPTH concentrations were followed closely during the 2 months of treatment.

While the serum calcium rose to normal levels after 30 days in one and after 10 days in the other patient, the iPTH decreased at a slower rate and reached the upper normal limit after 2 months only, when the trial had to be stopped because of shortage of the drug. The iPTH results plotted against the serum calcium concentrations are shown in Figure 4.1. The open symbols represent measurements in relapse, the closed symbols during effective treatment.

The increased iPTH values in the untreated child and the slow response to treatment correspond exactly to our observations in children with nutritional vitamin D deficiency (Fischer *et al.*, 1973). Figure 4.2 shows iPTH determinations in untreated nutritional rickets. Secondary hyperparathyroidism in both deficiency and pseudo-deficiency rickets is

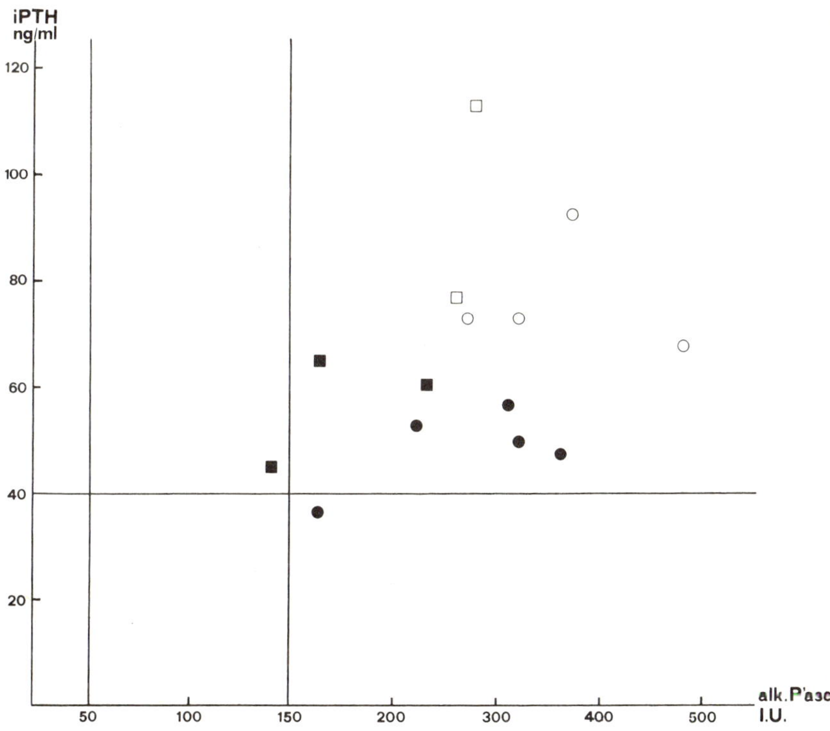

FIGURE 4.3 iPTH and serum alkaline phosphate in pseudovitamin D deficiency rickets. Symbols as in Figure 4.1.

beyond any doubt. Similar findings have been published by other investigators (Lequin *et al.*, 1970; Arnaud *et al.*, 1972; Arnaud *et al.*, 1970).

It is of particular interest, that iPTH in rickets is increased not only in hypocalcaemic but also in normocalcaemic patients. In hypocalcaemic patients the normalisation of iPTH takes longer than the normalisation of the serum calcium levels. The rate of normalisation of PTH corresponds to the slow decline of the alkaline phosphatase and therefore to the healing of the rickets rather than to the rapid rise of the serum calcium concentration. This phenomenon is shown on Figure 4.3, where iPTH in our two patients with pseudo-deficiency rickets is plotted against alkaline phosphatase measured in the same serum samples.

These observations might indicate that in both types of rickets hypocalcaemia is not the only stimulus for PTH secretion. Vitamin D may have a direct action on PTH secretion, vitamin D deficiency having a stimulating effect and vitamin D treatment a suppressing effect.

Familial hypophosphataemic vitamin D-resistant rickets (X-linked hypophosphataemia, phosphate diabetes)

The question whether hypophosphataemia was due to a secondary hyperparathyroidism following a primary disturbance of intestinal calcium absorption, or to a primary renal tubular phosphate leak, was hotly debated for many years. The determination of iPTH levels in the serum of these patients was therefore of particular interest. The answer was first given in 1971 by the work of Arnaud *et al.* (1971b), who found iPTH levels within or close to the normal range in untreated patients and in those treated with vitamin D. Patients receiving large therapeutic doses of oral phosphate had increased iPTH concentrations. Lewy *et al.*, (1972) and Reitz and Weinstein (1973) found slightly increased iPTH levels, however not sufficiently high to explain the severity of phosphaturia and hypophosphataemia in this disease.

Figure 4.4 shows our results in 11 patients aged 4–23 years (Fanconi *et al.*, 1974). iPTH is plotted against the serum calcium concentration. All the values are in the normal range, whether the patients were treated with vitamin D or not.

In two adult patients with the sporadic late onset type of hypophosphataemic vitamin D resistant osteomalacia, iPTH was also normal.

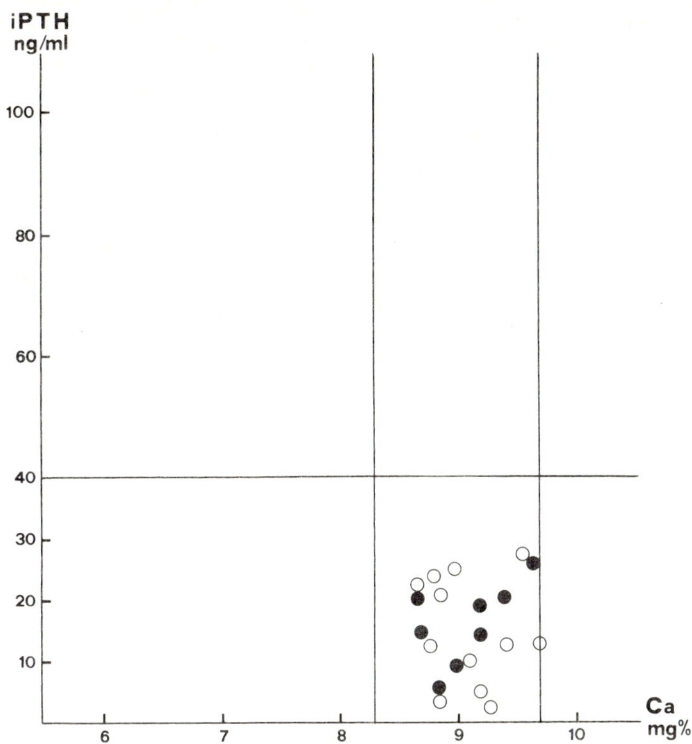

FIGURE 4.4 iPTH and serum calcium in familial hypophosphataemic vitamin D resistant rickets. 11 patients, 20 determinations, ○, Without vitamin D treatment; ●, With vitamin D treatment. The solid lines indicate the normal limits.

The effects of a single oral load with neutral sodium phosphate in three patients are shown on Figure 4.5. Although the serum phosphorus concentration rose by about 1 mg/100 ml, it failed to reach the normal range. The serum calcium decreased slightly, without however falling below normal levels. iPTH increased slightly within the normal range. These results demonstrate the sensitivity of the radioimmunoassay. The phosphate load however was too small to produce hyperparathyroidism. The same is true of two patients during long-term sodium phosphate treatment, 6 g/day in a child, and 10–15 g/day in an adult patient. However, iPTH concentrations rose from 15 to 122 ng/ml in our youngest patient, a boy of 3 months, when he was given 4 times 1 g neutral sodium phosphate per day. High dose phosphate treatment carries the risk of producing secondary hyperparathyroidism.

The fact that PTH is highly elevated in vitamin D deficiency and pseudo-deficiency rickets, but normal in familial hypophosphataemic rickets, is in agreement with older observations, that the former types of rickets are often associated with radiological signs of hyperparathyroidism whereas comparable findings are absent in untreated familial hypophosphataemia.

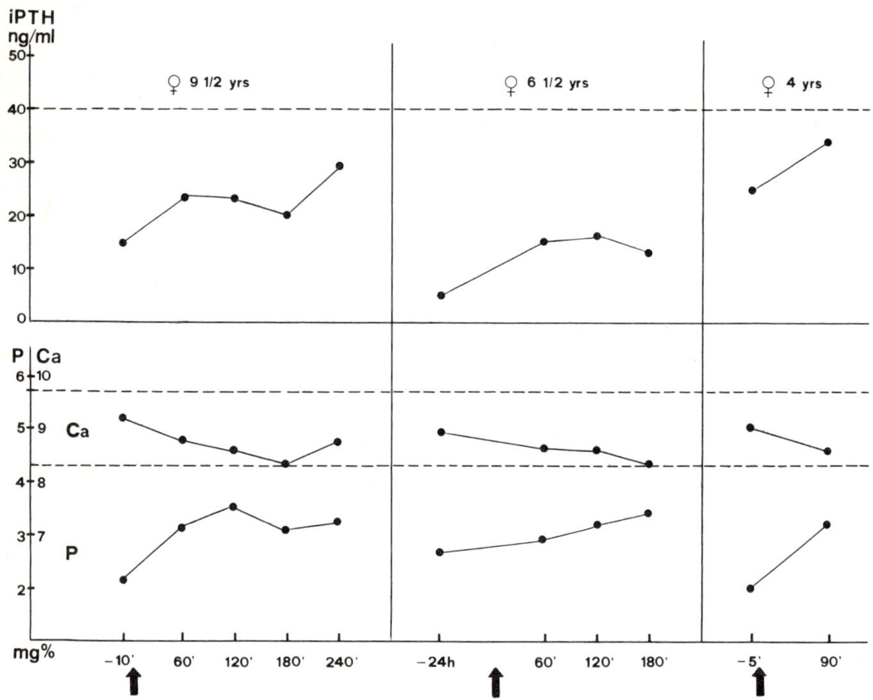

FIGURE 4.5 Effect of oral Na phosphate load (1000 mg/m²) on iPTH, serum calcium and serum phosphorus in three patients with familial hypophosphataemic rickets. The broken lines indicate the normal limits.

Pseudohypoparathyroidism

Figure 4.6 shows iPTH determinations plotted against serum calcium concentrations in patients with idiopathic hypoparathyroidism, pseudohypoparathyroidism, and pseudopseudohypoparathyroidism. In true idiopathic hypoparathyroidism, iPTH is not detectable or is very low, and there is no relationship to the serum calcium concentration. This finding is expected from the definition of the disease. Two normocalcaemic adults and a 12-year-old normocalcaemic girl with pseudopseudohypoparathyroidism had normal iPTH values.

The diagnosis in children with pseudohypoparathyroidism was based on the typical physical stigmata of Albright's osteodystrophy, hypocalcaemia, hyperphosphataemia, and insufficient urinary cyclic AMP responses to intravenous parathyroid extract (Stögmann and Fischer, 1975; Werder *et al.*, 1975). The iPTH values were elevated when the patients were not or were insufficiently treated and therefore hypocalcaemic. When the serum calcium returns to normal as the result of adequate vitamin D treatment, iPTH decreases into the normal range.

Two additional patients are of particular interest, since they demon-

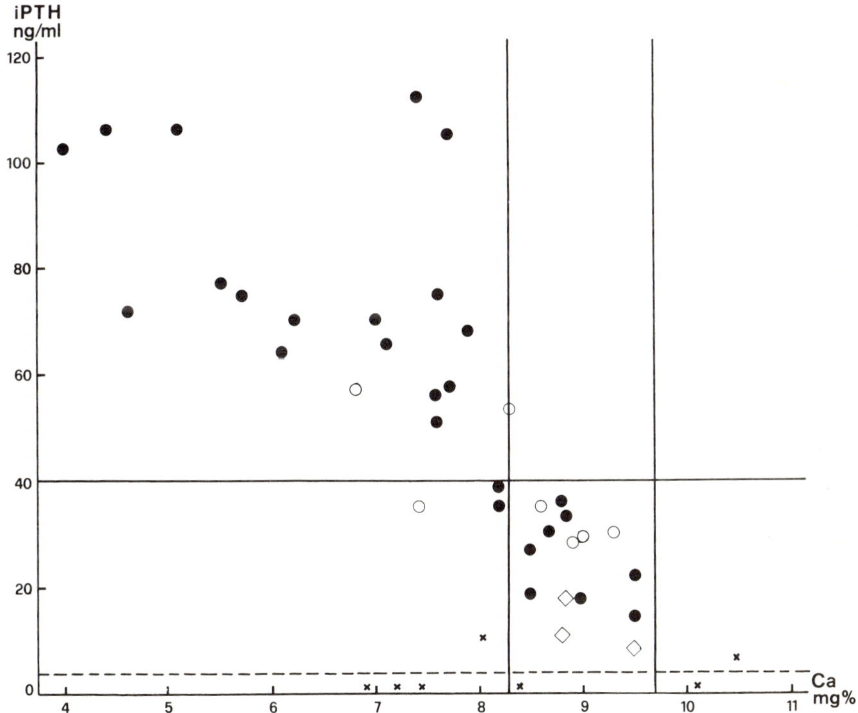

FIGURE 4.6 iPTH and serum calcium in pseudohypoparathyroidism, pseudopseudohypoparathyroidism and idiopathic hypoparathyroidism. ●, Pseudohypoparathyroidism (10 patients, 27 determinations); O, Pseudohypoparathyroidism without physical stigmata (two patients, seven determinations); □, Pseudopseudohyparathyroidism (three patients); ×, Idiopathic hypoparathyroidism (seven patients). The solid lines indicate the normal limits, the broken line the sensitivity limit of the iPTH assay.

strate the value of iPTH determinations for the diagnosis of pseudohypoparathyroidism. Both patients were previously diagnosed as cases of idiopathic hypoparathyroidism by their normal physical appearance and because they responded with an increase in the serum calcium concentration following intramuscular injections of parathyroid extract. Surprisingly, their iPTH levels were not low, but normal or even elevated. The diagnosis had therefore to be reconsidered. An intravenous injection of parathyroid extract (Parathormone Lilly 300 u.USP/1·73 m^2 body surface area) did not produce an increase of the urinary cyclic AMP excretion. The correct diagnosis is therefore pseudohypoparathyroidism without physical stigmata. Figure 4.7 is the photograph of

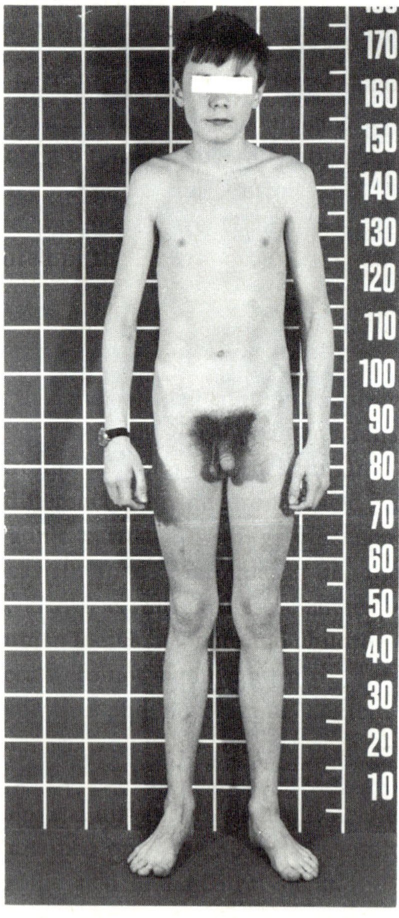

FIGURE 4.7 Fourteen-year-old boy with pseudohypoparathyroidism without physical stigmata of Albright's osteodystrophy.

one of these patients, a 14-year-old boy. The other patient is a girl, whose findings were published 10 years ago as 'clinical and biochemical hypoparathyroidism with radiological hyperparathyroidism' (Fanconi *et al.*, 1964). This apparently paradoxical combination which has been called 'hypo-hyperparathyroidism' by Costello and Dent (1963), has been described in at least eight published cases. In two of these (Frame *et al.*, 1972) the serum iPTH was also found to be elevated.

There exists therefore not only what we usually call Albright's osteodystrophy with or without hypocalcaemia (pseudo- and pseudo-pseudohypoparathyroidism), but also pseudohypoparathyroidism with or without the typical physical stigmata of Albright's osteodystrophy.

In untreated pseudohypoparathyroidism, the excessively secreted PTH might act on the bone structure producing radiological signs of hyperparathyroidism, but remain metabolically ineffective, since the renal tubule is unable to respond to the hormone in the expected way, and the serum calcium concentration remains low. However, after normalisation of the serum calcium and iPTH levels due to effective vitamin D treatment, an adequate hypercalcaemic and phosphaturic response to exogenous PTH has been demonstrated (Suh *et al.*, 1970; Kind *et al.*, 1973); Stögmann and Fischer, in press; Fanconi unpublished observation).

Summary

Serum immunoreactive parathyroid hormone is elevated in untreated vitamin D deficiency and pseudovitamin D deficiency rickets, whether these patients are hypocalcaemic or normocalcaemic. iPTH returns into the normal range when the rickets is healed and the alkaline phosphatase normalised.

In familial hypophosphateamic vitamin D resistant rickets, iPTH is normal, except when very high doses of phosphate are given. The hypophosphataemia is not the result of a secondary hyperparathyroidism, but rather of a primary defect of phosphate transport in the tubular cells.

Pseudohypoparathyroidism, whether associated with the stigmata of Albright's osteodystrophy or not, causes secondary hyperparathyroidism.

REFERENCES

ANDREATTA, R. H., HARTMANN, A., JOEHL, A., KAMBER, B., MAIER, R., RINIKER, B., RITTEL, W. and SIEBER, P. (1973). Synthese der Sequenz 1–34 von menschlichem Parathormon. *Helv. Chim. Acta*, **56**, 470

ARNAUD, C., MAIJER, R., READE, T., SCRIVER, C. R. and WHELAN, D. T. (1970). Vitamin D dependency. An inherited postnatal syndrome with secondary hyperparathyroidism. *Pediatrics*, **46**, 871

ARNAUD, C., TSAO, H. S. and LITTLEDIKE, E. T. (1971a). Radioimmunoassay of human parathyroid hormone in serum. *J. Clin. Invest.*, **50**, 21

ARNAUD, C., GLORIEUX, F. and SCRIVER, C. R. (1971b). Serum parathyroid hormone in X-linked hypophosphatemia. *Science*, **173**, 845

ARNAUD, C., GLORIEUX, F. and SCRIVER, C. R. (1972). Serum parathyroid hormone levels in acquired vitamin D deficiency of infancy. *Pediatrics*, **49**, 837

BREWER, H. B., FAIRWELL, T., RONAN, R., SIZEMORE, G. W. and ARNAUD, C. (1972). Human parathyroid hormone: amino-acid sequence of the amino-terminal residues 1–34. *Proc. Nat. Acad. Sci. USA.*, **69**, 3585

COSTELLO, J. M. and DENT, C. E. (1963). Hypo-hyperparathyroidism. *Arch. Dis. Child.*, **38**, 397

FANCONI, A., HEINRICH, H. G. and PRADER, A. (1964). Klinischer und biochemischer Hypoparathyreoidismus mit radiologischem Hyperparathyreoidismus. *Helv. Paediatr. Acta*, **19**, 181

FANCONI, A., FISCHER, J. A. and PRADER, A. (1974). Serum parathyroid hormone concentrations in hypophosphataemic vitamin D resistant rickets. *Helv. Paediatr. Acta*, **29**, 187

FISCHER, J. A., BINSWANGER, U., FANCONI, A., ILLIG, R., BAERLOCHER, K. and PRADER, A. (1973). Serum parathyroid hormone concentrations in vitamin D deficiency rickets of infancy. Effects of intravenous calcium and vitamin D. *Horm. Metab. Res.*, **5**, 381

FISCHER, J. A., BINSWANGER, U., RITTEL, W. and DIETRICH, F. M. (1974). Human parathyroid hormone: immunological characterisation of antibodies against the synthetic amino-terminal fragment 1–34 and their use in the determination of immunoreactive parathyroid hormone in human sera. In S. Taylor (ed.), *Endocrinology* **1973**, p. 229. (London : Heinemann)

FRAME, B., HANSON, C. A., FROST, H. M., BLOCK, M. and ARNSTEIN, A. R. (1972). Renal resistance to parathyroid hormone with osteitis fibrosa. 'Pseudohypohyperparathyroidism'. *Am. J. Med.*, **52**, 311

KIND, H. P., PARKINSON, D. K., SUH, S. M., FRASER, D. and KOOH, S. W. (1973). Parathyroid hormone response and effects of vitamin D in hypoparathyroidism and pseudohypoparathyroidism. *Endocrinology*, (*Suppl.*), **92**, 164

LEQUIN, R. M., HACKENG, W. H. L. and SCHOPMAN, W. (1970). A radioimmunoassay for parathyroid hormone in man. II. Measurement of parathyroid hormone concentrations in human plasma by means of a radioimmunoassay for bovine hormone. *Acta Endocrinol.*, **63**, 655

LEWY, J. E., CABANA, E. C., REPETTO, H. A., CANTERBURY, J. M. and REISS, E. (1972). Serum parathyroid hormone in hypophosphatemic vitamin D resistant rickets. *J. Pediatr.*, **81**, 294

REITZ, R. E. and WEINSTEIN, R. L. (1973). Parathyroid hormone secretion in familial vitamin D resistant rickets. *N. Engl. J. Med.*, **289**, 941

STOEGMANN, W. and FISCHER, J. A. (1975). Pseudohypoparathyroidism: Disappearance of the resistance to parathyroid extract during treatment with vitamin D. *Am. J. Med.*, **59**, 140

SUH, S. M., FRASER, D. and KOOH, S. W. (1970). Pseudohypoparathyroidism: responsiveness to parathyroid extract induced by vitamin D therapy. *J. Clin. Endocrinol.*, **30**, 609

WERDER, E. A., ILLIG, R., FISCHER, J. A., FANCONI, A., BERNASCONI, S., KIND, H. P. and PRADER, A. (1975). Excessive thyrotropin response to thyrotropin-releasing hormone in pseudohypoparathyroidism. *Pediatr. Res.*, **9**, 12

5

Parathyroid function in infants and children

Barbara E. Clayton, Angela Fairney, D. Flynn and Doreen Jackson

A radioimmunoassay for parathyroid hormone (iPTH) has been used to study some disturbances of calcium metabolism in children. Patients studied have included infants and children with hypocalcaemia, children with thalassaemia and some miscellaneous conditions.

Estimation of parathyroid hormone

The radioimmunoassay was an adaptation of the standard double antibody technique used for growth hormone (Morgan and Lazarow, 1963; Jackson *et al.*, 1968). It required only micro quantities of serum and used an antiserum known to cross-react with human parathyroid hormone (PTH).

Capillary or occasionally venous samples of blood were allowed to clot for less than 2 hours at room temperature; the sera were separated by centrifuging and stored at −20 °C in acid-washed glass bottles until required for assay.

ASSAY OF PARATHYROID HORMONE

Materials used included (1) for iodination (a) highly purified bovine PTH (bPTH), (Wilson Laboratories, Chicago, USA); (b) ^{125}I (Radiochemical Centre, Amersham, Bucks, UK); (2) for standards (a) bPTH, purified on Sephadex (2000MRC units/mg), (b) serum from a patient with primary hyperparathyroidism (kindly donated by Professor C. E. Dent); (3) for antiserum, anti-bPTH serum (guinea pig) batch AS 211/32 (supplied by Wellcome Research Laboratories, Beckenham, Kent and Division of Biological Standards, Mill Hill, London). This antiserum did not reveal an exclusive reaction with any portion of the parathyroid hormone molecule, either at the amino-terminal or the carboxy-terminal. (Cotes, 1974); (4) as precipitating serum, antiguinea-pig γ-globulin from rabbits; (5) three diluents were used in the system, A,

B, and C.: A was hypoparathyroid serum (kindly donated by Dr W. H. Taylor and Professor C. E. Dent) and was used for the standard curve and any test sera requiring further dilution; B was veronal buffer (0·1 M) + hypoparathyroid serum (6 : 1) and was used for the antiserum and labelled PTH; C consisted of 2 vol. diluent B, 1 vol. 0·1M EDTA and 1 : 1000 normal guinea-pig serum and was used to equalise incubation volumes. Parathyroid hormone was labelled with ^{125}I by a modified Hunter and Greenwood technique (Greenwood *et al.*, 1963; Yalow and Berson, 1966; Woodhead, 1971), stored in aliquots at −20 °C and diluted for the assay so that 30 μl labelled hormone gave 100 counts per second. The labelled material produced 75–80% counts bound in the presence of excess PTH antibody and less than 10% counts bound in the absence of PTH antibody. The assay procedure is shown in Table 5.1. The control incubation consisted of 'buffer blanks' composed of 400 μl diluent C + labelled hormone + precipitating serum. Two sera, one of known high PTH value and one of low, were included in each assay. When sufficient serum was available 'serum blanks' composed of a 1 : 2 dilution of serum to be assayed + diluent C + labelled hormone +

Table 5.1 *Assay procedure for iPTH*

Solution	*Volume* (μl)
Antiserum 1 : 40 000	100
Standard PTH : 50–3200 pg/ml bPTH or	
dilutions of primary hyperparathyroid serum	50
or patient samples	50
Diluent C	250
Preincubate at 4 °C for 24 hours	
[^{125}I]PTH	30
Incubate at 4 °C for 72 hours	
Precipitating serum	50
Incubate at 4 °C for 24 hours	

Procedure
Centrifuge twice at 1500 g for 15 minutes after washing with veronal buffer; count precipitate for 100 seconds.

Table 5.2 *Recovery of bPTH*

	Amount of bPTH added (pg)				
	50	150	300	600	1200
Mean amount recovered	56	149·5	355·6	627	1218
Mean % recovered	112	99	118	104	102
No. of experiments	4	4	4	4	4

precipitating serum were included for each patient. The reliability of the assay was assessed by performing recovery experiments (see Table 5.2). Most serum samples were assayed at two dilutions (25 and 50 μl/350 μl incubation volume), and values obtained agreed within 20%. For replicate determinations the interassay coefficients of variation for values above 300, 100 to 300 and less than 100 pg/ml were 7·9, 24·8 and 29·3% respectively. The lower limit of sensitivity for the assay was 39 pg/ml bPTH.

The reference range for iPTH during childhood

Concentrations of iPTH were determined in a series of healthy subjects which included (1) 14 cord bloods, (2) 14 infants at the sixth day of life, (3) 8 infants aged 4–36 weeks, (4) 15 children aged 1–6 years, (5) 3 children aged 7 years, (6) 13 children aged 8, 9 and 10 years, (7) 15 aged 11, 12 and 13 years, (8) 9 aged 14, 15 and 16 years and (9) 10 adults. The results are given in Figure 5.1. The iPTH concentration rose significantly ($P < 0{\cdot}01$) between birth and the sixth day of life but there was no significant further increase in the older infants or children aged 1–6 years. A further significant rise ($P < 0{\cdot}01$) was seen in the children aged 8, 9 and 10 years (mean concentration 403 pg/ml) compared with the levels in infants and children up to 6 years old. There was however no significant rise in the 11–16-year-olds compared with those under 6 years but the concentrations of iPTH were widely scattered. Perhaps comparison of the results against the stage of puberty rather than chronological age will clarify this when sufficient data are available. Levels in the adults were higher ($P < 0{\cdot}001$) compared with those in infants and children up to 6 years.

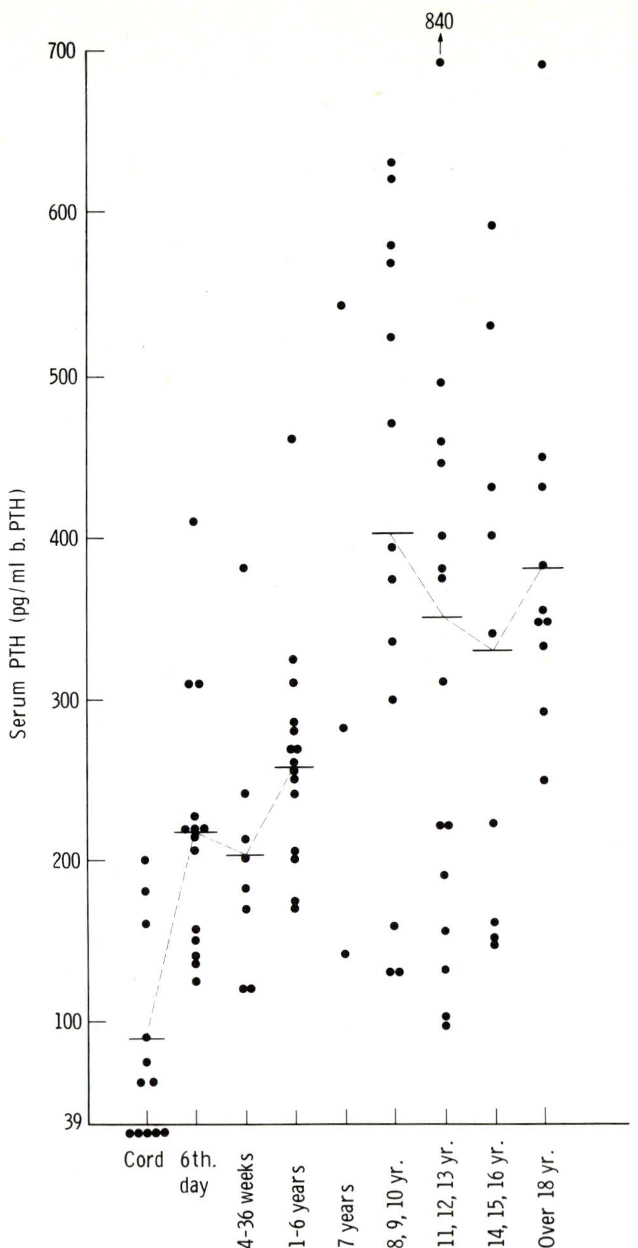

FIGURE 5.1 Concentrations of iPTH in terms of bPTH in normal children. (— indicates mean value for the age group)

Reports on the concentration of iPTH during childhood are somewhat conflicting. Other reports agree that it is low or undetectable in cord blood and rises during the first 9 days (David and Anast, 1974) and the first 2 years (Roof *et al.*, 1974) of life; the latter group also found higher levels in children than in adults. Arnaud *et al.* (1973) carried out an extensive study on iPTH concentrations in subjects aged 6 months to 20 years. They found that mean values were highest in the youngest children, decreased to a lower value at about 7–9 years and then increased to plateau at adolescence and the values at 14–20 years were similar to those of adults. They were able to measure iPTH in more than 94% of their subjects.

Differences in results are likely to be due to the use of a variety of antisera. Arnaud *et al.* (1973) pointed out that the parallel and decreasing concentrations of phosphorus and iPTH in children less than 6 years old are not consistent with the present understanding of the known effects of PTH, nor did they think that the lower concentrations which they found during middle childhood could be easily understood. In view of the problems associated with the heterogeneity of PTH, perhaps the differences between Arnaud's results and our own may provide an important clue to the reasons for some of the changes which occur during childhood.

Idiopathic hypercalcaemia

A wide spectrum of severity is seen in this condition which typically presents with failure to thrive, anorexia and vomiting, irritability, constipation and polyuria. In the severe form 'elfin' facies are present together with stenotic lesions of the aorta and renal arteries, nephrocalcinosis and mental retardation (Schlesinger *et al.*, 1952; Black *et al.*, 1963). The condition is now seen rather infrequently.

Concentrations of iPTH have been determined in three boys aged 10 weeks to 10 months, and eight girls aged 2 months to 5 years and 11 months. All had a typical early history and severely affected children had continued to attend the hospital. The results are shown in Table 5.3 and include the concentrations of total calcium at the time the blood samples for iPTH measurements were collected. Concentrations of iPTH were low in no less than seven of the children and in all except one of these there were severe features of the condition, i.e. typical facies and/or heart lesions and/or brain damage. It appears that

Table 5·3 *Idiopathic hypercalcaemia*

Patient	*Age Years*	*Age months*	*Fasting Ca‡ (mg/100 ml plasma)*	*iPTH (pg/ml bPTH) Value*	*iPTH (pg/ml bPTH) Normal N or Low L*	*Typical* facies*	*Heart* lesion*	*Other lesions*
Boys								
1		2.5	10·9	215	N	—†	—	Supernumary digit
2		7	10·6	< 40	L	—	+	—
		8	10·9	< 40	L			
3		10	12·0	400	Upper N	—	—	—
Girls								
1		2	10·6	255	N	—	—	—
2		3	10.8	45	L	—	—	Laryngomalacia
3		8	13·6	205	N	—	—	Hiatus hernia
		9	9·4	140	N			
4		11	11·6	135	Low N	+	—	Recurrent urinary tract infection; hiatus hernia
5	1	0	15·6	85	L	+	+	Microcephaly
6	1	1	13·1	75	L	+	+	—
7	3	0	10·7	145	L	—	—	Mentally retarded
8	5	0	12·6	92	L	+	+	Mental retardation
9	5	11	9·6	62	L	+	—	Slow development

* + = present; — = absent.
† Facies odd but not typical of idiopathic hypercalcaemia
‡ at time of study

concentrations of iPTH can fall in response to increased circulating calcium in the condition. In spite of this, plasma calcium levels may remain raised, suggesting that another mechanism is responsible for the increase.

Immunoreactive PTH was measured in an interesting patient with persistent hypercalcaemia for which the cause could not be established. She had shown slow development and failure to thrive since birth. She had always been constipated and had had episodes of vomiting. Hypercalcaemia was diagnosed at 7 months of age, no cause for it was found and in spite of treatment with steroids and very severe restriction of dietary calcium the child did not improve. Concentrations of iPTH at 16, 17 (twice), 18 and 23 months of age were 290, 600, 335, 375 and 330 pg/ml respectively, and concentrations of calcium throughout this period were 12–13 mg/100 ml plasma. All except one of the values for iPTH were similar to those in normal children. She had not heart lesion nor typical facies. This child who was under the care of Dr T. M. Barratt and later Professor C. E. Dent had four normal parathyroids removed. This operation resulted in marked improvement in her general condition and mental state, the plasma calcium concentration being controlled with vitamin D.

Hypocalcaemia

The incidence of hypocalcaemia of infancy appears to have been increasing (Baum *et al.*, 1968; Begum *et al.*, 1968; Eades, 1968; Pugh, 1968; Cockburn *et al.*, 1973). It is very rare in the breast-fed infant; breast milk contains less calcium, magnesium and phosphorous than cow's milk but the calcium to phosphorous ratio is much higher. A number of other aetiological factors have been implicated. These include a poor intake of vitamin D and possibly calcium by the Asian mother and high parity of the mother (Watney *et al.*, 1971; Roberts *et al.*, 1973). Hypocalcaemic fits have a tendency to occur more in boys (Saville and Kretchmer, 1960). the infants tend to be of average or above average birth weight (Baum *et al.*, 1968).

Infants with hypocalcaemia admitted to the Hospital for Sick Children tend to be from a somewhat selected and unusual group, often with many complicating features. Since it is a referral hospital there is frequently an interval between the age at which hypocalcaemia has been first diagnosed and admission to our hospital and hypocalcaemia may

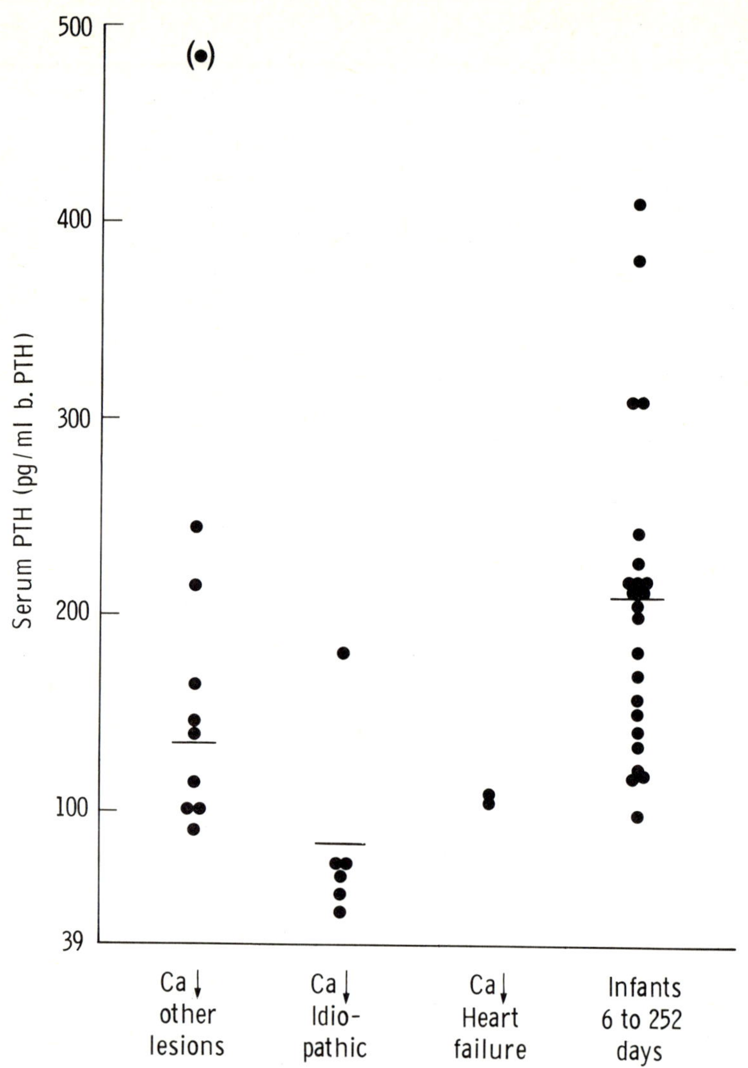

FIGURE 5.2 Concentrations of iPTH in terms of bPTH in infants with hypocalcaemia. (— indicates mean value for the age group)

have been intermittently corrected by treatment. Eighteen infants have been studied. In 10 of them there were serious associated lesions, for example:

Infant 1, male: atrial septal defect + ventricular septal defect + preductal coarctation + partial anomolous venous drainage.

Infant 2, male: right diaphragmatic hernia + left cleft-lip and palate.

Infant 3, female: transposition of the great arteries + ventricular septal defect + mental retardation.

Infant 4, female: oesophageal atresia without tracheo-oesophageal fistula + lactose intolerance.

Infant 5, female: tracheo-oesophageal fistula.

Associated lesions were not present in six of the infants. In two further infants the presentation was heart failure and they were referred from their hospitals with possible congenital heart disease. This was not present and correction of the plasma calcium led to normal cardiac function. The concentrations of iPTH in these infants (see Figure 5.2) were not significantly different whether or not associated lesions were present, but the values were significantly lower compared with those found in healthy infants (for those with lesions present and for those without lesions, compared with normal infants, $P < 0{\cdot}02$ and $< 0{\cdot}001$ respectively).

The cause of the findings is not known. Recently David and Anast (1974) have also demonstrated undetectable or very low values for iPTH in hypocalcaemic infants in the first 9 days of life, a finding which they did not see in 'sick' newborns. We wonder if there could be a functional immaturity of the enzymes concerned with the formation of secreted PTH or its peripheral degradation and thus changes in the heterogeneity of the material which we are measuring.

Some other interesting patients with hypocalcaemia have given the results shown in Table 5.4. Coeliac disease with severe hypocalcaemia is now uncommon. In the two infants studied, concentrations of iPTH were not raised. In 1972, Joffe *et al.* reported that a patient with nutritional rickets and Kwashiorkor did not show the expected increase in the concentration of iPTH. Perhaps severe malabsorption in the young may interfere with the formation of iPTH as measured with some antisera. In a further two children with hypocalcaemia associated with prolonged treatment with phenytoin the values for iPTH were within the normal range. Estimations of iPTH were performed on many occasions in an infant with primary hypomagnesaemia. When the calcium and magnesium levels in the blood were low concentrations of iPTH were low also. Unlike the iPTH concentrations reported by Suh *et al.* (1973) and Anast *et al.* (1972), no rise was observed when calcium and magnesium levels were being well-controlled with large oral supplements of magnesium. Our patient was very young whereas the other two were 8 and 16 years old when iPTH levels were studied. Suh *et al.* (1973) and Anast *et al.* (1972) concluded that in magnesium depletion the synthesis and/or secretion of parathyroid hormone is impaired and that if magnesium is given, the ability of the parathyroid glands to respond is restored. It will be of interest to measure iPTH in our infant as he grows older.

Endocrinological function has been studied in thalassaemia major, a hereditary disorder characterised by impaired formation of normal adult haemoglobin so that a large proportion of the haemoglobin is present in the foetal form. Although life is prolonged by repeated blood transfusions, the children are likely to develop transfusion siderosis resulting in impaired liver function, endocrine abnormalities and cardiac failure; the overload which is responsible for these abnormalities may be somewhat reduced by chelating agents (Barry *et al.*, 1974). In a group of patients at the Hospital for Sick Children the occurrence of isolated

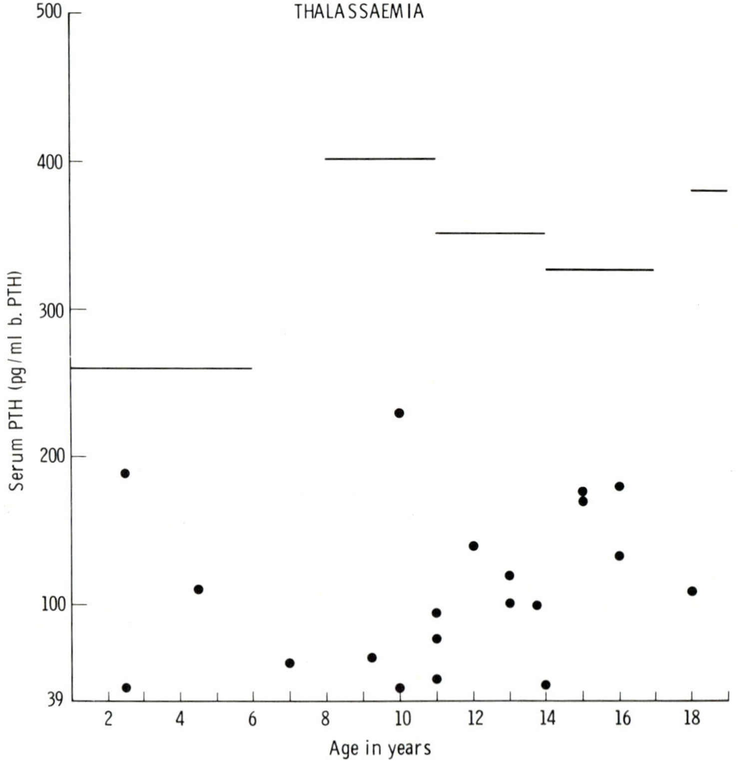

FIGURE 5.3 Concentrations of iPTH in terms of bPTH in children with thalassaemia. (— indicates mean value for the age group)

cases of diabetes, hypoparathyroidism and short stature prompted us to look more closely at endocrinological function in many of the children. Investigations were performed 3 weeks after the last blood transfusion. Thirty-one subjects were available for study but not all of them had complete investigations of endocrine function. Although clinical evidence of hypothyroidism was not seen, serum thyroxine was significantly reduced ($P < 0{\cdot}001$) and serum thyroid stimulating hormone raised ($P < 0{\cdot}001$). Six of the group were below the third percentile in height; four of these had a Bovril stimulation test (Jackson *et al.*, 1968) with a good response so growth hormone deficiency did not appear to be a problem. Most of the children had delayed puberty ratings for their chronological ages, and raised excretion of luteinising hormone but not follicle stimulating hormone with respect to their stage of puberty. This suggests a failure of ovarian function. Six children developed diabetes mellitus and showed an abnormal glucose tolerance test and impaired insulin response. In 15 other patients without clinical symptoms no biochemical features of the condition were present.

Only two of the children had clinical hypoparathyroidism, but low values of iPTH were found in many of the others and indeed of the 20 children

Table 5.4 *Some patients with hypocalcaemia*

Age	*Sex*	*Fasting Ca* (mg/100 ml *plasma*)	*iPTH* (pg/ml *bPTH*) *Value*	*Normal N or Low L*	*Fasting Mg* (mg/100 ml *plasma*)
Coeliac disease					
4 months	Female	7·6	130	Low N	
5 months	Female	6·5	110	L	
Prolonged Phenytoin					
3 months	Male	7·8	290	N	
9 years	Male	7·4	240	N	
Primary hypomagnesaemia					
3 months	Male	8·2	105	L	0·58
		8·3	40	L	0·54
3 months later		10·1	< 40	L	2·14
		9.8	< 40	L	1.7

in whom the estimation was done none of them had a concentration of iPTH higher than the mean for their age group (see Figure 5.3). In spite of the low concentrations of iPTH, the plasma calcium measurements (using a Perkin Elmer 290 B Atomic Absorption Spectrophotometer) were within the reference range for subjects of these ages but it should be noted that the children were not fasting when blood was collected. Table 5.5 shows some examples of serial determinations. Seventeen children had measurements of both serum iPTH and the contents of iron in the liver but the correlation was poor ($P < 0{\cdot}10$).

The metabolism of parathyroid hormone is complex. The principal secretory product of the parathyroid glands is the intact hormone which then undergoes cleavage, and it is fragments of the hormone which are responsible for most of the immunoreactive material which is measured in the assay (Segre *et al.*, 1974). The amount of iPTH which is measured will depend upon which circulating fragments are recognised by the particular antiserum used, as well as on the actual concentrations of fragments present. A variety of antisera are used by different workers and this would explain discrepancies in results from different laboratories (Arnaud *et al.*, 1974).

Table 5.5 *Serial estimations of iPTH in three patients with thalassaeima*

Patient	*Age* *Years*	*Months*	*iPTH* (pg/ml *bPTH*)
1	13	2	225
	13	4	75
	13	5	<40
	13	8	<40
2	13	10	160
	14	2	170
	14	5	85
	15	0	100
3	11	0	45
	11	5	140
	11	8	135

REFERENCES

ANAST, C. S., MOHS, J. M., KAPLAN, S. L. and BURNS, T. W. (1972). Interrelationship of magnesium metabolism and parathyroid function in man. *Pediatr. Res.*, **6**, 350

ARNAUD, C. D., GOLDSMITH, R. S., BORDER, P. J., SIZEMORE, G. W., LARSEN, J. A. and GILKINSON, J. (1974). Influence of immunoheterogeneity of circulating parathyroid hormone on results of radioimmunoassays of serum in man. *Am. J. Med.*, **56**, 785

ARNAUD, S. B., GOLDSMITH, R. S., STICKLER, G. B., MCCALL, J. T. and ARNAUD, C. D. (1973). Serum parathyroid hormone and blood minerals: interrelationships in normal children. *Pediatr. Res.* **7**, 485

BARRY, M., FLYNN, D. M., LETSKY, E. A. and RISDON, R. A. (1974). Long-term chelation therapy in thalassaemia major: effect on liver iron concentration, liver histology and clinical progress. *Br. Med. J.*, **2**, 16

BAUM, D., COOPER, L. and DAVIES, P. A. (1968. Hypocalcaemic fits in neonates. *Lancet*, **i**, 598

BEGUM, R., YUDKIN, S. and DORMANDY, T. L. (1968). Hypocalcaemic fits in neonates. *Lancet*, **i**, 690

BLACK, J. A. and BONHAM CARTER, R. E. (1963). Association between aortic stenosis and facies of severe infantile hypercalcaemia. *Lancet*, **ii**, 745

COCKBURN, F., BROWN, J. K., BELTON, N. R. and FORFAR, J. O. (1973). Neonatal convulsions associated with primary disturbances of calcium, phosphorous and magnesium metabolism. *Arch. Dis. Child.*, **48**, 99

COTES, M. (1974). Personal communication from J. T. Potts Jr.

DAVID, L. and ANAST, C. S. (1974). Calcium metabolism in newborn infants. The interrelationship of parathyroid function and calcium, magnesium and phosphorous metabolism in normal, 'sick' and hypocalcemic newborns. *J. Clin. Invest.*, **54**, 287

EADES, S. (1968). Hypocalcaemic fits in neonates. *Lancet*, **i**, 644

GREENWOOD, F. C., HUNTER W. M. and GLOVER, J. S. (1963). The preparation of ^{131}I-labelled human growth hormone of high specific radioactivity. *Biochem. J.*, **89**, 114

JACKSON, D., GRANT, D. B. and CLAYTON B. E. (1968). A simple oral test of growth hormone secretion in children. *Lancet*, **ii**, 373

JOFFE, B. I., HACKENG, W. H. L., SEPTEL, H. C. and HARTDEGEN, R. G. (1972). Parathyroid hormone concentrations in nutritional rickets. *Clin. Sci.*, **42**, 113

MORGAN, C. R. and LAZAROW, A. (1963). Immunology of insulin; two antibody system. *Diabetes*, **12**, 115

PUGH, R. J. (1968). Hypocalcaemic fits in neonates. *Lancet*, **i**, 644

ROBERTS, S. A., COHEN, M. D. and FORFAR, J. O. (1973). Antenatal factors associated with neonatal hypocalcaemic convulsions. *Lancet*, **ii**, 809

ROOF, B. S., PIEL, C. F., RAMES, L., POTTER, D. and GORDAN, G. S. (1974). Parathyroid Function in uremic children with and without osteodystrophy. *Pediatrics*, **53**, 104

SAVILLE, P. D. and KRETCHMER, N. (1960). Neonatal tetany: and report of 125 cases and review of the literature. *Biol. Neonate.*, **2**, 1

SCHLESINGER, B., BUTLER, N. and BLACK, J. (1952). Chronische hypercalcämie: Londoner Fall. *Helv. Paediatr. Acta.*, **7**, 335

SEGRE, G. V., NIALL, H. D., HABENER, J. F. and POTTS, J. T. Jr. (1974). Metabolism of parathyroid hormone. *Am. J. Med.*, **56**, 774

SUH, S. M., TASHJIAN, A. H. Jr., MATSUO, N., PARKINSON, D. K. and FRASER, D. (1973). Pathogenesis of hypocalcemia in primary hypomagnesemia: normal end-organ responsiveness to parathyroid hormone, impared parathyroid gland function. *J. Clin. Invest.* **52**, 153

WATNEY, P. J. M., CHANCE, G. W., SCOTT, P. and THOMPSON, J. M. (1970). Maternal factors in neonatal hypocalcaemia: a study in three ethnic groups. *Br. Med. J.*, **2**, 432

WOODHEAD, J. S. (1971). Personal communication

YALOW, R. S. and BERSON, S. A. (1966). Purification of ^{131}I parathyroid hormone with microfine granules of precipitated silica. *Nature (London)*, **212**, 357

6

Use of 1,25-dihydroxycholecalciferol ($1,25(OH)_2D_3$) in the treatment of hypoparathyroidism and pseudohypoparathyroidism

H. P. Kind, A. Prader and H. F. DeLuca

The serum hypercalcaemic effect of $1,25(OH)_2D_3$ and $1\alpha OHD_3$ in hypoparathyroidism has recently been demonstrated by Russel *et al.* (1974). We would like to present our own experience with $1,25(OH)_2D_3$ in two patients, one with idiopathic hypoparathyroidism (HP) and one with pseudohypoparathyroidism (PHP).

An 11-year-old girl was referred to the hospital with a history of recurrent carpopedal spasms, headache, occasional vomiting and abdominal cramps. At admission she had positive Trousseau and Chvostek signs and pronounced papilloedema but no other signs of increased intracranial pressure. Obesity, round face and impaired intellectual capacity were stigmata suggesting PHP. Short metacarpals, however, were absent. The initial laboratory results showed a low serum calcium of 6·6 mg/100ml and an elevated serum phosphorus of 6·1 mg/100ml. All other electrolytes, alkaline phosphatase, protein, creatinine, blood gases as well as thyroid and adrenal function tests were within the normal range. At the time when her serum calcium was 6·6 mg/100ml, immunoreactive plasma PTH (iPTH) was undetectable. Urinary 3′,5′-AMP excretion before and after one single intravenous injection of bovine PTE (Lilly) was determined using the protocol described by Chase *et al.* (1969). Our patient showed an immediate and marked rise in 3′,5′-AMP excretion as usually seen in patients with idiopathic hypoparathyroidism. In addition, she demonstrated a prompt and dramatic rise in serum calcium, following 8-hourly intramuscular injections of PTE (200 IU PTE Lilly/m^2). This effect is shown on the left part of Figure 6.1. Serum calcium increased from 6·6 to 11·5 mg/100 ml with four injections of PTE. These results established a diagnosis of idiopathic HP (Kind *et al.*, 1973).

Subsequently the girl was started on a therapeutic trial with syn-

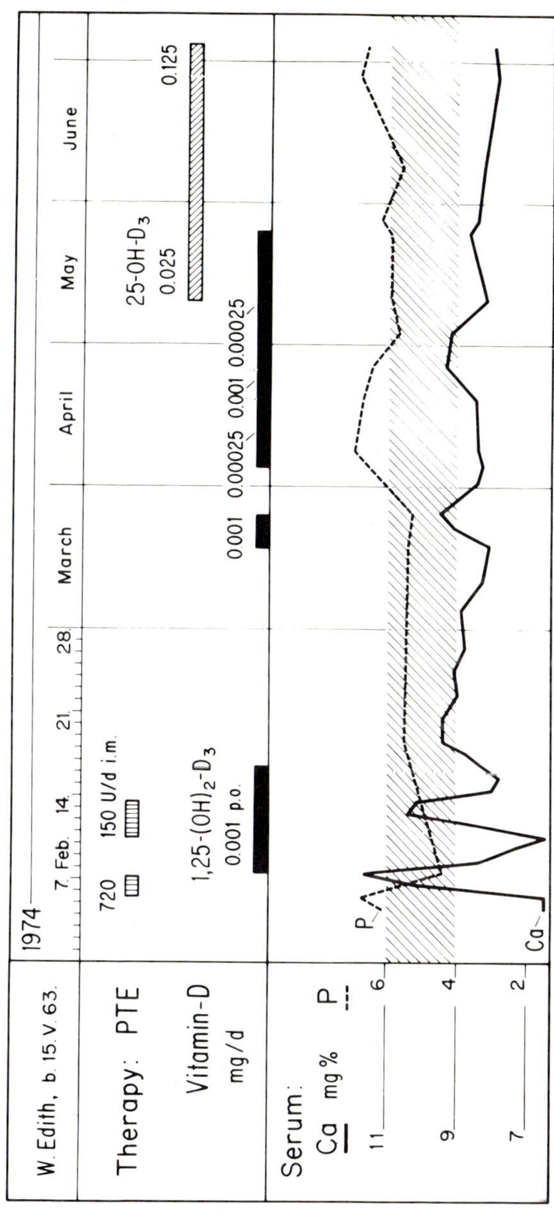

FIGURE 6.1 Effect of various doses of 1,25(OH)$_2$D$_3$, 25(OH)D$_3$ and PTE on serum calcium and phosphorus in an 11-year-old girl with idiopathic hypoparathyroidism.

thetic 1,25$(OH)_2D_3$, 0·001 mg dissolved in propylene glycol being given daily by mouth in a single morning dose. During the investigation period she was kept on a normal hospital diet without supplementary calcium. After the effect of intramuscular PTE had vanished and after 4 days of 1,25$(OH)_2D_3$ treatment, her serum calcium dropped to the pretreatment level of 6·6 mg/100 ml. Because symptoms of tetany reappeared, additional support of serum calcium by exogenous PTE was necessary. The effect of 1,25$(OH)_2D_3$ on serum calcium was therefore initially blurred. After 10 doses the metabolite was discontinued when serum calcium was 8·8 mg/100 ml. Two and 5 days after the last oral dose, serum calcium was 9·4 mg /100 ml and serum phosphorus 5·2 mg/100 ml Subsequently serum calcium fell slowly but continuously. During normocalcaemia, all symptoms, including papilloedema, had disappeared. The girl was discharged from hospital and subsequently controlled as an out-patient twice weekly.

Four weeks after the initial treatment period, the girl's serum calcium was 8·1 mg/100 ml. Moderate symptoms of hypocalcaemia reappeared. She was again put on 1,25$(OH)_2D_3$ in order to confirm its hypercalcaemic effect, this time, however, without the blurring effect of exogenous PTE. With six doses on subsequent days, her serum calcium quickly rose to normocalcaemic levels (9·5 mg/100 ml).

Further investigations were done to establish the minimal dose of the metabolite affecting serum calcium. After discontinuation of therapy and relapse to hypocalcaemia, 0·00025 mg of 1,25$(OH)_2D_3$ ($\frac{1}{4}$ of the previous dose) was given for 15 days. This therapy was ineffective. Serum calcium remained low and serum phosphorus high. However, serum calcium did not decrease any further. Subsequently, the girl was brought back to normocalcaemia (9·3 mg/100 ml) with six doses of 0·001 mg of 1,25$(OH)_2$-D_3. Restarted on 0·00025 mg it was evident that this dose was too small to maintain normocalcaemia. Serum calcium fell to 8·2 mg/100 ml within 15 days. At this point the girl was started on 25$(OH)D_3$. Low doses of 0·025 mg of 25$(OH)D_3$ given for 6 weeks with an initial overlap of low doses of 1,25$(OH)_2D_3$ for 17 days and of 0·125 mg of 25$(OH)D_3$ for 10 days were ineffective. The patient is now taking vitamin D_3 in a dose of 2·5 mg/day and is normocalcaemic.

The results of our therapeutic trials with 1,25$(OH)_2D_3$ in this patient with idiopathic HP show that 0·001 mg by mouth per day normalise serum calcium within a week to 10 days, even if no supplementary oral calcium is given, and that lower doses than 0·001 mg/day have no effect on hypocalcaemia and do not prevent a relapse from normo- to hypocalcaemia. These results are in accordance with those of Russel *et al.* (1974) who demonstrated that small and presumably physiological doses of $1,25(OH)_2D_3$ and in their cases $1\alpha(OH)D_3$ as well are capable to normalise plasma calcium in patients with hypoparathyroidism. The balance studies (Russel *et al.*, 1974) and results of animal experiments presented today by DeLuca suggest that increased intestinal absorption of calcium is responsible for the major part of this rise.

A similar investigation was performed in a girl with pseudohypoparathyroidism (PHP). This study was done very recently and therefore has not been mentioned in our abstract. We have so far not been aware of any reports regarding the effect of $1,25(OH)_2D_3$ on serum calcium in PHP.

The 9-year-old girl demonstrated all the typical physical features of PHP (Albright *et al.*, 1952). In addition the diagnosis was proven biochemically by a low serum calcium, an elevated serum phosphorus, excessively elevated iPTH, defective excretion of urinary 3′, 5′-AMP after intravenous PTE and unresponsiveness of serum calcium to repeated intramuscular injections of PTE (Kind *et al.*, 1973). $1,25\text{-}(OH)_2D_3$ in a dose of 0·001 mg was given orally for a total of 15 days (Figure 6.2). The girl was kept on a normal hospital diet without

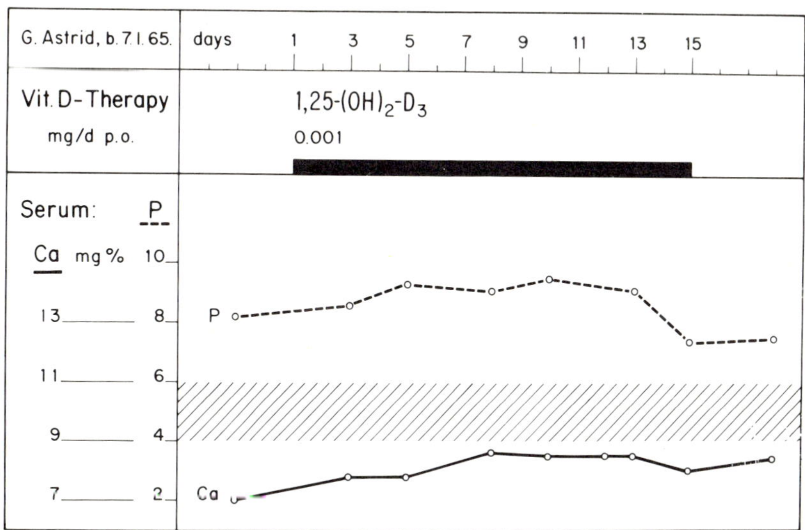

FIGURE 6.2 Effect of $1,25(OH)_2D_3$ (0·001 mg/day) in a 9-year-old girl with pseudohypoparathyroidism.

supplementary oral calcium. Within the period of therapy, serum calcium and serum phosphorus were only slightly influenced. Serum calcium rose about 1 mg/100 ml but only transiently. Normocalcaemia or normophosphataemia was never achieved. In short, $1,25(OH)_2D_3$ in our patient with PHP was uneffective.

The differences in responsiveness to $1,25(OH)_2D_3$ between our two patients are not easy to explain. It has been suggested that in hypoparathyroidism production of $1,25(OH)_2D_3$ is defective (Garabedian *et al.*, 1972; Rasmussen *et al.*, 1972; Fraser and Kodicek, 1973; Galante *et al.*, 1972). This could either be directly due to the lack of endogenous PTH or indirectly due to elevated plasma and therefore possibly intracellular phosphorus levels (Tanaka and DeLuca, 1973). If inorganic phosphorus concentration is the only important compound triggering $1,25(OH)_2D_3$ synthesis, the production of the active metabolite would also be impaired in PHP, irrespective of the presence of high PTH. Unresponsiveness to $1,25(OH)_2D_3$ in PHP therefore remains unexplained. Measurements of circulating $1,25(OH)_2D_3$ may help to answer this question (Brumbaugh *et al.*, 1974) and hopefully provide further insight into the pathophysiology of PHP.

REFERENCES

Albright, F. G., Forbes, A. P. and Hennemann, H. (1952). Pseudo-pseudohypoparathyroidism. *Trans. Assoc. Am., Physicians*, **65**, 337

Brumbaugh, P. F., Haussler, D. H., Bressler, R. and Haussler, M. R. (1974). Radioreceptor assay for 1α, 25-dihydroxyvitamin D_3. *Science*, **183**, 1089

Chase, L. R., Melson, G. L. and Aurbach, S. D. (1969). Pseudohypoparathyroidism: Defective excretion of 3′, 5′-AMP in response to parathyroid hormone. *J. Clin. Invest.*, **48**, 1832

Fraser, D. R. and Kodicek, E. (1973). Regulation of 25-hydroxycholecalciferol-1-hydroxylase activity in kidney by parathyroid hormone. *Nature* (*New Biol.*), **241**, 163

Galante, L., MacAnley, S. J., Colston, K. W. and MacIntyre, I. (1972). Effect of parathyroid extract on vitamin D metabolism. *Lancet*, **i**, 985

Garabedian, M., Holick, M. F., DeLuca, H. F. and Boyle, I. T. (1972). Control of 25-hydroxycholecalciferol metabolism by parathyroid glands. *Proc. Natl. Acad. Sci. USA*, **69**, 1673

Kind, H. P., Parkinson, D. K., Suh, S. M., Fraser, D. and Kooh, S. W. (1973). Parathyroid hormone response and effects of vitamin D in hypoparathyroidism and pseudohypoparathyroidism (abstract). *Endocrinology*, (*Suppl.*), **92**, 164

Rasmussen, H., Wong, M., Bikle, D. and Goodman, D. B. P. (1972). Hormonal control of the renal conversion of 25-hydroxycholecalciferol to 1,25-dihydroxycholecalciferol. *J. Clin. Invest.*, **51**, 2502

Russel, R. G. G., Smith, R., Walton, R. J., Preston, C., Basson, R., Henderson, R. G. and Norman, A. W. (1974). 1,25-dihydroxycholecalciferol and 1A-hydroxycholecalciferol in hypoparathyroidism. *Lancet*, **ii**, 14

Tanaka, T. and DeLuca, H. F. (1973) The control of 25-hydroxyvitamin-D metabolism by inorganic phosphorus. *Arch. Biochem. Biophys.*, **154**, 566

7

Calcitonin : Recent advances in genetic and physiological aspects

I. MacIntyre, P. B. Greenberg, C. J. Hillyard, O. Ljungberg and J. F. Dymling

Calcitonin in familial medullary carcinoma

INTRODUCTION

Medullary thyroid carcinoma, a tumour of the calcitonin secreting 'C' cells of the thyroid, can occur sporadically or as an inherited disease. This neoplasm occurs frequently in some families, often in association with phaeochromocytoma, and clinical observations indicate that the pattern of inheritance is autosomal dominant (Ljungberg, 1972). The trait is more commonly expressed as asymptomatic hypercalcitoninaemia than as a palpable thyroid tumour (Melvin *et al.*, 1972; Jackson *et al.*, 1973). The association of medullary thyroid carcinoma and phaeomochromocytoma has been termed familial chromaffinomatosis (Ljungberg *et al.*, 1967).

We have studied a large family living in Sweden and found hypercalcitoninaemia in many of the healthy members (Greenberg *et al.*, 1974).

PATIENTS AND METHODS

Calcitonin radioimmunoassay

Heparinised blood samples were stored in ice for up to 6 hours before centrifugation and plasma was separated, immediately frozen and stored at −18 °C until assayed.

Plasma immunoreactive calcitonin was measured as previously described (Coombes *et al.*, 1974). Normal circulating levels of calcitonin are undetectable using this assay (< 0·1 ng/ml).

Whisky test

(a) Screening test:

After a minimum fast of 4 hours, blood was drawn for calcitonin assay before and 10–15 minutes after the ingestion of 50 ml whisky.

(b) Complete test:

Fasting blood samples were taken 15 and 3 minutes before and 3, 15, 30 and 60 minutes after ingestion of 50 ml whisky.

Calcium infusion

A standard 4-hour intravenous calcium infusion of 15 mg of calcium (as gluconate) per kilogramme of body weight in 1 litre of isotonic glucose was given to subjects after an overnight fast. Blood samples were drawn 5 minutes before and 30, 60, 120, 180 and 240 minutes after the start of the infusion and finally, 120 minutes after ending the infusion.

Patients

Basal calcitonin levels were analysed in 80 members of a family with familial chromaffinomatosis aged 9–67 years and in 82 healthy hospital employees aged 20–67 years.

A screening whisky test was performed in 64 of the family members and all the healthy volunteers.

Fifteen of the family members with elevated calcitonin levels were admitted to hospital for further investigations. A complete whisky test was performed on these 15 patients and a calcium infusion was performed on the six patients whose basal calcitonin levels in the initial screen were above 1·0 ng/ml.

RESULTS

Screening test

In all the healthy volunteers, calcitonin was undetectable. Thirteen of the family members had basal calcitonin levels above 1·0 ng/ml, 18 had levels between 0·1 and 1·0 ng/ml and the remaining 49 had undetectable circulating calcitonin.

Sixty-four members were given 50 ml whisky. Following ingestion 33 of these still had undetectable levels and of those with measurable basal calcitonin, 19 had levels above 1·0 ng/ml (including one subject in whom a basal determination was not performed) and six had levels between 0·1 and 1·0 ng/ml. However, six of the family members whose basal levels were undetectable had levels of 0·19, 0·20, 0·28, 0·36, 0·54, and 1·05 ng/ml respectively 10–15 minutes after whisky ingestion (Table 7.1).

Table 7.1 *Basal plasma calcitonin levels in 80 members of a family with familial chromaffinomatosis and post-whisky levels in 63 of these and 1 family member on whom no basal level was obtained*

Plasma calcitonin (ng/ml)	*Basal Level*	*Post-whisky Level*
>1·0	13	20
0·1–1·0	18	11
<0·1	49	33
	80	64

The mean increase in plasma calcitonin over basal was 181% 10–15 minutes after whisky ingestion.

Complete whisky test

All 15 subjects tested showed an increase in plasma calcitonin levels after alcohol, the maximum increase being reached after 3–15 minutes (Figure 7.1, Table 7.2). The increases observed at 3 and 15 minutes were statistically significant ($P < 0{\cdot}001$). The mean maximum increase of 444% of basal was reached 15 minutes after whisky ingestion.

Calcium infusion

Calcium caused an increase in circulating calcitonin in all six patients tested, but only one of these showed a greater response to calcium than to whisky (Figure 7.2, Table 7.3).

Elevated levels of calcitonin were found in 36% of the family studied and the incidence of either hypercalcitoninaemia, medullary carcinoma or phaeochromocytoma in branches of the family where either a parent or sibling has had surgically proven medullary carcinoma or phaeochromocytoma, was estimated to be 41–77 per cent, which is consistent with an autosomal dominant inheritance (Figure 7.3). Not all the relatives were available for study

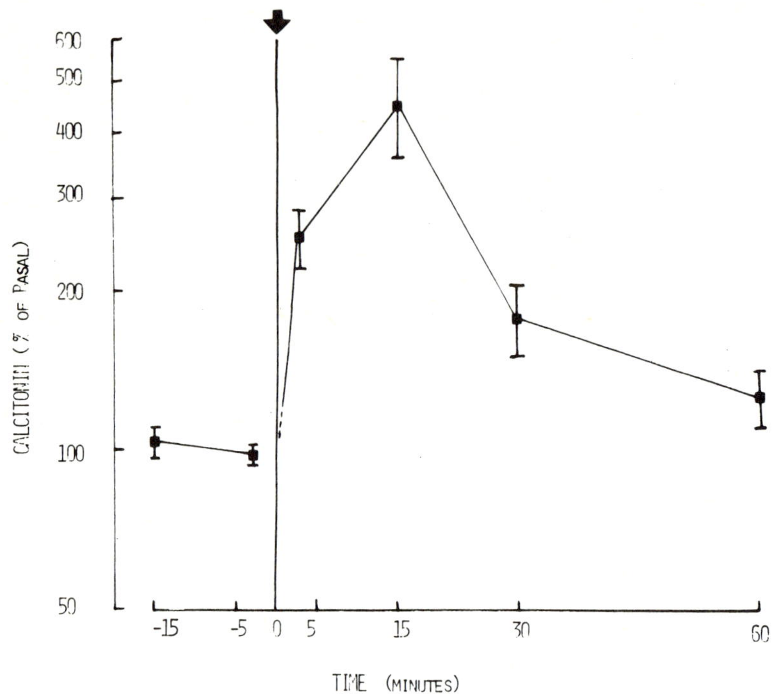

FIGURE 7.1 Response of plasma calcitonin to a single oral dose of whisky in 15 members of a family with familial chromaffinomatosis. Calcitonin as a percentage of the basal level is plotted on a log scale on the ordinate and time in minutes on the abscissa. 50 ml of whisky was given at time 0.

Calcitonin in non-thyroid cancers

INTRODUCTION

Immunoreactive calcitonin is detectable in the plasma of patients with medullary thyroid carcinoma (Clark *et al* , 1969; Tashjian *et al.*, 1970; Deftos *et al.*, 1971; Sizemore *et al.*, 1973; Samaan *et al.*, 1973; Milhaud *et al.*, 1974) and calcitonin assays are commonly used in the diagnosis and management of this disease. Elevated levels of calcitonin have also been found in patients with the Zollinger-Ellison syndrome (Sizemore *et al.*, 1973) in patients with tumours of cells derived from the

Table 7.2 *Results of the complete whisky test, and the clinical diagnoses of 15 members of a family with familial chromaffinomatosis admitted to hospital. Tabulation is based on the calcitonin levels 15 minutes after whisky.*

Name	*Sex*	*Age*	*Calcitonin* (ng/ml) *Time in minutes after 50 ml whisky*						*Diagnosis*
			−15	−3	+3	+15	+30	+60	
SS	M	64	<0.1	<0.1	0.66	<0.1	<0.1	<0.1	Healthy
SN	F	47	0.36	0.25	0.59	0.32	0.22	0.24	Healthy
TJ	M	38	<0.1	<0.1	0.33	0.34	<0.1	<0.1	Healthy
RJ	M	30	0·15	0·13	0·33	0·48	0·13	0·30	Healthy
BMA	F	18	0·24	0·27	0·78	0·50	0·22	0·21	Healthy
SJ	M	29	0·47	0·53	0·80	0·61	0·42	0·36	Healthy
GS	M	50	0·33	0·13	0·13	0·93	0·46	0·37	Healthy
GS	M	52	0·62	0·67	1·45	0·98	0·90	0·78	Healthy
MP	F	23	0·39	0·41	0·47	1·05	0·52	0·38	Healthy
BJ	M	33	0·16	0·16	0·70	1·08	0·94	0·42	Phaeochromocytoma
BJ	M	40	0·26	0·24	0·44	1·92	0·24	0·26	Phaeochromocytoma
NS	M	56	1·75	2·77	3·38	7·55	1·73	1·33	Medullary carcinoma
KG	M	53	3·95	3·63	18·00	12·50	7·13	5·13	C-cell proliferation
JG	M	57	2·73	2·57	7·50	15·00	5·43	2·91	Medullary carcinoma phaeochromocytoma
AL	F	48	0·93	—	2·38	18·00	4·38	0·43	Phaeochromocytoma

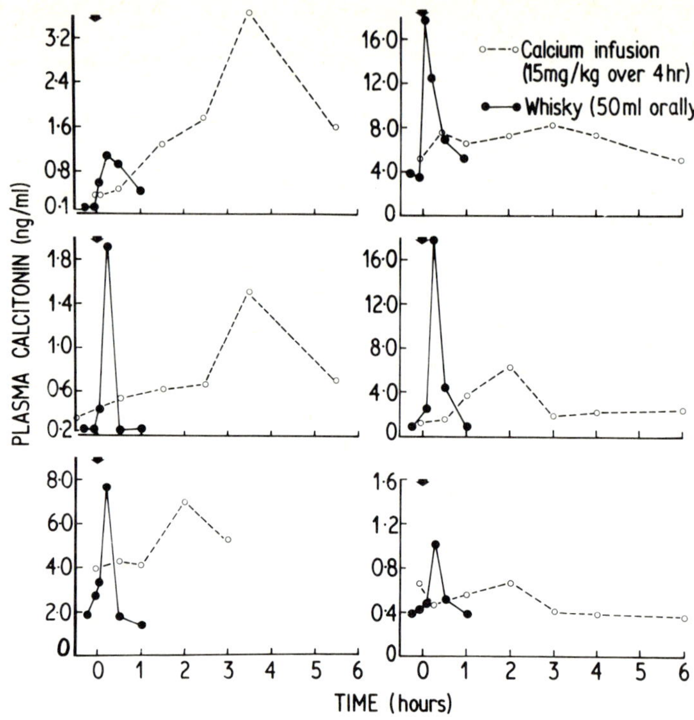

FIGURE 7.2 Comparison of the responses produced by oral whisky (●——●) and intravenous calcium infusion (O- -O) in six members of a family with familial chromaffinomatosis.

neural crest, such as carcinoid (Milhaud *et al.*, 1974) and in oat cell carcinoma of the lung (Silva *et al.*, 1973; Whitelaw and Cohen, 1973; Milhaud *et al.*, 1974). We have found that plasma calcitonin is often detectable in patients with a variety of non-thyroid cancers.

Patients

Forty-six patients with primary or metastatic tumours were studied. Venous blood was drawn and stored in ice for up to 1 hour, plasma was separated and stored at −18 °C until assayed. Twenty-one patients were fasting.

RESULTS

In samples taken from 32 non-fasting control patients (aged 23–79) with conditions not known to be associated with hypercalcitoninaemia or diseases of the skeleton, calcitonin was undetectable.

Table 7.3 *Results of the calcium infusions and the clinical diagnoses of 6 members of a family with familial chromaffinomatosis. Tabulation is based on the basal calcitonin levels.*

Name	*Sex*	*Age*	*Plasma calcitonin* (ng/ml) *Time in minutes after beginning of infusion*							*Diagnosis*
			−5	+30	−60	+120	+180	+240	+360	
KG	M	53	5·5	7·26	6·76	7·13	8·26	7·26	5·20	C-cell proliferation
NS	M	56	3·93	4·33	4·03	6·95	5·25	—	—	Medullary carcinoma
AL	F	48	1·15	1·59	3·57	6·07	1·85	2·01	2·29	Phaeochromocytoma
MP	F	23	0·65	0·46	0·55	0·67	0·41	0·39	0·36	Healthy
BJ	M	33	0·36	0·44	0·53	0·61	0·65	1·50	0·70	Phaeochromocytoma
BJ	M	40	0·39	0·39	0·47	1·32	1·76	3·63	1·6	Phaeochromocytoma

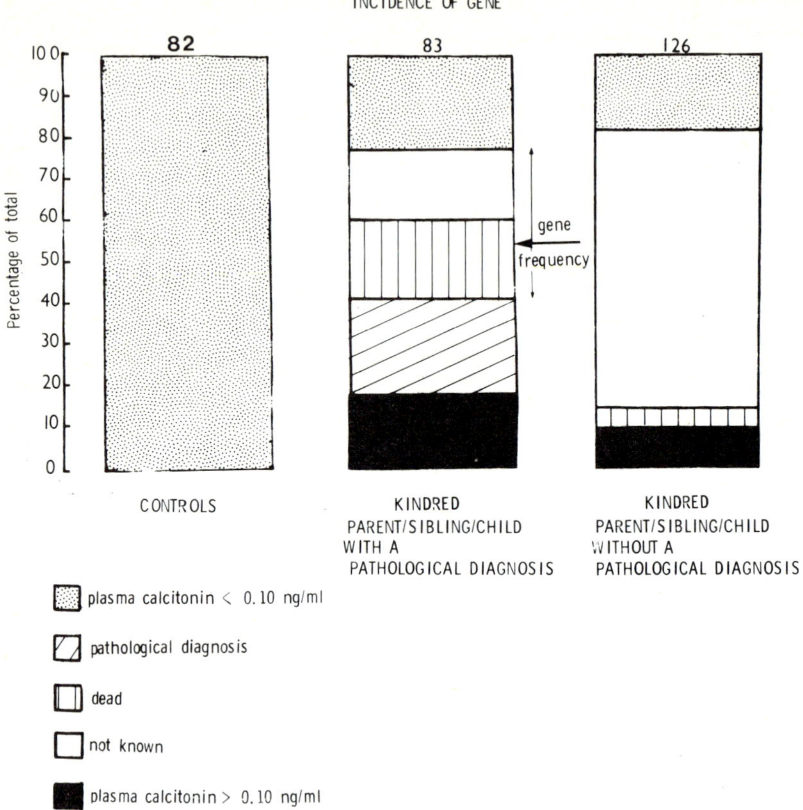

FIGURE 7.3 Probable incidence of the gene in members of the family with familial chromaffinomatosis.

In the patients with tumours, immunoreactive calcitonin was found in 21 patients (aged 42–84) in concentrations of 0·16–7·4 ng/ml (Figure 7.4). Most notably, eight of the 11 patients with oat cell carcinoma of the lung and all eight patients with breast cancer had raised plasma levels of calcitonin. Calcitonin was detected more frequently in patients with skeletal metastases.

Characterisation of the nature of the immunoreactive material in plasma is incomplete, but two of its properties closely resemble those of human calcitonin; the inhibition of binding of ^{125}I-labelled calcitonin to antibody produced by the plasma samples from patients with tumours paralleled that produced by synthetic human calcitonin in calcitonin-free plasma (Figure 7.5) and immunoreactive material could be com-

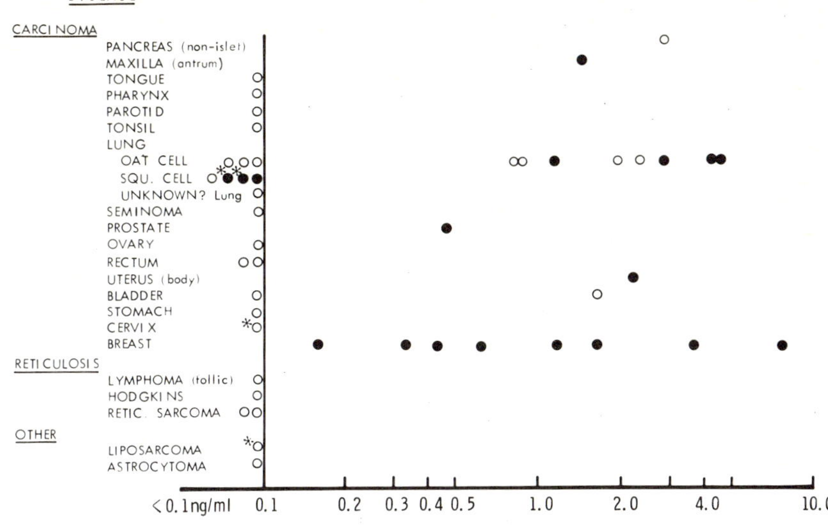

FIGURE 7.4 Plasma immunoreactive calcitonin in patients with a variety of neoplasia. ●, with skeletal metastases; O, no skeletal metastases; *, hypercalcaemic. Reproduced by kind permission of the *Lancet*).

pletely removed by extraction with spherosil, which has previously been shown to remove calcitonin from plasma (Coombes *et al.*, 1974).

Discussion

Calcitonin assays, previously used almost exclusively in the diagnosis and management of medullary thyroid carcinoma have now been shown to have a much broader application. They can be used in familial chromaffinomatosis to indicate which family members possess the gene and may also be useful in the management of breast, lung and possibly other non-thyroid carcinomas.

The need for a provocative test for latent hypercalcitoninaemia became apparent when the basal levels of members of a family with familial chromaffinomatosis were found to vary considerably from day to day, some of those with lower values occasionally becoming undetectable. Oral whisky was chosen for study as a provocative agent, after observing an increase in plasma calcitonin in a patient with medullary carcinoma whose clinical symptoms were precipitated by the social ingestion of alcohol (Cohen *et al.*, 1973). The pilot study showed

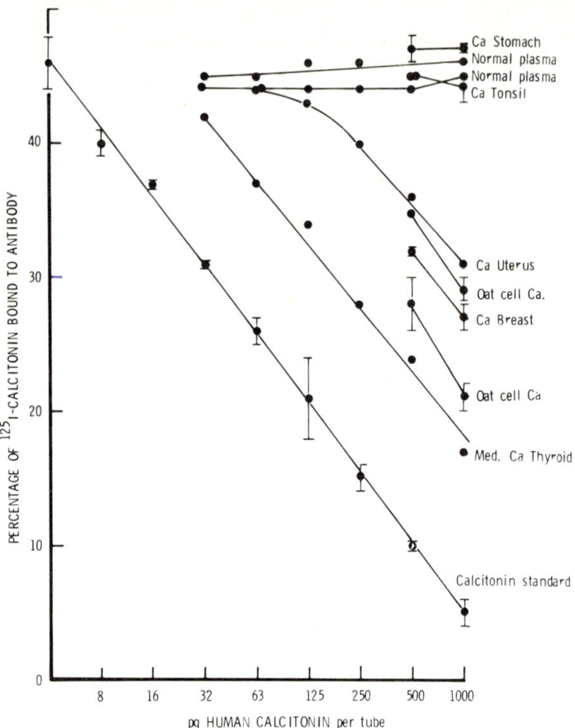

FIGURE 7.5 Comparison of displacement of ^{125}I-labelled calcitonin from antibody by increasing amounts of synthetic calcitonin standard and by dilutions of plasma taken from patients with various carcinomas.

that whisky increased plasma calcitonin in 13 patients with medullary carcinoma (to be published), hence a screening test procedure was devised. When the screening whisky test was applied to 64 members of a family with familial chromaffinomatosis, six members whose basal levels were undetectable had measurable calcitonin after whisky ingestion. In this family, some branches showed no evidence of hypercalcitoninaemia, medullary carcinoma or phaeochromocytoma, whereas in others, hypercalcitoninaemia was common even in branches in whom a pathological diagnosis of disease has not been made for several generations. The management of the asymptomatic subjects is still a matter of dispute (Tashjian *et al.*, 1974; Greenberg and MacIntyre, 1974).

The complete whisky test, which was performed in 15 members of the family with familial chromaffinomatosis showed that oral whisky was a most effective stimulus of calcitonin secretion, causing a rise in plasma calcitonin at 3 minutes after ingestion. Whisky was found to be comparable to a calcium infusion in the six subjects tested, but it lacks the disadvantages of a 4-hour intravenous infusion.

The mechanism of whisky-induced calcitonin secretion remains to be determined, but it may be mediated by the release of gastrointestinal hormones. Gastrin (Care *et al.*, 1971a), pancreozymin (Care *et al.*, 1971b) and enteroglucagon (Swaminathan *et al.*, 1973) can all increase plasma calcitonin levels.

Our recent results indicate that calcitonin is quite common also in non-thyroid cancers. The source of this calcitonin is as yet unclear, but recently Silva *et al.* (1974) reported that calcitonin can be released *in vivo* by oat cell carcinoma of the lung; and electron microscopy of such tumours has demonstrated intracellular neurosecretory granules (Hattori *et al.*, 1972). Ectopic synthesis and secretion of calcitonin may well be responsible for the elevated plasma calcitonin levels in patients with these non-thyroid cancers; hypersecretion of calcitonin by the thyroid gland and subsequent uptake by the tumour is unlikely as we have been unable to stimulate the normal thyroid to secrete calcitonin in sufficient amounts to enable detection in plasma, but this cannot yet be ruled out.

These findings have important practical implications. A raised plasma calcitonin can no longer be considered pathognomonic of medullary thyroid carcinoma and other causes of hypercalcitoninaemia must be excluded before thyroid surgery is contemplated.

Acknowledgements

We thank Dr Imogen Evans for helpful criticism and advice. The work was supported in part by the Medical Research Council and the Wellcome Trust. P. B. G. was in receipt of an overseas scholarship of the Royal Australasian College of Physicians. Synthetic Human Calcitonin was supplied by Ciba-Geigy Ltd.

REFERENCES

Care, A. D., Bates, R. F. L., Swaminathan, R. and Ganguli, P. C. (1971a). The role of gastrin as a calcitonin secretagogue. *J. Endocrinol.*, **51**, 735

Care, A. D., Bruce, J. B., Boelkins, J., Kenny, A. D., Conaway, H. and Anast, C. S. (1971b). Role of pancreozymin-cholecystokinin and structurally related compounds as calcitonin secretagogues. *Endocrinology*, **89**, 262

Clark, M. B., Boyd, G. W., Byfield, P. G. H. and Foster, G. V. (1969). A Radio-immunoassay for human calcitonin M. *Lancet*, **ii**, 74

Cohen, S. L., MacIntyre, I., Grahame-Smith, D. and Walker, J. G. (1973). Alcohol-stimulated calcitonin release in medullary carcinoma of the thyroid. *Lancet*, **ii**, 1172

Coombes, R. C., Hillyard, C. J., Greenberg, P. B. and MacIntyre, I. (1974). Plasma immunoreactive calcitonin patients with non-thyroid tumours. *Lancet*, **i**, 1080

Deftos, L. J., Bury, A. E., Habener, J. F., Singer, F. R., Potts, J. T. Jr. (1971). Immunoassay for human calcitonin. II Clinical Studies. *Metabolism*, **20**, 1129

Greenberg, P. B., Hillyard, C. J., Ljungberg, O., Dymling, J. F. and MacIntyre, I. (1974). Immunoreactive plasma calcitonin in medullary cell carcinoma (MCCT) of the thyroid and in asymptomatic members of a kindred with familial MCCT. *Eur. J. Clin. Invest.*, **4**, 338.

Greenberg, P. B. and MacIntyre, I. (1974). Serum calcitonin and thyroid carcinoma. *Br. Med. J.*, **3**, 256

Hattori, S., Matsuda, M., Tateishi, R., Nishihara, H. and Hoari, T. (1972). Oat-cell carcinoma of the lung: Clinical and morphological studies in relation to its histogenesis. *Cancer*, **30**, 1014

Jackson, C. E., Tashjian, A. H. Jr. and Block, M. A. (1973). Detection of medullary thyroid cancer by calcitonin assay in families. *Ann. Intern. Med.*, **78**, 845

Ljungberg, O. (1972). On medullary carcinoma of the thyroid. *Acta Path. Microbiol. Scand.* (*A*), **231**, 1

Ljungberg, O., Cederquist, E. and Von Studnitz, W. (1967). Medullary thyroid carcinoma and phaeochromocytoma: A familial chromaffinomatosis. *Br. Med. J.*, **1**, 279

Melvin, K. E. W., Tashjian, A. H. Jr. and Miller, H. H. (1972). Studies in familial (medullary) thyroid carcinoma. *Recent Prog. Horm. Res.*, **28**, 399

Milhaud, C., Calmette, C., Taboulet, J., Julienne, A. and Moukhtar, M. S. (1974). Hypersecretion of calcitonin in neoplastic conditions. *Lancet*, **i**, 462

Samaan, N. A., Stratton-Hill, C., Beceiro, J. R. and Schulz, P. M. (1973). Immunoreactive calcitonin in medullary carcinoma of the thyroid and in maternal and cord serum. *J. Lab. Clin. Med.*, **81**, 671

Silva, O. L., Becker, K. L., Primack, A., Doppman, J. and Snider, R. H. (1973). Ectopic production of calcitonin. *Lancet*, **ii**, 317

Sizemore, G. W., Go, V.-L. M., Kaplan, E. L., Sanzenbacher, L. J., Holtermuller, K. H. and Arnaud, C. D. (1973). Relations of calcitonin and gastrin in the Zollinger–Ellison syndrome and medullary carcinoma of the thyroid. *N. Engl. J. Med.*, **288**, 641

Swaminathan, R., Bates, R. F. L., Bloom, S. R., Ganguli, P. C. and Care, A. D. (1973). The relationship between food, gastrointestinal hormones and calcitonin secretion. *J. Endocrinol.*, **59**, 217

Tashjian, A. H. Jr., Howland, B. G., Melvin, K. E. W. and Stratton Hill, C. (1970). Immunoassay of human calcitonin. Clinical measurement, relation to serum calcium and studies in patients with medullary carcinoma. *N. Engl. J. Med.*, **283**, 890

Tashjian, A. H. Jr., Wolfe, H. J. and Voelkel, E. F. (1974). Human calcitonin. Immunologic assay, cytologic localisation and studies on medullary thyroid carcinoma. *Am. J. Med.*, **56**, 840

Whitelaw, A. G. L. and Cohen, S. L. (1973). Ectopic production of calcitonin. *Lancet*, **ii**, 443

8

Aspects of growth and bone structure in hypophosphataemic rickets

R. Steendijk

Hypophosphataemic rickets, X-linked hypophosphataemia, primary vitamin D-resistant rickets and phosphate diabetes are synonyms for a type of rachitic bone disease, which is characterised by subnormal levels of serum P, normal values for serum Ca and absence of vitamin D deficiency. The disease is predominantly familial, although sporadic cases are not rare (Burnett *et al.*, 1964). The mode of inheritance is X-linked dominant, except in one pedigree recently described by Bianchine *et al.* (1971), where the inheritance was autosomal dominant. Consequently the disease is more often seen in girls than in boys. The frequency has been estimated at 1 : 25 000 (Prader, 1960) or 1 : 20 000 (Burnett *et al.*, 1964). Cases in which hypophosphataemia is present without clinically apparent bone disease may escape detection however; therefore the actual incidence may be higher.

The low serum P concentration results from an impairment of the renal tubular reabsorption of inorganic phosphate. According to Glorieux and Scriver (1972) this phosphate leak is caused by the loss of a parathyroid hormone-sensitive component of phosphate transport. Recently Short *et al.* (1974) reached opposite conclusions however. In their patients they found evidence for a hypersensitivity to the phosphaturic effect of parathyroid hormone. This controversy will not be be further discussed here.

The concentration of parathyroid hormone in plasma has usually been found normal (Arnaud *et al.*, 1971; Fanconi *et al.*, 1974). Other authors have reported minor elevations (Lewy *et al.*, 1972; Reitz and Weinstein, 1973). In this respect the disease differs from vitamin D-deficient rickets, in which secondary hyperparathyroidism is present with markedly elevated concentrations of parathyroid hormone in plasma (Fischer *et al.*, 1973). A disturbance in the metabolism of vitamin D has been postulated (DeLuca *et al.*, 1967) but could not be confirmed (Brickman *et al.*, 1973). The serum P level does not rise, nor do the rachitic lesions heal upon administration of 1,25-dihydroxycholecalciferol (Brickman *et al.*, 1973; Glorieux *et al.*, 1973).

In a number of patients large doses of vitamin D or dihydrotachysterol, bordering on quantities that provoke hypercalcaemia, cause a slight rise in serum P and have a favourable effect on the rachitic lesions. The disease cannot be cured in this manner however. This effect of vitamin D is possibly caused by the increased renal excretion of calcium by which it is accompanied and which enhances tubular reabsorption of phosphate (Steendijk *et al.*, 1968; Glorieux and Scriver, 1972).

Several comprehensive reviews of hypophosphataemic rickets have appeared recently (Stickler *et al.*, 1970; Parfitt, 1973). In this paper, attention will be focused exclusively on the linear growth of the patients and on the morphological aspects of bone in this disease.

Growth in hypophosphataemic rickets

Rickets and growth in stature are interrelated. On the one hand, rickets affects normal growth and development of the skeleton. In any type of rachitic bone disease, whether vitamin D deficient or hypophosphataemic, the rate of growth is impaired and the shape of the developing bones becomes abnormal. On the other hand growth is a necessary condition for the clinical and roentgenographic expression of rickets. Other factors being equal, rachitic bone disease is more severe in rapidly growing children than in slowly growing children. This effect of growth on rickets is mainly apparent in the chronic types such as hypophosphataemia, in which the rachitic lesions are present over long periods of time with changing rates of growth.

In familial hypophosphataemic rickets various aspects of growth have been studied by several authors. In the following paragraphs some of the results obtained will be discussed and a few new data will be added. It will be shown that although children with this disease are short, their height varies as much as in normal children. Skeletal deformities, which contribute to the shortness of stature, may be absent or very extensive. The response to treatment also varies widely. Usually it is limited, but some patients show conspicuous improvement, whereas others do not seem to react at all. Some of the conflicting opinions found in the literature on the effect of treatment on growth probably result from this wide range of individual variation. Conclusions drawn from the observation of one or two cases sometimes erroneously have been considered valid in the majority of patients.

GROWTH IN INFANCY

Usually hypophosphataemic rickets does not become clinically apparent before the end of the first year of life and only a small number of observations on height of affected infants are available. Harrison *et al.* (1966) studied three children from birth onward and found that they grew normally during the first 6 months. In the course of the second half of the first year the growth rate decreased too rapidly, whilst rachitic bone lesions appeared. Tapia *et al.* (1964) reported the case of a boy who measured 57 cm at birth and who was said to grow normally until he was 9 months old. At that time growth rate decreased abruptly and became very slow for the following 6 years at the end of which stature was only 100 cm. Treatment had not been given. Schoen and Reynolds (1970) compared this boy to one of their own patients who had been treated from the age of 3 months and whose height was at the 50th centile when he was 5 years old. These authors suggested that early treatment might prevent severe curtailment of height. From the description of their case however it appears that it was not very severe since treatment with moderately high doses of vitamin D resulted in virtually complete disappearance of the roentgenographic signs of rickets. This can only be accomplished in a minority of the cases.

Finally, Stickler (1960) in a study of nine patients which included the cases described by Harrison *et al.* (1966) concluded that growth retardation began at the age of 7–12 months. This suggested a relation with the age of weight-bearing. Furthermore he found that treatment, regardless of the age at which it began, did not seem to have a favourable influence on growth.

According to Harrison *et al.* (1966) the normal growth rate during the first half year may be related to the normal serum P levels which prevail in these months. From the more elaborate study of Stickler (1969) however it appears that serum P is already below the normal range in the first months of life and even—in one patient—in the first week. Both Stickler and Harrison *et al.* found that the serum P level declines during infancy, as is the case in normal children. Whether serum P is normal or low in early infancy, it appears to be sufficiently high to prevent the occurrence of rickets. In older infants however it has become too low for normal bone growth and development to proceed.

SERUM PHOSPHATE AND GROWTH

Here it is appropriate to point out that in normal children the average level of serum P is related to the average rate of growth. Both are higher in infancy than in childhood and there is evidence to suggest that a rise in serum P occurs during the adolescent growth spurt (Morse *et al.*, 1949; de Wijn, 1965). Once growth has ceased serum P declines still further. The concentration in adults (3–4·5 mg/100 ml) is one-half to two-thirds of the concentration in early childhood. The importance of this relation is illustrated by the fact that the bone of children becomes rachitic when serum P falls to 3·0 mg/100 ml, whereas in adults this concentration does not result in the development of osteomalacia, provided the level of serum Ca is normal. The higher turnover of bone tissue during growth apparently requires a higher serum P for proper mineralisation.

The mechanism responsible for the changing level of serum P in childhood and adolescence is not known, but probably growth hormone and the sex hormones are involved (Tanner, 1962). It is of interest that similar changes in serum P are observed in patients with hypophosphataemic rickets. It has already been mentioned that the level is higher in infancy than in childhood. Serum P in adults with hypophosphataemic osteomalacia is still lower and may be below 1·0 mg/100 ml (Nagant de Deuxchaisnes and Krane, 1967).

In individual children with hypophosphataemic rickets evidence for a relation between height and serum P could not be found. This lack of relationship will be discussed in the following paragraphs.

HEIGHT IN CHILDHOOD AND ADOLESCENCE

In 1971 Steendijk and Latham published an extensive study on height in untreated patients. They recorded the height of 23 girls and 14 boys, 1·2 and 12·9 years old. The data were derived from the literature and from patients under the care of the authors.

The values for height and serum P were expressed as SDS (the difference between the height of the patient and the average height of normal boys or girls of equal age, divided by the standard deviation for height at the age of the patient). Patients with serum P values < −1·8 SDS were excluded. Mean values and standard deviations of these data are shown in Table 8.1. It is of interest that the standard deviations for height and for serum P approach the normal value of 1, indicating that the variations in height and in serum P were the same as in normal children. Apparently other factors influencing height and serum P were normally active. A positive value for height—SDS was found in none of the patients. In seven of the 14 boys and in 12 of the 23 girls stature fell within the normal range (0 — Height—SDS > −2).

Table 8.1 *Mean values and standard deviations (in brackets) for height—SDS and serum P—SDS for boys and girls with hypophosphataemic rickets*

	Boys (14)	*Girls* (23)	*Boys + girls* (37)
Height—SDS	−1·91 (0·97)	−2·06 (1·09)	−2·01 (1·04)
Serum P—SDS	−4·16 (1·21)	−4·01 (0·85)	−4·06 (0·99)

Height and serum P were not related (Figure 8.1) and the serum P value in untreated patients therefore does not seem to be a useful parameter for the prediction of future growth in stature. Height and age were also unrelated in these patients ($r = -0{\cdot}01$). Since the severity of the deformities is known to vary during growth, it is important to point out that these results were obtained without taking into account the absence or presence of deformities. It is difficult to measure the contribution of the deformities to the shortness of stature, but from an attempt made in this direction by McNair and Stickler (1969) a relation between the extent of the leg deformities and the deviation from normal height could not be found. Eleven years earlier, Winters *et al.*, (1958) had reached similar conclusions.

These investigations were cross-sectional. Longitudinal data on growth in untreated children are rare, since most patients receive vitamin D as soon as the diagnosis has been established, and accurate data on growth in the preceding years usually are not available. Therefore it is unknown whether the deviation of height from the normal mean in the untreated condition may change spontaneously during the childhood years. Since the rachitic lesions are most severe during the

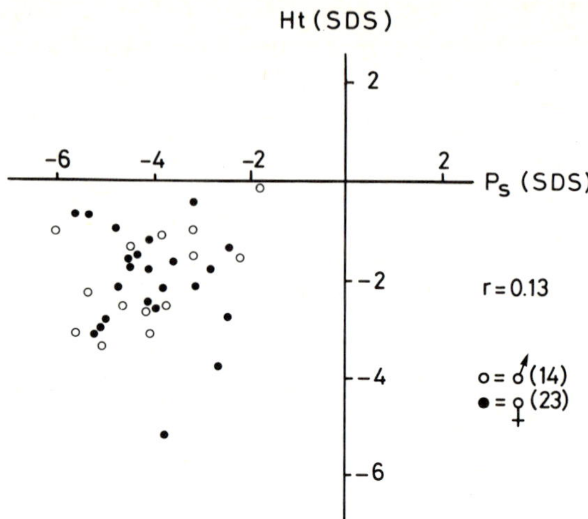

FIGURE 8.1 Relation between serum P and height (expressed as SDS) in 37 children with hypophosphataemic rickets.

period of rapid growth such spontaneous changes might entail some recovery of height during the years between early childhood and puberty.

The shortness of stature appears to be mainly if not exclusively to result from shortness of the legs, whether or not deformities are present (Steendijk, 1962; McNair and Stickler, 1969). The length of the spine was found to be insignificantly reduced, whereas the length of the arms (span) was in the low–normal range. The unequal reductions in leg length, arm length and spine length can be explained by an inhibiting effect of weight bearing on growth of the legs.

A number of adult relatives of patients with X-linked hypophosphataemic rickets or osteomalacia were found to have low serum P levels without bone disease (Winters *et al.*, 1958). The height of these people was less than the average height of their normophosphataemic siblings. From these observations it seems that hypophosphataemia *per se* is associated with shortness of stature. Investigations by Travis *et al.* (1971) and by Card and Brain (1973) revealed that the levels of adenosine triphosphate and 2,3-diphosphoglycerate in the red blood cells fall when serum P is low. As a result, the haemoglobin–oxygen dissociation curve shifts to the left. Glorieux *et al.* (1972) postulated that this might cause a fall in the release of oxygen to the tissues of sufficient magnitude to impair growth. Alternatively the absence of rachitic bone disease in a number of hypophosphataemic people could be more apparent than real. Clinically and roentgenographically, mild osteomalacia in adults may be undetectable and bone biopsies are required to find the rachitic changes. Until it has been shown that apparently non-rachitic hypophosphataemic patients with short stature have normal bone structure it cannot be excluded that a minimal degree of rickets has been responsible for the impairment of growth in such cases.

THE EFFECT OF TREATMENT ON GROWTH

It is well known that treatment with large doses of vitamin D or dihydrotachysterol does not cure the rachitic lesions. Serum P usually rises to less subnormal values and some improvement is visible on X-ray examination of the metaphyseal areas of the long bones. The roentgenographic signs of rickets vanish almost completely only in the least severe cases (Figure 8.2).

Since rickets persists, the effect on growth of this type of treatment is not satisfactory. In 1960 Prader stated that the occurrence of deformities and the progression of deformities that were already present could be prevented by vitamin D in high doses. A growth-promoting effect was doubtful however. In a study of 36 patients McNair and Stickler (1969) found that neither growth nor deformities were favourably affected by vitamin D. They agreed with Prader (1960) that such treatment might at best prevent an aggravation of the signs and symptoms. In the experience of others however (Fraser and Salter, 1958; Tapia *et al.*, 1964; and Harrison *et al.*, 1966) in a number of patients treatment is followed by improvement of existing deformities of the legs. According to these authors the effects on growth are disappointing; occasionally some improvement could be achieved, although the average height of normal children was not attained and stature in most cases remained below the 3rd centile.

These observations leave no doubt as to the persistence of growth failure. Still, the paucity of longitudinal studies with accurate measurements of height at regular intervals does not permit proper evaluation of the effect of treatment on growth in individual cases. Tapia *et al.* (1964) published longitudinal growth curves of six children. At least two of these grew slightly better during therapy than before. The case presented by Parfitt (1972) is another example of an increased rate of growth during uninterrupted therapy with vitamin D. The height of this

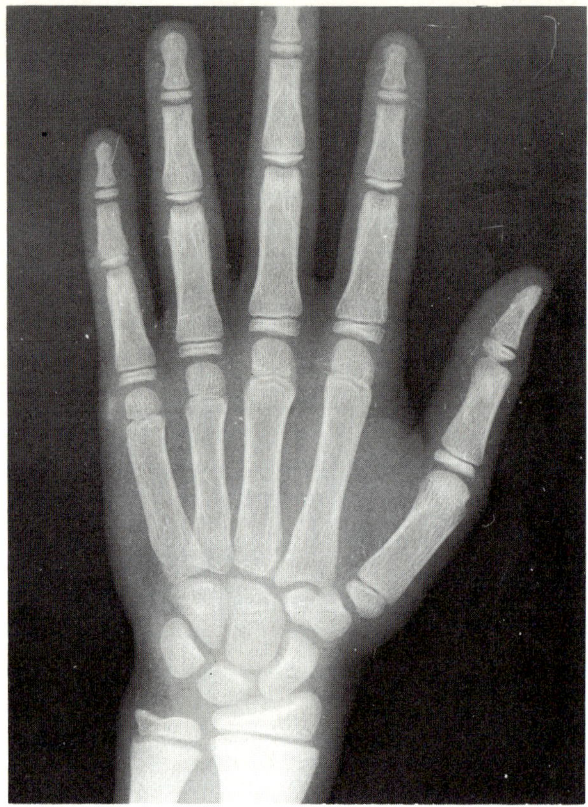

FIGURE 8.2 Radiograph of the left hand of an 11·3-year-old boy with hypophosphataemic rickets. Note minimal signs of rickets at ulnar metaphysis, and coarse trabecular structure in all bones. The growth curve of this boy is presented in Figure 8.3.

patient moved from the 3rd to the 50th centile in the course of 8 years. Comparable improvement occurred in one of my patients (Figure 8.3). This boy had been treated continuously first with vitamin D and later with dihydrotachysterol from his first birthday. The slight deformities that were present at the beginning of treatment disappeared in a few years. X-ray evidence of rickets soon became minimal (Figure 8.2). The height of the boy followed the 3rd centile until age 5 years. During the next 5 years it moved up to the 50th centile and presumably adult height will be just above the 50th centile. The rather sudden increase of growth rate at the age of 5 years is unexplained. It did not coincide with a change in the daily dose of vitamin D or with a rise in serum P. The average level of serum P (66 estimations in 15 years) was 3·2 mg/100 ml.

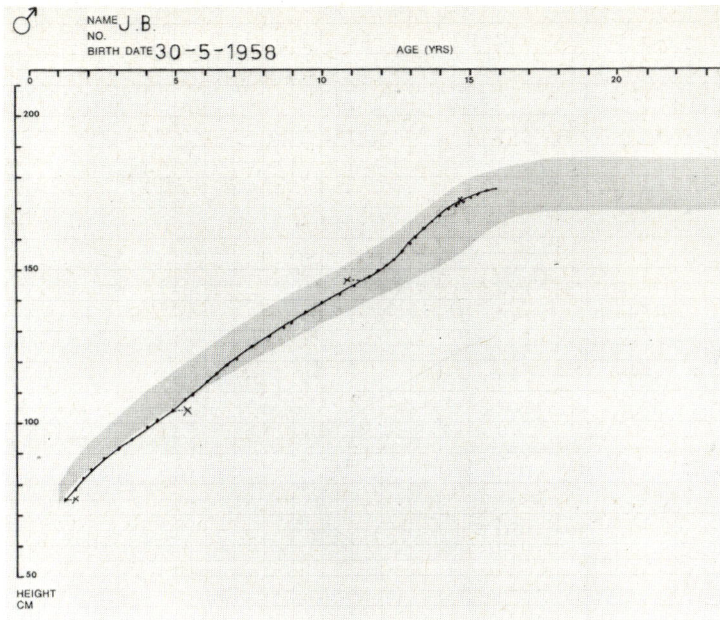

FIGURE 8.3 Growth curve of a boy (J.B.) with mild hypophosphataemic rickets. Note advance in height between the ages of 5 and 10. (In Figures 8.3, 8.4 and 8.5 the grey area represents the space between the 10th and 90th centiles of height of the normal population. Skeletal age is indicated by 'X').

The growth curve in Figure 8.4 is from a boy who also had mild rickets (Steendijk, 1962). He received vitamin D or dihydrotachysterol from the age of 5 years. Initially, his lower legs were slightly bowed. These deformities disappeared slowly and they were no longer present at puberty. Roentgenographic evidence of rickets during the years of treatment was very slight. He grew along the 3rd centile and his adult height was a little above the 10th centile. This late advance in height probably was the result of a slight delay in the onset of puberty and prolonged growth rather than to an effect of vitamin D. The average serum P concentration (53 determinations in 11 years) was 3·1 mg/100 ml.

Finally, Figure 8.5 shows the growth curve of a girl who was more severely affected. Bilateral genu valgum persisted in spite of continuous therapy with high doses of vitamin D for 11 years. Between the ages of 7 and 18 height—SDS was approximately −2·5. After adult height had been reached osteotomies were performed on both lower legs to correct the deformities. The average serum P level (45 determinations in 11 years) was 2·8 mg/100 ml.

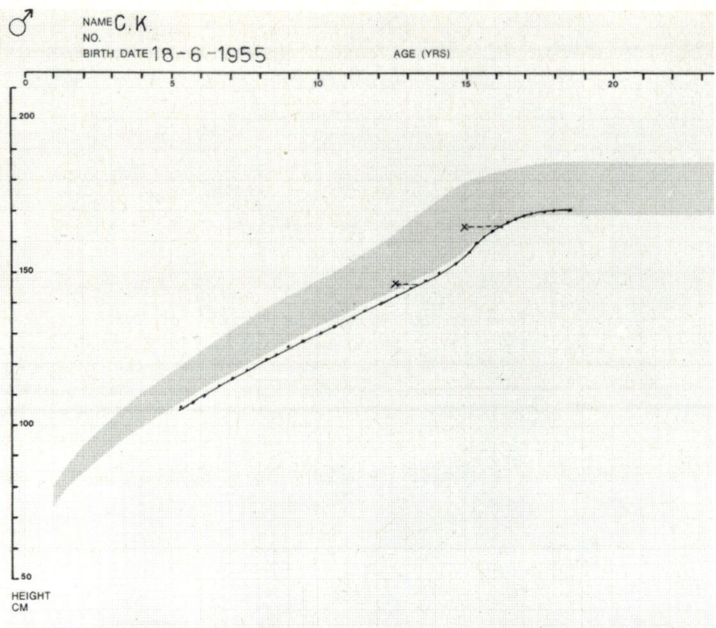

FIGURE 8.4 Growth curve of a boy (C.K.) with mild hypophosphataemic rickets. Note slight advance in height during the pubertal growth spurt.

These very short case-histories and the accompanying growth charts may serve as examples of the different degrees of severity and the varying responses to treatment encountered in this type of rickets.

Contrary to the findings of Tapia *et al.* (1964) a pubertal growth spurt is observed in all patients (Figures 8.3–8.5). In nine of my patients height was measured regularly before, during and after puberty. From these data the peak height velocity (PHV) during the growth spurt was calculated in the manner described by Tanner *et al.* (1966). The findings are presented in Table 8.2, which in addition contains the age at which PHV occurred, the height attained at this age and the serum P level at that time. Adult height in the patients who had stopped growing and the age at menarche in the girls are also presented in Table 8.2. It was found that the range of PHV was wide, as in normal children. Its mean value was low and the age at which PHV occurred, though perhaps slightly delayed, fell within the normal range (Tanner *et al.*, 1966; Marshall and Tanner, 1969). Age at menarche was normal.

By comparing the patients J.B. (Figure 8.3), M.M. (Figure 8.5) and others like them one sometimes gets the impression that the response to

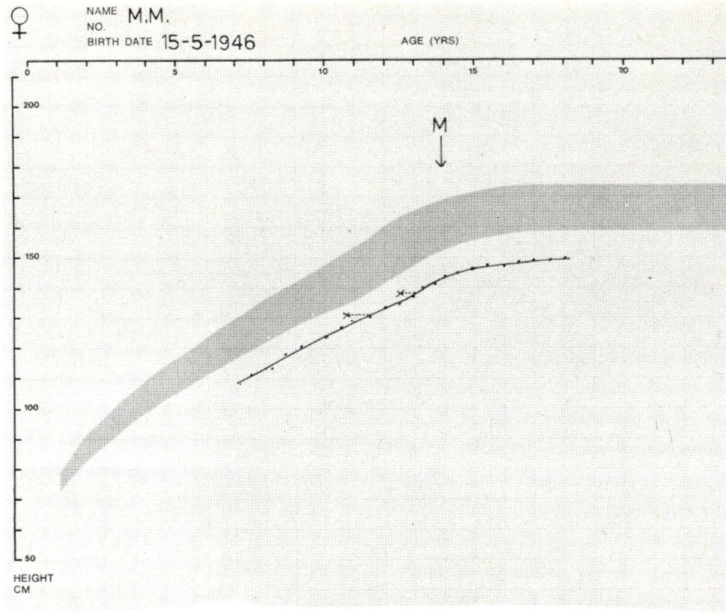

FIGURE 8.5 Growth curve of a girl (M.M.) with moderate hypophosphataemic rickets. Note absence of advance in height.

treatment in terms of growth, deformities and the X-ray findings improves when it is possible to raise serum P to values above 3·0 mg/100 ml. If so, such improvement is limited and it is not observed in all patients. In eight of the nine children from Table 8.2 serum P was between 3·0 and 3·3 mg/100 ml at the time of PHV and in four of them (P.N., M.A.V. and P.S.) the deformities became worse when growth accelerated during puberty (see below).

On the other hand the results of treatment have recently been improved by the use of phosphate either alone or in addition to high doses of vitamin D (Moncrieff and Chance, 1969; McEnery *et al.*, 1972; Glorieux *et al.*, 1972). By oral administration of large amounts of inorganic phosphate five times per day at regular intervals it is possible to raise serum P to normal values for the better part of the day. The roentgenographic signs of rickets vanish and growth accelerates. In the few cases reported until now the improvement in the rate of growth usually has been slight but persistent and stature advanced gradually over a number of years. True catch-up growth with a sudden con-

Table 8.2 *Peak height velocity (PHV) during the pubertal growth spurt, age, height and serum P at PHV, age at menarche and adult height in children with hypophosphataemic rickets, treated with vitamin D or dihydrotachysterol. The normal values are from Tanner* et al. *(1966) and from Marshall and Tanner (1969)*

Initials	*Sex*	*Age at PHV* (years)	*PHV* (cm/year)	*Height at PHV* (cm)	*Height at PHV* (SDS)	*Serum P at PHV* (mg/100 ml)	*Age at menarche*	*Adult Height* (cm)
P.N.	Male	16·3	6·6	148·8	−3·6	3·0		157·3
C.K.	Male	15·5	10·0	160·2	−1·3	3·1		171·0
P.V.	Male	15·3	5·9	147·9	−2·6	2·5		152·0
J.B.	Male	13·4	10·7	162·8	+0·6	3·1		
Average		15·1	8·3	153·6	−1·7			
Normal mean		14·1	10·3					
Normal range		12·0–16·0	7·0–15·5					
I.K.	Female	13·5	7·2	142·3	−2·6	3·2	14·3	152·2
M.K.	Female	13.0	8·4	153·3	−0·5	3·2	13·6	165.3
M.M.	Female	12·8	5·9	137·4	−2·6	3·1	13·9	149·2
A.V.	Female	12·7	8·2	141·3	−2·0	3·3	13·1	152·0
P.S.	Female	12·7	6·6	134·5	−3·0	3·1	13·7	143·1
Average		13·0	7·3	141·8	−2·1		13·7	
Normal mean		12·1	9·0				13·5	
Normal range		10·5–13·5	6·2–11·0					

spicuous rise in growth rate has also been recorded however (Glorieux *et al.*, 1972).

The combination of vitamin D and oral phosphate at present seems to be the treatment of choice for those patients who respond insufficiently to vitamin D alone.

THE EFFECT OF GROWTH ON RICKETS

It has been mentioned already that in a number of patients the enhanced growth rate during puberty is accompanied by the development or aggravation of the leg deformities. This is an example of the effect of growth on rickets. It may happen in a few months' time and therefore it cannot be caused by increased bowing of the long bones of the legs. Rather it appears to be the result of partial collapse of the proximal epiphyseal plate of the tibia and sometimes perhaps also of the distal epiphyseal plate of the femur (Steendijk, 1971). It occurs in spite of uninterrupted treatment with high doses of vitamin D. Presumably the wide and irregularly shaped growth plate is unstable. Changes occurring in the plate when growth accelerates, such as an additional increase in width, may further decrease its stability and bring about the observed collapse. Postpubertal deceleration of growth usually is not accompanied by spontaneous correction of this deformity and the legs may have to be straightened by osteotomies. The possibility of an increase of the deformities at puberty is a strong argument against early surgical correction of any deformities that have occurred before that time. Reoperation may then be necessary. If possible osteotomies should be postponed until adult height has been reached.

Occasionally children are reported who seem to acquire rickets at the time of puberty. They have no distinct physical signs of the disease until the onset of sexual maturation, when deformities of the legs appear. The stature of such children usually is short and sometimes the patients belong to families which carry the hypophosphataemic gene (Christansson, 1958). Presumably these children have been hypophosphataemic all the time but because of the absence of overt signs of rickets no attention is drawn to the disease until it is unmasked by the increased rate of growth at puberty.

Morphological features of hypophosphataemic rickets

ROENTGENOGRAPHIC FINDINGS

The changes in growth and development of bone described in the foregoing paragraphs result from structural changes of bone tissue. Rachitic bone tissue is primarily characterised by incomplete mineralisation of the organic collagenous matrix. Histologically, much uncalcified osteoid is found and the degree of mineralisation of calcified bone appears to be low (Steendijk and Boyde, 1973). Therefore it is surprising to find in treated as well as in untreated patients that the roentgenographic density of the bones is increased (Steendijk, 1962; Steinbach and Noetzli, 1964) (Figure 8.6). In addition, the trabecular

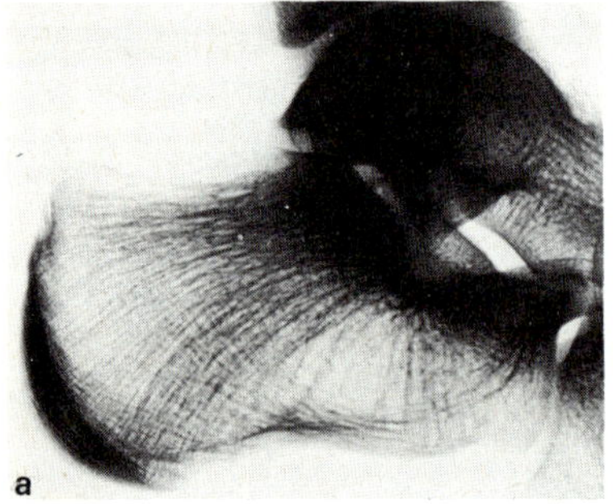

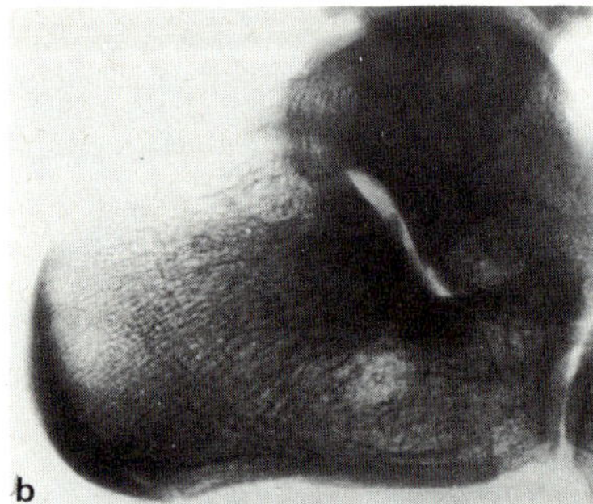

FIGURE 8.6 X-ray photographs of the os calcis of a normal adolescent boy (a) and of a boy of the same age with severe hypophosphataemic rickets (b). (From Steendijk, R. (1962), *Helv. Paediatr. Acta*, **17**, 65, with kind permission of the publisher.)

structure is conspicuously coarse (Figure 8.2). This feature offers an explanation for the high mineral density, since it implies the presence of an increased amount of bone tissue: in spite of incomplete mineralisation, the total amount of bone mineral may thus be uncommonly large.

The roentgenographic signs of rickets at the metaphyses of the long bones are similar to those seen in other types of rickets. Usually these are mild, although the degree of severity differs widely. Signs of hyperparathyroidism are not encountered. In some patients extensive localised overgrowth of bone occurs in the form of ossicles, spurs and exostotic growths (Steinbach and Noetzli, 1964). These phenomena are not seen in other types of rickets.

MICROSCOPICAL FINDINGS

Microradiography of thin, undecalcified sections of bone tissue is a good method for the study of bone structure in this disease. It reveals an increased porosity of cortical bone; in addition, there are many areas of decreased mineral density (Jowsey, 1963). The porosity results from the presence of large amounts of unmineralised matrix (osteoid), which is not visible on the microradiographs. It must be distinguished from true osteoporosis in which the amounts of matrix and mineral are reduced proportionally. In normal bone tissue osteoid is almost exclusively present at mineralising surfaces and it begins to take up bone salt a few days after its deposition. In rickets, the layer of osteoid at such surfaces is many times thicker than in the normal condition (Figure 8.7a). Moreover, it often remains unmineralised for long periods of time.

The mineral density of bone tissue is decreased in parts of the cement lines surrounding the osteones, and also around a number of osteocyte lacunae and their canaliculi (Figure 8.7b). This latter feature is very conspicuous. Whereas unmineralised cement lines occur in all types of rachitic bone disease, the circumlacunar lack of bone mineral has not been encountered in vitamin D-deficient rickets or in renal osteodystrophy. It does occur however in two apparently unrelated conditions: in chronic fluorosis (Adams and Jowsey, 1965) and in the bone of parathyroidectomised dogs (Burkhart and Jowsey, 1966). The area of low mineral density is mainly localised on the side of the lacunae which is directed towards the nearest bone surface, usually the central canal of an osteone (Figure 8.7b). Bone matrix is present in these lesions, but its structure is abnormal. This becomes visible upon treatment of decalcified bone sections with precipitating stains such as Schmorl's azure II–picric acid stain and Bodian's silver stain (Steendijk, Jowsey, Van den Hooff and Nielsen, 1967) as shown in Figure 8.8. The normal lamellar architecture of the matrix is interrupted at these sites, and at higher magnifications it appears that the matrix has taken up these stains in a globular fashion.

Initially, it was not clear whether the matrix lesion was the result of a primary insufficient mineralisation of the matrix, whether there was some abnormal feature of the matrix which rendered adequate mineralisation impossible, or whether there had been secondary demineralisation in these lesions, in the sense of a leaching out of bone salt from an area which had previously been well mineralised. The first of these possibilities seemed to be the most likely one since the lesions were already present in the most recently mineralised bone at the inner edge of growing osteones. This view was substantiated by

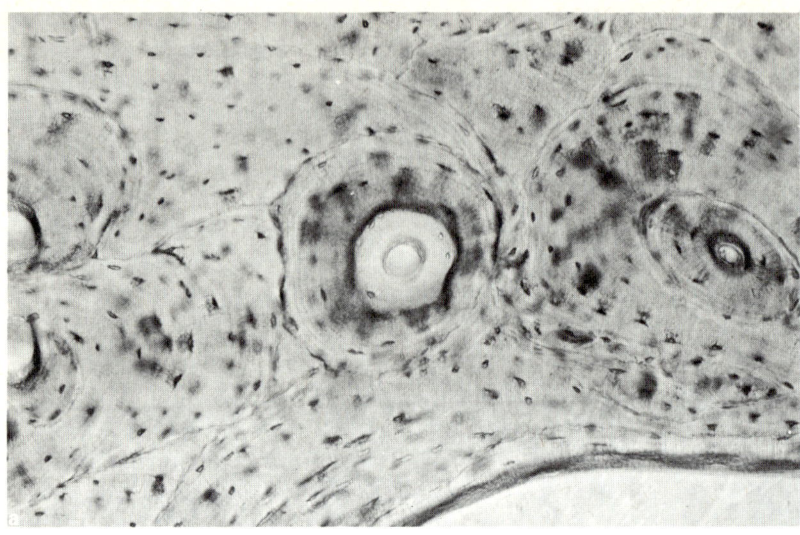

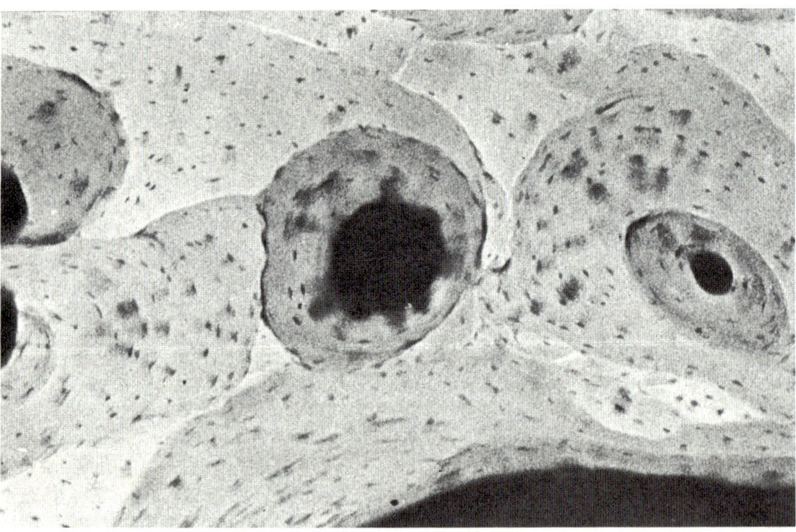

FIGURE 8.7 (a) Undecalcified unstained cross-section (100 μm thick) of fibula from a patient with hypophosphataemic rickets (× 112). Note wide osteoid band in Haversian system. (b) Microradiograph from section (a). Note circumlacunar deficit of bone mineral, most conspicuous in the recently formed Haversian system. The area of mineral deficit is mainly on the side of the lacunae towards the nearest surface. Bone mineral is also lacking in parts of the cementlines.

examination of bone from patients with hypophosphataemic rickets in the scanning electron microscope (Steendijk and Boyde, 1973). The

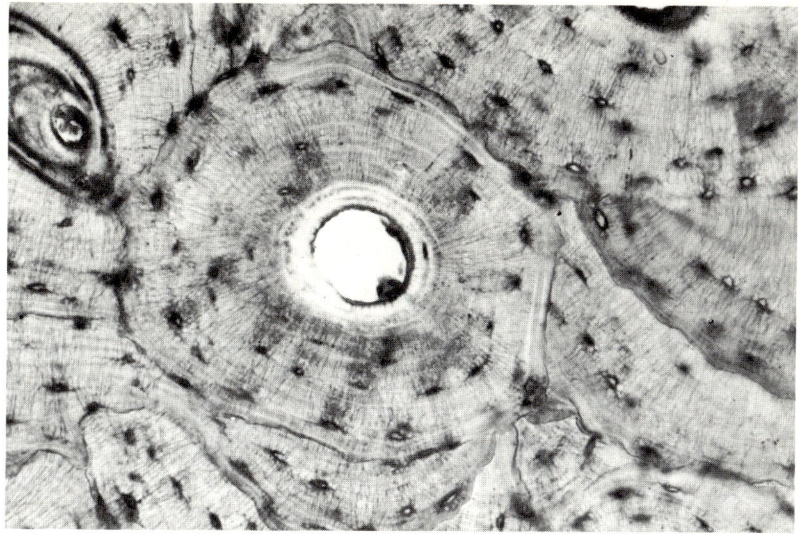

FIGURE 8.8 Decalcified cross-section (10 μm thick) of fibula from a patient with hypophosphataemic rickets (× 180). Schmorl's stain. The matrix is more heavily stained in the circumlacunar areas of low mineral density.

circumlacunar area appeared as a conglomeration of mineral particle clusters, each cluster measuring 1–3 μm in diameter (Figure 8.9). This appearance closely resembles a mineralising front where new bone is being laid down. Here, mineral deposition occurs in a large number of clusters which grow and finally fuse to form a solid mineralised mass (Boyde and Hobdell, 1969; Figure 8.10). It was concluded from these observations that the circumlacunar lesions appeared to result from interrupted mineralisation of bone. The structural change in the matrix at these sites presumably represents a secondary phenomenon.

The presence of the circumlacunar lesions may indicate that osteocytes have an inhibiting effect on the mineralisation of bone tissue, which is greatest in their immediate vicinity (Steendijk and Boyde, 1973). Such an effect would not be discernible in normal conditions, but might be revealed by a disorder of mineralisation such as hypophosphataemic rickets. It cannot be explained why the mineral defect is more extensive on one particular side of the lacuna.

Microscopic examination of bone from several patients with hypophosphataemic rickets has revealed that the number of lacunae surrounded by incompletely mineralised bone varies greatly. In some patients almost all lacunae were involved, whereas in others most

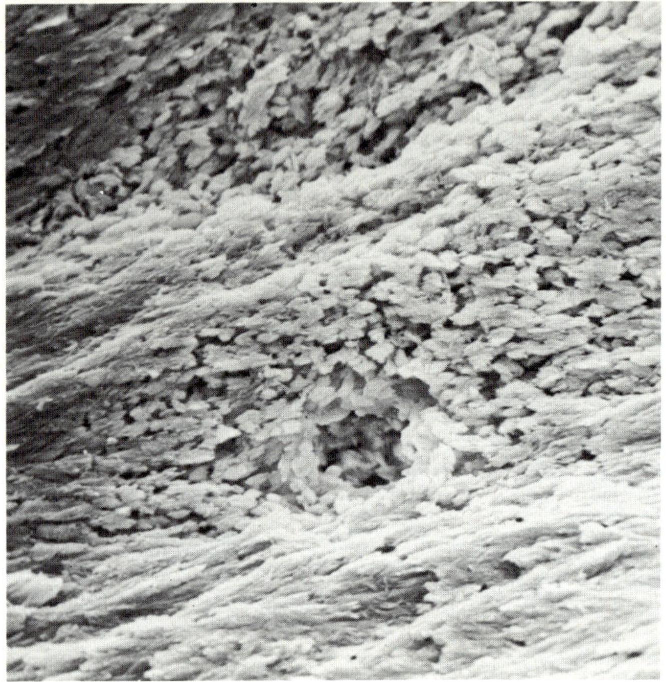

FIGURE 8.9 Scanning electron microscopic picture of osteocyte lacuna with circumlacunar mineral deficit. The area of low mineral density is traversed by a band of interlamellar substance, which is more heavily mineralised. (Fracture surface, anorganic bone; width of the picture: 57 μm.)

lacunae appeared normal (Steendijk *et al.*, 1967). It appeared that the frequency of the lesions varies in conjunction with other features of the bone such as the average width of the osteoid layers and the number of osteoid-covered osteones. There was however no apparent relation between the clinical severity of the disease (height of the patients, deformities of the legs) and the degree of bone disease as revealed by these microscopic studies (Steendijk, 1971). Apparently, the deformities are brought about by a number of interrelated factors, among which the histologically determined extent of the disorder is only one. It is also possible that the histological expression of the disease may change over the years. In a patient with severely deformed legs and only slight histological rickets for instance, bone structure may have improved spontaneously since the time when the deformities appeared. This assumption would be in agreement with the observations in at least a number of patients that the circumlacunar lesions appear to be more

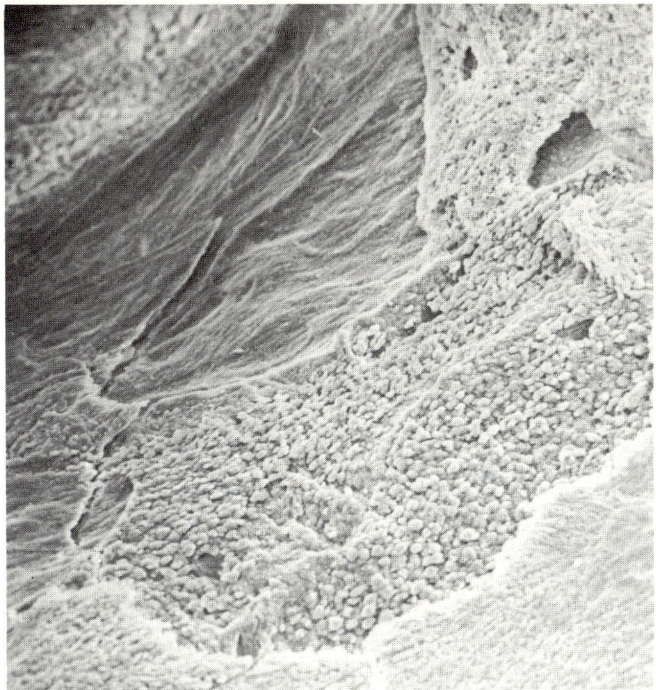

FIGURE 8.10 Scanning electron microscopic picture of resorbing area of bone from a patient with hypophosphataemic rickets. New bone is being deposited in the lower half of this area. Its aspect resembles the circumlacunar lesion (Figure 8.9). (Fracture surface anorganic bone; width of picture: 230 μm.)

numerous and more extensive in recently deposited bone. Interstitial bone, which is at least several years old, sometimes contains very few lesions, whereas they are abundantly present in new Haversian systems. This difference, which has not yet been worked out quantitatively, is illustrated in Figure 8.7b.

During treatment with large doses of vitamin D the lesions persist and fresh ones continue to appear as bone is being deposited. The effect of the combined vitamin D–phosphate treatment on the microscopic bone lesions has not yet been elucidated.

Summary

In this review on hypophosphataemic rickets two aspects of this disease have been discussed: growth in height of the patients and the morphological and structural changes of bone tissue.

Growth. From cross-sectional studies in 37 patients it appeared that the average stature was equal to the 3rd centile of normal children, whereas the standard deviation for height was not different from the normal value. Longitudinal studies revealed that some catch-up may occur in mild cases perhaps as a result of treatment with high doses of vitamin D or dihydrotachysterol.

Bone tissue was studied with the aid of microradiography, histology and scanning electron microscopy. The most conspicuous lesion is a deficiency of bone mineral around the osteocyte lacunae, mainly at the side of the lacunae towards the nearest bone surface. It appeared that this lesion is the result of impaired mineralisation of bone matrix.

Acknowledgements

I am indebted to Dr Alan Boyde for Figures 8.9 and 8.10 and to Dr A. van den Hooff for critical evaluation of the manuscript.

REFERENCES

Adams, P. H. and Jowsey, J. (1965). Sodium fluoride in the treatment of osteoporosis and other bone diseases. *Ann. Intern. Med.*, **63**, 1151

Bianchine, J. W., Stambler, A. A. and Harrison, H. E. (1971). Familial hypophosphataemic rickets showing autosomal dominant inheritance. *Birth Defects*, **5**

Boyde, A. and Hobdell, M. H. (1969). Scanning electron microscopy of lamellar bone. *Z. Zellforsch.*, **93**, 213

Brickman, A. S., Coburn, J. W., Kurokawa, K., Bethune, J. E., Harrison, H. E. and Norman, A. W. (1973). 1,25-dihydrocholecalciferol in hypophosphatemic vitamin D-resistant rickets. *N. Engl. J. Med.*, **289**, 495

Burkhart, J. M. and Jowsey, J. (1966). Morphological evidence of osteomalacia in dogs. *Mayo Clin. Proc.*, **41**, 663

Burnett, C. H., Dent, C. E., Harper, C. and Warland, B. J. (1964). Vitamin D-resistant rickets. Analysis of twenty-four pedigrees with hereditary and sporadic cases. *Am. J. Med.*, **36**, 222

Card, R. T. and Brain, M. C. (1973). The 'anemia' of childhood. *N. Engl. J. Med.*, **288**, 388

Christiansson, G. (1958). Emergence of primary vitamin D resistant rickets at puberty. *Acta Paediatr.*, **47**, 288

DeLuca, H. E., Lund, J., Rosenbloom, A. and Lobeck, C. C. (1967). Metabolism of tritiated vitamin D_3 in familial vitamin D-resistant rickets with hypophosphatemia. *J. Pediatr.*, **70**, 828

Fanconi, A., Fischer, J. A. and Prader, A. (1974). Serum parathyroid hormone concentrations in hypophosphataemic vitamin D resistant rickets. *Helv. Paediatr. Acta*, **29**, 187

Fischer, J. A., Binswanger, U., Fanconi, A., Illig, R., Baerlocher, K. and Prader, A. (1973). Serum parathyroid hormone concentrations in vitamin D deficiency rickets of infancy. *Horm. Metab. Res.*, **5**, 381

Fraser, D. and Salter, R. B. (1958). The diagnosis and management of the various types of rickets. *Pediatr. Clin. N. Am.*, **5**, 417

Glorieux, F. and Scriver, C. R. (1972). Loss of a parathyroid hormone-sensitive component of phosphate transport in X-linked hypophosphatemia. *Science*, **175**, 997

Glorieux, F. H., Scriver, C. R., Reade, T. M., Goldman, H. and Roseborough, A. (1972). Use of phosphate and vitamin D to prevent dwarfism and rickets in X-linked hypophosphatemia. *N. Engl. J. Med.*, **287**, 481

Glorieux, F., Scriver, C. R., Holick, M. F. and DeLuca, H. E. (1973). X-linked hypophosphataemic rickets: inadequate therapeutic response to 1,25-dehydroxycholecalciferol. *Lancet*, **ii**, 287

HARRISON, H. E., HARRISON, H. C., LIFSHITZ, F. and JOHNSON, D. (1966). Growth disturbance in hereditary hypophosphatemia. *Am. J. Dis. Child.*, **112**, 290

JOWSEY, J. (1963). Microradiography of bone resorption. In R. F. Sognnaes (ed.), *Mechanisms of Hard Tissue Destruction*, p. 447 (Washington : Am. Assoc. Adv. Sci.)

LEWY, J. E., CABANA, E. C., REPETTO, H. A., CANTERBURY, J. M. and REISS, E. (1972). Serum parathyroid hormone in hypophosphatemic vitamin D-resistant rickets. *J. Pediatr.*, **81**, 294

MARSHALL, W. A. and TANNER, J. M. (1969). Variations in pattern of pubertal changes in girls. *Arch. Dis. Child.*, **44**, 291

McENERY, P. T., SILVERMAN, F. N. and WEST, G. D. (1972). Acceleration of growth with combined vitamin D-phosphate therapy of hypophosphatemic resistant rickets. *J. Pediatr.*, **80**, 763

McNAIR, S. and STICKLER, G. B. (1969). Growth in familial hypophosphatemic vitamin D-resistant rickets. *N. Engl. J. Med.*, **281**, 511

MONCRIEFF, M. W. and CHANCE, G. W. (1969). Nephrotoxic effect of vitamin D therapy in vitamin D refractory rickets. *Arch. Dis. Child.*, **44**, 571

MORSE, M., SCHULTZ, F. W. and CASSELS, D. E. (1949). Relation of age to physiological responses of the older boy (10–17 years) to exercise. *J. Appl. Physiol.*, **1**, 683

NAGANT DE DECHAISNES, C. and KRANE, S. M. (1967). The treatment of adult phosphate diabetes and Fanconi syndrome with neutral sodium phosphate. *Am. J. Med.*, **43**, 508

PARFITT, M. (1972). Hypophosphatemic vitamin D refractory rickets and osteomalacia. *Orthop. Clin. N. Am.*, **3**, 653

PRADER, A. (1960). Die hereditäre hypophosphatämische vitamin D-resistente Rachitis (Phosphatdiabetes). *Mod. Probl. Paediatr.*, **6**, 337

REITZ, R. E. and WEINSTEIN, R. L. (1973). Parathyroid hormone secretion in familial vitamin D resistant rickets. *N. Engl. J. Med.*, **289**, 941

SCHOEN, E. J. and REYNOLDS, J. B. (1970). Severe familial hypophosphatemic rickets. *Am. J. Dis. Child.*, **120**, 58

SHORT, E., SEBASTIAN, A., SPENCER, M. and MORRIS, R. C. (1974). Hyperresponsiveness to the phosphaturic effect of parathyroid hormone in X-linked hypophosphatemic vitamin D-resistant rickets. *J. Clin. Invest.*, **53**, 75a (Abstr.)

STEENDIJK, R. (1962). Studies on growth in refractory rickets. *J. Pediatr.*, **60**, 340

STEENDIJK, R. (1962). On the pathogenesis of vitamin D deficient rickets and primary vitamin D resistant rickets. *Helv. Paediatr. Acta*, **17**, 65

STEENDIJK, R., JOWSEY, J., VAN DEN HOOFF, A. and NIELSEN, H. K. L. (1967). Microradiographic and histological studies in vitamin D-resistant rickets. In D. J. Hioco (ed.), *L'Ostéomalacie*, p. 127 (Paris : Masson & Cie)

STEENDIJK, R., NIELSEN, H. K. L. and KRAAI, A. (1968). Osteotomy, vitamin D and the metabolism of calcium and inorganic phosphate in vitamin D-resistant rickets and osteomalacia. *Helv. Paediatr. Acta*, **23**, 627

STEENDIJK, R. (1971). Metabolic bone disease in children. *Clin. Orthop.*, **77**, 247

STEENDIJK, R. and LATHAM, S. C. (1971). Hypophosphataemic vitamin D-resistant rickets; an observation on height and serum inorganic phosphorus in untreated cases. *Helv. Paediatr. Acta*, **26**, 179

STEENDIJK, R. and BOYDE, A. (1973). Scanning electron microscopic observations on bone from patients with hypophosphataemic (vitamin D resistant) rickets. *Calcif. Tissue Res.*, **11**, 242

STEINBACH, H. L. and NOETZLI, M. (1964). Roentgen appearance of the skeleton in osteomalacia and rickets. *Am. J. Roentgenol.*, **91**, 955

STICKLER, G. B. (1969). Familial hypophosphatemic vitamin D resistant rickets. *Acta Paediatr. Scand.*, **58**, 213

STICKLER, G. B., BEABOUT, J. W. and RIGGS, B. L. (1970). Vitamin D-resistant rickets: Clinical experience with 41 typical familial hypophosphatemic patients and 2 atypical nonfamilial cases. *Mayo Clin. Proc.*, **45**, 197

TANNER, J. M. (1962). *Growth at Adolescence*, p. 190 (Oxford : Blackwell)

TANNER, J. M., WHITEHOUSE, R. H. and TAKAISHI, M. (1966). Standards from birth to maturity for height, weight, height velocity and weight velocity: British children, 1965. *Arch. Dis. Child.*, **41**, 454

TAPIA, J., STEARNS, G. and PONSETTI, I. V. (1964). Vitamin D-resistant rickets. *J. Bone Joint Surg. (Am.)*, **46A**, 935

Travis, S. F., Sugerman, H. J., Ruberg, R. L., Dudrick, S. J., Delivoria-Papadopoulos, M., Miller, L. D. and Oski, F. A. (1971). Alterations of red-cell glycolytic intermediates and oxygen transport as a consequence of hypophosphatemia in patients receiving intravenous hyperalimentation. *N. Engl. J. Med.*, **285**, 763

Winters, R. W., Graham, J. B., Williams, T. F., McFalls, V. W. and Burnett, C. H. (1958). A genetic study of familial hypophosphatemic vitamin D resistant rickets with a review of the literature. *Medicine* (Baltimore), **37**, 97

Wijn, J. F. de (1965). Growth and chemical growth of adolescent boys, related to physique and somatotype. *Helv. Paediatr. Acta*, **20**, 497

9

Pseudovitamin D deficiency (vitamin D dependency)

A. Prader, H. P. Kind and H. F. DeLuca

The terms pseudovitamin D deficiency rickets (Prader *et al.*, 1961) and vitamin D dependency rickets (Scriver, 1970) are synonymously used as descriptive terms for a disease that is caused by an inborn error of vitamin D metabolism. The condition mimics all the clinical, radiological and biochemical features of vitamin D deficiency rickets. However, only pharmacological doses of vitamin D bring about complete healing of rickets, and the patient depends on a lifelong intake of vitamin D in high doses in order to prevent a relapse. The metabolic defect is inherited as an autosomal recessive trait. The high frequency of consanguinity (Fanconi and Prader, 1969) suggests that the mutation is relatively rare. The disease is much less frequent than familial X-linked hypophosphataemic refractory rickets.

At birth, the patients are healthy, The clinical symptoms usually appear within the first year of life. They include muscular hypotonia, retarded growth and development, hypocalcaemic tetany (later followed by enamel defects of the permanent teeth), and rarely anaemia and respiratory difficulties (Balsan *et al.*, 1972). Clinical examination and X-ray studies show severe rickets, sometimes associated with fractures. Plasma chemistry is characterised by low calcium, low or normal phosphorus, elevated alkaline phosphatase, high concentration of iPTH (Arnaud *et al.*, 1970; Fanconi and Fischer, 1975) and mild hyperchloraemic acidosis. Intramuscular PTE has no effect on the mobilisation of calcium from bone (Fanconi and Prader, 1969). The intestinal absorption of calcium is decreased (Hamilton *et al.*, 1970). Tubular reabsorption of phosphorus (TRP) is decreased, and there is hypocalciuria and generalised hyperaminoaciduria. The acidosis, the hyperaminoaciduria and the decreased TRP can be interpreted as proximal tubular insufficiency, possibly caused by the secondary hyperparathyroidism (Fraser *et al.*, 1967). All the symptoms and signs mentioned are also present in nutritional vitamin D deficiency.

In the following we wish to present our experiences with three patients, all of whom we have studied for many years (Fanconi and Prader, 1969). They demonstrate the *natural history* of the disease from birth to adulthood and show the *effect of vitamin-D_3, of vitamin-D-metabolites and of some vitamin-D-analogues* which will allow us to speculate about the primary enzymatic block and its effect on prenatal and postnatal calcium metabolism.

Daniela, now 8 years old, was referred to us at the age of 16 months with severe rickets which so far had not responded to treatment with vitamin D. She had severe muscular hypotonia, was unable to sit or stand and showed considerable retardation of growth and psychomotor development. X-rays of the long bones exhibited severe rickets and several fractures. She had hypocalcaemia, hypophosphataemia, elevated alkaline phosphatase and generalised hyperaminoaciduria. Therapy was started with a daily oral dose of 0·25 mg (10 000 IU) of vitamin-D_3 given for 4 weeks. This dose did not affect the bone lesions. Figure 9.1 shows the effect of D_3 during the first year of treatment. Serum calcium, phosphorus and alkaline phosphatase only became normal after a daily dose of 1 mg (40 000 IU) of D_3 was given for several months. Nine months

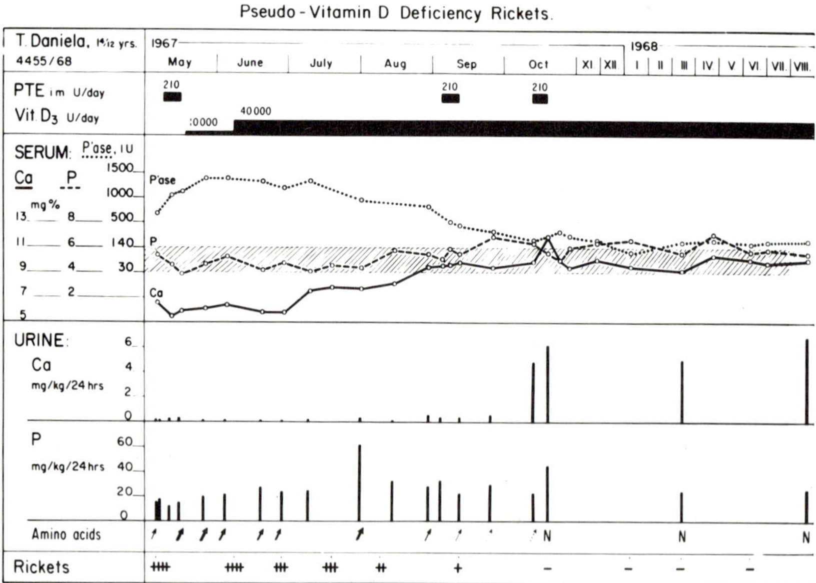

FIGURE 9.1 The effect of PTE and D_3 on serum and urine chemistry, aminoaciduria and radiological rickets during the first year of treatment in patient Daniela (from Fanconi and Prader, 1969).

after initiation of treatment, the rickets was cured. Before, and twice during treatment an intramuscular PTE test was performed for a total of 6 days each (PTE 200 U/m_3 8 hourly). A normal response with a continuous rise of serum calcium only was observed in the last test, when all biochemical parameters were normalised and the rickets was cured. Later, at the age of 3 years, treatment was withheld for a period of 8 months. This lead to a full biochemical relapse with radiologically moderate rickets. Treatment was then reinstituted using now 25(OH)D_3 (Figure 9.2). A daily dose of 0·025 mg given for 2 months had no effect.

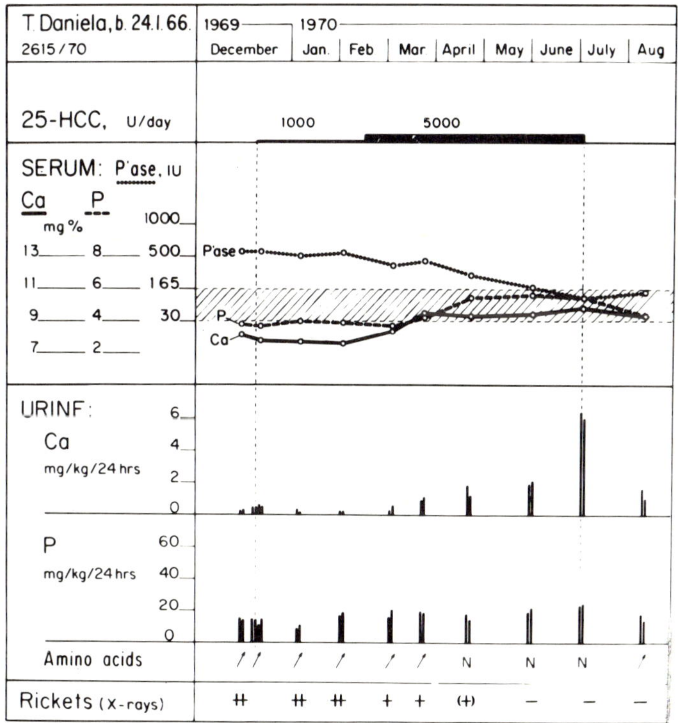

FIGURE 9.2 The effect of 0·025 and 0·125 mg of 25(OH)D_3 on serum and urine chemistry, aminoaciduria and radiological rickets in patient Daniela.

With a daily dose of 0·125 mg rickets was cured within a period of 3 months.

Recently when the girl was 7 years old and at a time when moderate rickets was present, we had the opportunity to test 1,25$(OH)_2D_3$. First

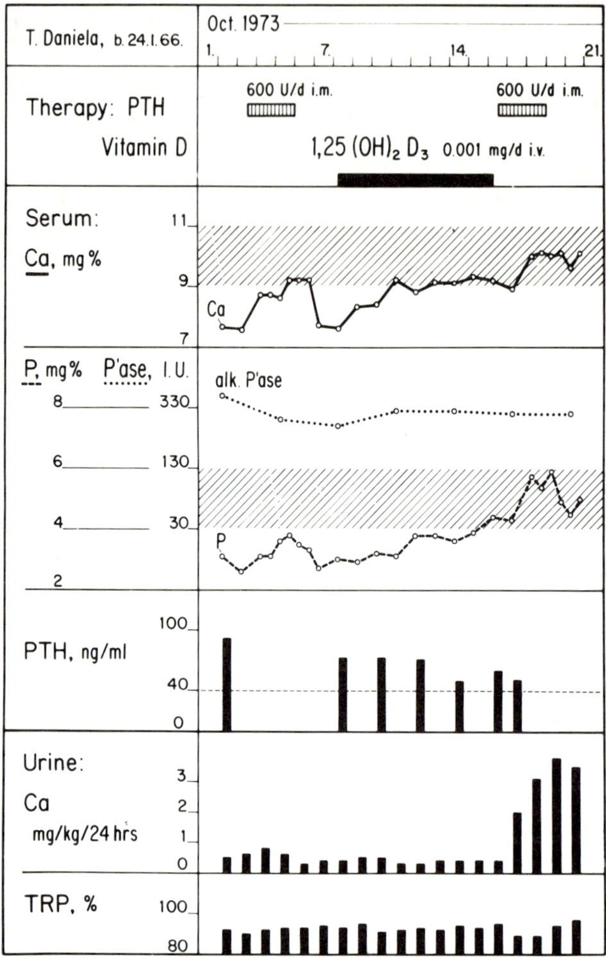

FIGURE 9.3 The effect of PTE and i.v 0·001 mg of $1{,}25(OH)_2D_3$ on serum and urine chemistry, on plasma PTH and on TRP in patient Daniela.

a dose of 0·001 mg daily was given i.v. for 8 days (Figure 9.3). Serum calcium and phosphorus increased and became low normal after 6 days. Alkaline phosphatase and iPTH remained high. After several months without therapy, $1{,}25(OH)_2D_3$ was given orally at the same dose of 0·001 mg/day for a total of 75 days (Figure 9.4). Before the initiation of treatment biochemical and radiological findings were typical for a moderate relapse. Serum calcium and phosphorus level became normal within a few weeks. Alkaline phosphatase slowly decreased to nearly normal levels and the iPTH concentration returned to normal values. Radiological rickets improved greatly but did not disappear completely within this treatment period.

Figure 9.4 summarises our experience with oral D_3, DHT, 25(OH)D_3 and 1,25$(OH)_2D_3$ in this patient during the last 7½ years. A relapse occurred whenever treatment was interrupted. The maintenance dose of D_3 seems to be 1 mg or possibly 0·75 mg. DHT was effective in a dosage of 0·46 and 0·33 mg whereas a relapse occurred with a dosage of 0·66 mg. 25(OH)D_3 in a dosage of 0·025 mg did not correct the abnormal findings while 0·125 mg was effective as was 1,25$(OH)_2D_3$ in a

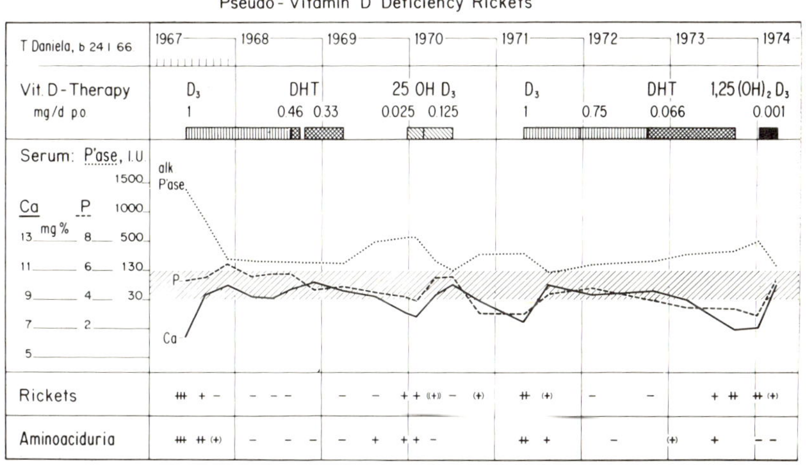

FIGURE 9.4 The effect of D_3 DHT, 25(OH)D_3 and 1,25$(OH)_2D_3$ on serum chemistry, aminoaciduria and radiological rickets in patient Daniela, during the observation period of 7½ years.

dosage of 0·001 mg. It may be concluded that the following daily dosage is necessary for this patient: D_3, 1 mg; DHT, 0·4 mg; 25(OH)D_3, 0·125 mg; and 1,25$(OH)_2D_3$, 0·001 mg. The dosage of D_3, DHT and 25(OH)D_3 is in the pharmacological range whereas the dosage of 1,25$(OH)_2D_3$ is in the presumed physiological range.

At the time when the diagnosis of pseudovitamin D deficiency rickets was made, the girl's height was below 3rd percentile. Under treatment catch-up growth occurred (Figure 9.5), and after the age of 3–4 years her height remained above the 50th percentile. This is one of the most beautiful examples of catch-up growth we have ever seen, and provides the best evidence that treatment was fully effective.

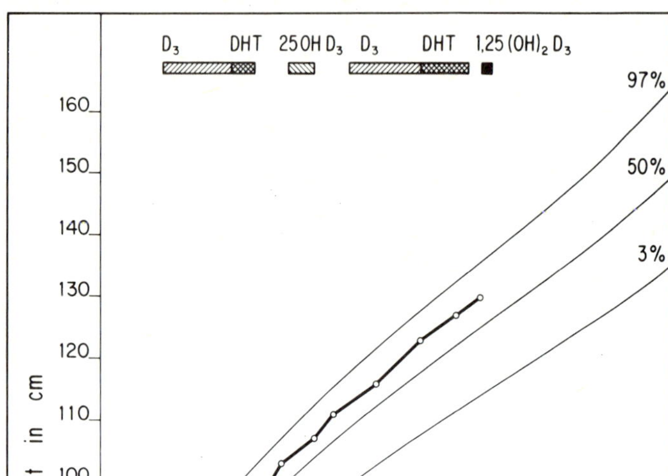

FIGURE 9.5 Catch-up growth in patient Daniela during the period shown in Figure 9.4.

The patient's younger sister, Laura, now 7 years old, underwent the same investigations. She demonstrated identical responses to D_3, $25(OH)D_3$ and DHT therapy. In contrast to her sister she was given $1\alpha(OH)D_3$ instead of $1,25(OH)_2D_3$ for the same period of 75 days. Her daily oral dose was 0·002 mg. Figure 9.6 shows the positive effect upon serum calcium, phosphorus, alkaline phosphatase, iPTH and amino-aciduria. Rickets was cured.

Our experience with these two patients demonstrates that $1,25(OH)_2D_3$ *and* $1\alpha(OH)D_3$ *are fully effective in a daily dosage of 0·001 or 0·002 mg by mouth, whereas* D_3, *DHT and* $25(OH)D_3$ *are only effective in doses 100 to 1000 times higher*. This confirms the study of Fraser *et al.*, (1973) who

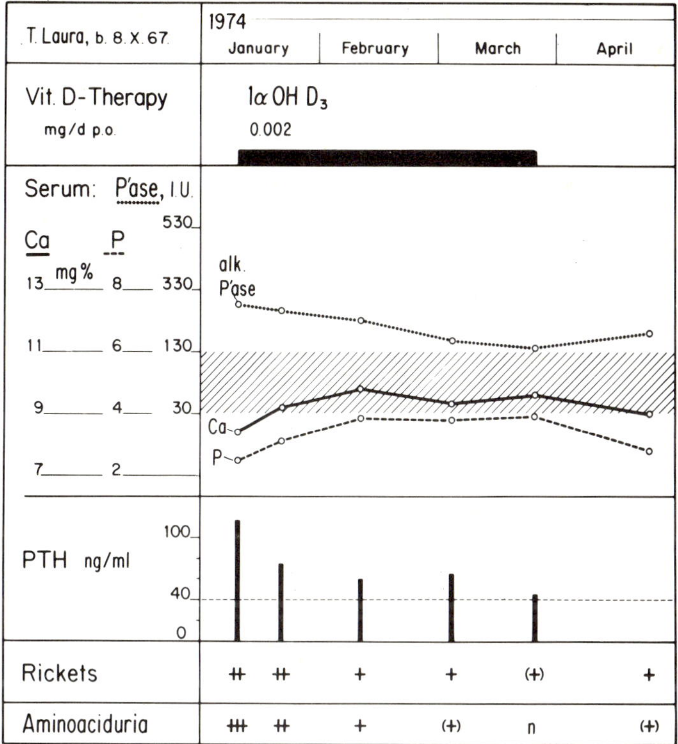

FIGURE 9.6 The effect of 0·002 mg of 1α(OH)D_3 on serum and urine chemistry, plasma PTH and radiological rickets in patient Laura.

have treated one patient with i.v. 1,25$(OH)_2D_3$, and is similar to the unpublished experience of Dr Balsan in Paris and Dr Scriver in Toronto. The results suggest that the primary metabolic defect is a *hereditary block of the 25(OH)D_3 1α-hydroxylase in the kidney*. This hypothesis has still to be proven by direct measurements of the activity of this enzyme. The fact that D_3 is effective if given at a dosage 1000 times higher suggests that the metabolic block is not complete. It is rather disappointing that DHT which is an analogue of 1,25$(OH)_2D_3$ is so much less effective than 1α(OH)D_3 and 1,25$(OH)_2D_3$. It his apparently only a chemical and not a biological analogue.

Another problem is the question of *genetic heterogeneity*. In inborn errors of metabolism, the same phenotype may be caused by different genotypes, i.e. different defects of the same enzyme and/or defects of different enzymes in the same metabolic pathway. Different defects of the 25(OH)D_3 — 1α-hydroxylase and a primary defect of the D_3- 25-hydroxylase in the liver would probably produce the same phenotype. In the hypothetical case of a D3-25-hydroxylase deficiency, a physiological dosage of 25(OH)D_3 should be fully effective.

A further problem to be discussed is the fact that the disease does not become manifest in the *neonatal period*. Our patient Laura has been followed since birth. D3 was given in the routine prophylactic dose of 0·02 mg (800 IU) daily. The first findings, hyperaminoaciduria and unresponsiveness of serum calcium to intramuscular PTE, were found at the age of 2 months. Rickets developed at the age of 4 months, and therapy with high doses of D_3 was started at 5 months of age. Since one can assume that the metabolic defect is present at birth, a mechanism that protects the affected foetus and newborn from the development of hypocalcaemia and rickets must be postulated. The most likely mechanism is placental transfer of 1,25$(OH)_2D_3$ from the mother to the foetus.

Very little is known about the development of the disease in *adult patients*. Case 4 in our earlier paper (Fanconi and Prader, 1969) is now 32 years old. He had discontinued treatment himself at the age of 21. Over the following years he had a slow relapse, starting with pain in the back, hips, ribs and sternum and with biochemical but not radiological rickets. He recovered with DHT and later with D_3 in a dose of 1·5 mg/day. Two years ago, at the age of 30, he discontinued treatment again and still feels perfectly well, despite severe hypocalcaemia (serum calcium 6·5 mg%), elevated alkaline phosphatase, elevated iPTH and generalised hyperaminoaciduria. The X-rays are normal. This patient at the age of 32 is proving that vitamin D dependency is lifelong. In the mature skeleton a relapse, however, develops very slowly, leading first to biochemical rickets and then to bone pains, but not necessarily to radiologically apparent osteomalacia.

REFERENCES

ARNAUD, C., MAIJER, R., READE, T., SCRIVER, C. R. and WHELAN, D. T. (1970). Vitamin D dependency: An inherited postnatal syndrome with secondary hyperparathyroidism. *Pediatrics*, **46**, 871

BALSAN, S., GARABEDIAN, M. and LE BOUADEC, L. (1972). Le rachitisme vitamino-résistant pseudocarential hypocalcémique. *Arch. Fr. Pédiatr.*, **29**, 287

FANCONI, A. and FISCHER, J. A. (1975). Parathyroid hormone in hereditary diseases of mineral metabolism. This symposium, p. 53.

FANCONI, A. and PRADER, A. (1969a). Die hereditäre Pseudomangelrachitis. *Helv. Paediatr. Acta*, **24**, 423

FANCONI, A. and PRADER, A. (1969b). Pseudo-vitamin D deficiency rickets. In D. Barltrop and W. L. Burland (eds.), *Mineral Metabolism in Paediatrics*, p. 19. (Oxford and Edinburgh : Blackwell Scientific Publications)

FRASER, D., KOOH, S. W., KIND, H. P., HOLICK, M. F., TANAKA, Y. and DELUCA, H. F. (1973). Pathogenesis of hereditary vitamin-D-dependent rickets. *N. Engl. J. Med.*, **289**, 817

FRASER, D., KOOH, S. W. and SCRIVER, C. R. (1967). Hyperparathyroidism as the cause of hyperaminoaciduria and phosphaturia in human vitamin D deficiency. *Pediatr. Res.*, **1**, 425

HAMILTON, R., HARRISON, J., FRASER, D., RADDE, I., MORECKI, R. and PAUNIER, L. (1970). The small intestine in vitamin D dependent rickets. *Pediatrics*, **45**, 364

PRADER, A., ILLIG, R. and HEIERLI, E. (1961). Eine besondere Form der primären Vitamin-D-resistenten Rachitis mit Hypocalcämie und autosomal-dominantem Erbgang : die hereditäre Pseudo-Mangelrachitis. *Helv. Paediatr. Acta*, **16**, 452

SCRIVER, C. R. (1970). Vitamin D dependency. *Pediatrics*, **45**, 361

10

Metabolic forms of rickets (and osteomalacia)

The Third Milner Lecture delivered at the Twelfth Annual Meeting

C. E. Dent

The final discovery that most cases of rickets were due to a nutritional defect and that the disease could be cured either by cod liver oil or by exposure of the skin to sunlight was made soon after World War I (Mellanby, 1919; Chick *et al.*, 1922; Medical Research Council, 1923). This important historic event led to another important medical advance that could hardly have been anticipated by the original nutritional workers, namely the definition and study of a group of other diseases, sometimes remarkably similar to if not identical with rickets, but which were not cured by cod liver oil or sunlight.

I was asked to review all these diseases in 1969 (Dent, 1969) to mark the fiftieth anniversary of Mellanby's classical dog experiments. I found it easier to consider the remarkable progress of these 50 years by dividing them into approximately 10-year periods. In the first, good descriptions of coeliac and of renal rickets were published and it became possible to distinguish some of the other diseases, such as the chondrodystrophies, that were not true forms of rickets because the defective calcification was not a generalised one throughout the skeleton but only affected bone formed from calcified cartilage. The second decade was important for the discovery of a new form of renal rickets in which the disease affected renal tubular dysfunction rather than glomerular filtration. The original patients of Debré, de Toni and Fanconi were all shown sooner or later to belong to a remarkably homeogeneous disease, cystinosis, in which large deposits of crystalline cystine (up to 3% of the wet weight of the spleen for instance) occurred throughout the body (Reviewed by McCune *et al.*, 1943). In the same decade came the important description of 'Vitamin D resistant' rickets by the Albright group (Albright *et al.*, 1937) The third decade (which was when your lecturer entered the field) saw a further development of disease descriptions. Renal tubular dysfunction practically identical with that in cystinosis was described in an adult patient whose tissues did not contain cystine crystals (Dent, 1947; Stowers and Dent, 1947) and who also had cirrhosis of the liver. He was described as having 'Adult Fanconi syndrome' and the fact that he was retrospectively rediagnosed as having Wilson's disease (Dent and Stowers, 1965) does not detract from the importance of the finding that cystinosis was not necessarily linked with this particular combination of renal tubular reabsorptive defects. The same decade saw another extension of paediatrics to adult medicine when McCance (1947) described a girl of 16 years with a form of vitamin D resistance rather similar to that described in Albright's child.

The real explosion of new knowledge in this field began in the fourth decade. Much greater study was made of the detail of the renal tubular dysfunction causing rickets. The common feature was that they all showed a poor reabsorption of phosphate. In the Albright *et al.*, and McCance forms this was the only defect and there were no other long term consequences with regard to renal function (as with renal glycosuria). In the so-called Fanconi syndromes the dysfunction also involved many substances other than phosphate—amino acids, glucose and the minerals sodium and potassium. There was also a gross inability to concentrate the urine and a defect of urine acidification leading to chronic acidosis. It was clear that the dysfunction here was of a more blundering nonspecific kind so it was hardly surprising that many other causes of the same dysfunction would be discovered. Furthermore in all cases the renal tubular dysfunction was associated with progressive glomerular damage, most of all in the children with cystinosis who had good glomerular filtration when the first classic descriptions were made in early infancy but who all died (and still die) in uraemia before the age of 10. New diseases described in this decade were of child 'Fanconi syndrome' without cystinosis (Saville *et al.*, 1955; Illig and Prader, 1961), idiopathic adult Fanconi syndrome without the liver cirrhosis of the first described patient (Dent and Harris, 1951) the oculocerebrorenal (Lowe's) syndrome (Lowe *et al.*, 1952) and many similar diseases obviously acquired as the result of some toxin, such as a heavy metal, which could damage the renal tubule in this way. The same decade saw the realisation that adult coeliac disease, sensitive to gluten as in the paediatric disease, also occurred and could produce osteomalacia, and there were also other odd descriptions of other causes, for instance, ureterocolostomy, chronic liver disease, and rarely primary hyperparathyroidism (for references see Dent, 1969).

By this time I am sure I could be forgiven for being mighty puzzled at the way things were going. Here were two manifestations of one bone disease, rickets and its adult equivalent osteomalacia, both showing at different ages the same highly specific calcification defect. This could be precisely defined in pathological terms, as a disorder of calcification either of the matrix of endosteal bone, or of the primary cartilage, in endochondral bone. Furthermore the clinical accompaniments were nearly always similar bearing in mind obvious modifications due to the state of the skeleton at the age of onset. The X-ray signs were also very characteristic and similar. Biochemical changes in the plasma levels of Ca, P and alkaline phosphatase were similar. Finally in most cases a partial, not always complete cure of the disease could be achieved with varying but always large doses of one of the vitamin Ds. Nevertheless the fact had to be faced that this apparently similar bone disease could be the result not only of dietary vitamin D lack but also of a wide variety of metabolic causes, ranging from hereditary defects of many kinds to seemingly quite unrelated conditions such as chronic liver

Table 10.1 *The kinds of rickets (and osteomalacia) discovered since Mellanby (1919). The diseases have been arranged in five columns relating to the 10-year periods shown. The arrows show how particular 'diseases' have later been divided into further separate diseases*

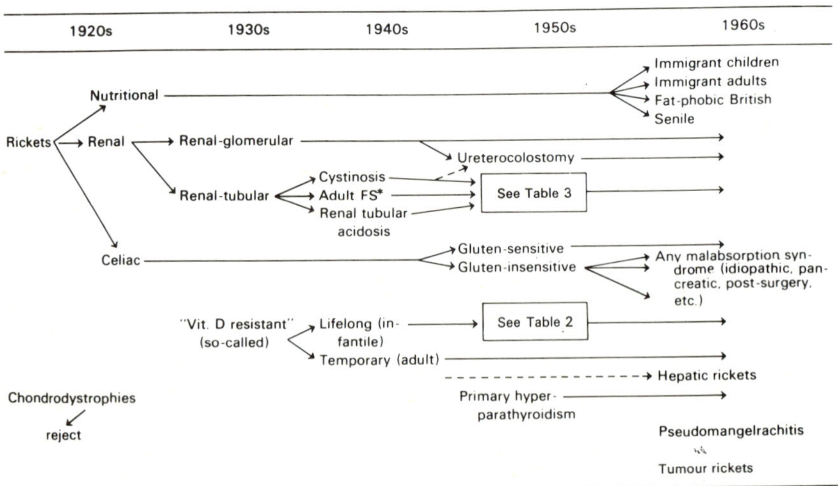

* Fanconi Syndrome

disease, various malabsorption syndromes, a wide range of renal dysfunctions and other seemingly irrelevant diseases. The plot was thickening.

The fifth decade kept up the momentum imparted by its predecessors. There were further subdivisions of known disease aetiologies. There were important new descriptions such as that of vitamin D dependant rickets (Pseudomangelrachitis—Prader *et al.*, 1961) and of tumour rickets (Prader *et al.*, 1959) with still further forms of 'Fanconi syndrome' and of hypophosphataemic rickets. I have tried to summarise this complicated data, using the division into five decades in Tables 10.1–10.3. The subject still continues to grow however and a small revision was later made (Dent, 1971) and still more and more is seen in the current journals.

Table 10.2 *Detail from Table 10.1 (q.v.), showing how further forms of hypophosphataemic rickets have been uncovered. In the text we suggest that this table should now include tumour rickets and rickets with fibrous dysplasia*

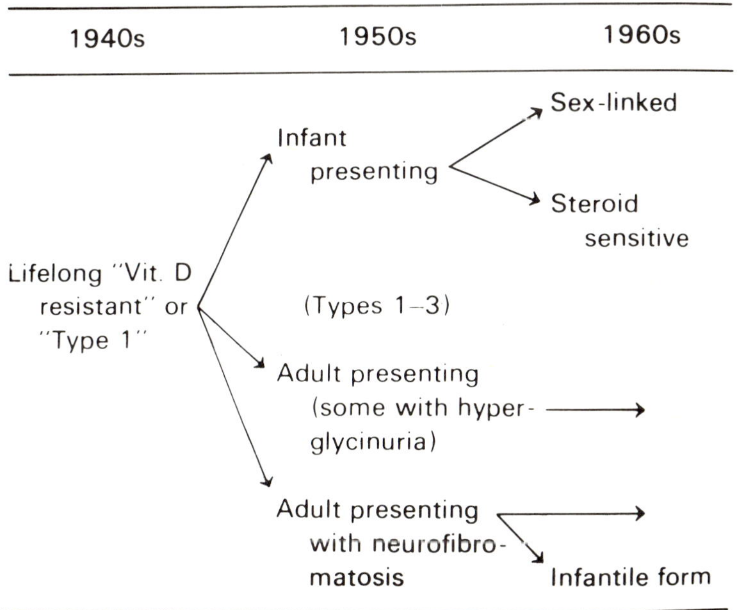

Clearly the recent stimulus to much of this work comes from the increasing and consistent interest in vitamin D and bone metabolism. The fifth decade mentioned above (and the few years following) also coincided with the discovery and identification of calcitonin, with the purification of parathyroid hormone and more recently but most importantly with the now classic identifications of the vitamin D metabolites. For all these too there have been more or less adequate assay methods applicable to the human in chosen situations. It is surely my duty as Milner lecturer to a conference of this kind to give examples of the problems in human disease which should benefit from a further study by the appropriate scientist. I judge the present moment in medical history to be that in which further enormous advances can be made by applying this new theoretical knowledge to the huge sum of human illness which we now know exists in the various forms of rickets and osteomalacia.

First I owe it to you to say a little more about a few diseases I have mentioned only in passing in my previous reviews and which so far have not been adequately described.

Table 10.3. *Detail from Table 10.1 (q.v.). The type numbers refer to a previous classification (Dent, 1952), now clearly outdated, for types 1 and 4 in particular are now known to include several diseases*

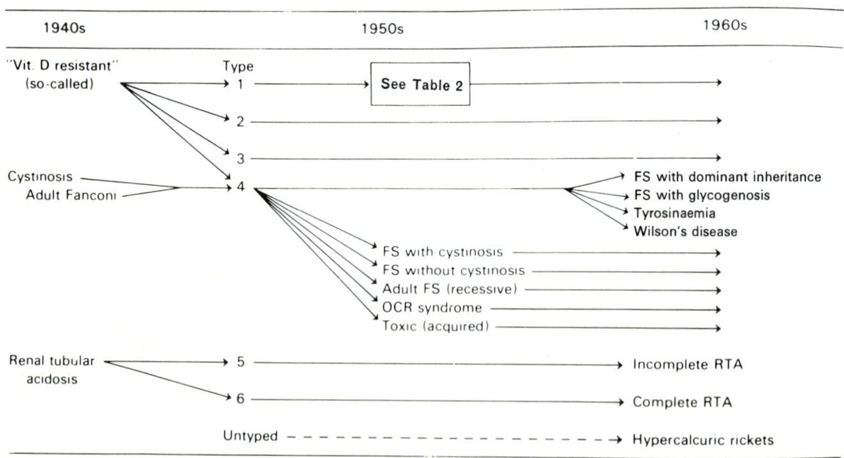

FS = Fanconi Syndrome
OCR = Oculocerebrorenal Syndrome
(Tables 1-3 from *Proc. Roy. Soc. Med.*, **63**, 401. 1970 with permission of the editor.)

'Steroid sensitive' hypophosphataemic rickets (Table 10.2)

John D. came to us aged 10 years 9 months for investigation of knock-knee found radiologically to be due to hypophosphataemic rickets. His parents were not consanguinous and he was one of six children, the others all being healthy. Although his knock-knee was recent a study of family group photographs showed clear evidence of longer duration growth retardation. At 5 years of age his height seemed to be normal as against his older and younger sibs. By the age of 10 years he was clearly dwarfed and was now smaller than his next younger brother and this continued till we first saw him. This unusual age of presentation was linked with another oddity. The finger and long bone X-rays showed characteristic subperiosteal erosions, a feature rarely seen in other forms of hypophosphataemic rickets of unknown cause. The plasma chemistry was unremarkable, normal Ca, low P, raised alkaline phosphatase. When admitted he had a high fever (up to 103 °F) which had begun on his train journey to hospital and which continued for several days. This was attributed to an upper respiratory infection. During the next few days while other investigations were temporarily suspended we noted a gradual rise and fall in his plasma P without appreciable change in urine P (Figure 10.1). During his previous hospital admissions elsewhere he had always been grossly hypophosphataemic. I wondered if this change to almost normal in renal PO_4 clearance would have been due to some stress reaction from his high fever. When the plasma P had reached low levels again he was given a course of cortisone to see if the fever effect could be mimicked artificially. This was exactly what happened. His plasma P rose at about the same rate as before, to reach a peak of 5·6 mg/100 ml only falling a little as the dose of cortisone was later reduced. Again there was no appreciable change in urine P. As his Ca and P balances had become strongly positive on the cortisone and a dose of vitamin D_2 (0·25 mg) relatively small for any of these hypophosphataemic forms of rickets I sent him home on the reduced dose of cortisone (12·5 mg b.d.) and the same amount of vitamin D_2 which was later raised to 1·0 mg daily. During the next 6 years of follow-up his rickets and secondary hyperparathyroidism quickly healed and remained healed and he grew from below the 3rd percentile to reach the 20th. He was also normophosphataemic throughout. By this time I had introduced cautious trials of the same steroid/vitamin D regime to a few other cases of hypophosphataemic rickets without doing any good (or harm) to them so it was discontinued in these latter, and the decision made to tail off the cortisone in John D. Unfortunately he then failed to attend for regular follow-up but was sent to me in mid-1966 by the doctors of the Royal Marine Corps which he had then joined. He was then strong and well, taking no treatment with no symptoms and

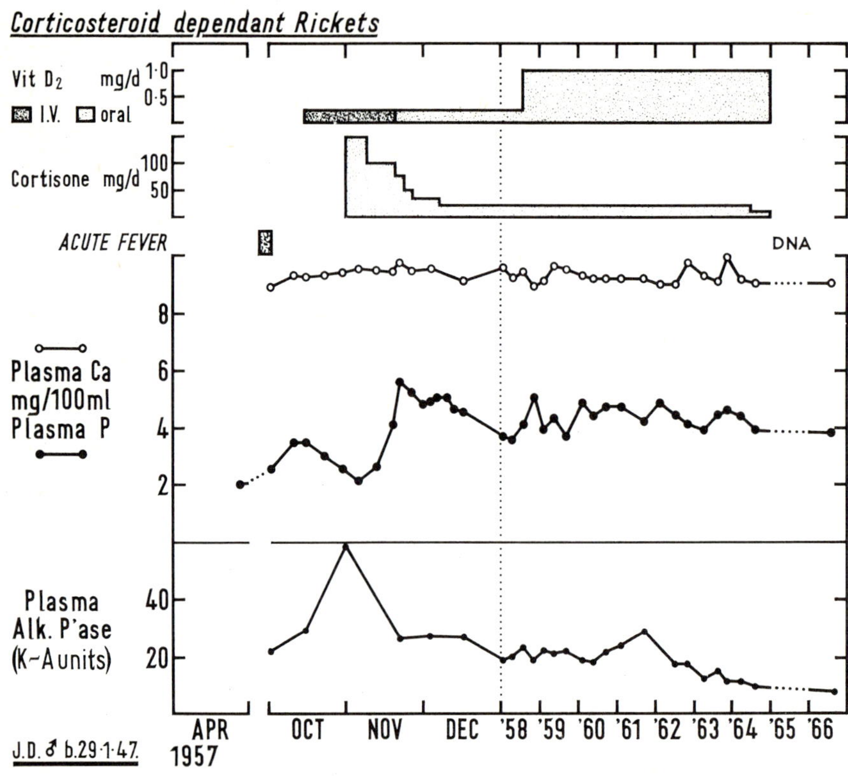

FIGURE 10.1 John D. Steroid dependent rickets. Biochemical findings and response to treatment. (Further details in text.)

with normal bone X-rays and normal plasma levels. Unfortunately he deserted from the Marines soon after and became a fugitive and presumably was not later arrested as I asked to be told if he was for I wanted to check up on his bones, What on earth was wrong with this boy? Needless to say other known causes of rickets were eliminated on his first admission.

Tumour rickets

This particularly fascinating cause of rickets while very rare, has a reasonable literature (reviewed by Salama *et al.*, 1970). I greatly admire the judgement of Professor Prader who, in the first described case where florid rickets co-existed with a rib tumour thought to be an osteoclastoma, decided to remove the tumour and not do anything else at the same time such as beginning treatment with vitamin D (Prader *et al.*, 1959). In the event the child's rickets healed fully and the new entity came into being. Of interest too is McCance's (1947) original case of hypophosphataemic rickets in a girl of 16 years. She had a tumour in her femur which the pathologists had difficulty in identifying. The tumour was removed while she was given a short course of high-dosage vitamin D. She recovered fully and I understand has needed no more vitamin D to the present time. Clearly this was a case of tumour rickets which presumably would have healed without vitamin D .These cases mimic hypophosphataemic rickets closely and any case of this occurring sporadically must be searched carefully for occult bone tumours. I must now add that a recent patient of ours (Mrs Gladys N.) aged 58 years was confidently diagnosed as having adult presenting hypophosphataemic rickets and responded well to our current treatment with vitamin D and oral sodium phosphate. Only recently did we discover that 2 years before she came to us she had had a 'haemangioma' removed, unfortunately incompletely, from her nasopharynx which in retrospect was probably the cause of all her trouble. The nature of this tumour effect is clearly worth studying as illustrating yet another metabolic abnormality induced by tumour growth (Reviewed by Omenn, 1971). I presume the histology of the tumour need not be too specific. My colleague Dr R. Nassim showed me a lady with adenocarcinoma of the breast and local metastases. There was a lesion in a pubic ramus that looked like a Looser zone and the plasma chemistry was rachitic. On radical mastectomy with subsequent local radiotherapy the Looser zone fully healed, and the chemistry became normal, no other treatment being given.

Senile osteomalacia

This is another disease mentioned in passing in my previous reviews and not yet properly described, We have had about six cases in old women and one in an old man, all of whom developed all signs and symptoms of osteomalacia for no clear reason. The disease was not of nutritional origin as it did not heal quickly with ordinary antirachitic doses of vitamin D (50 μg of D_2), but it did heal quickly with larger doses and when healed it could be maintained healed on about 0·25 mg of vitamin D_2 daily. The essential data in a recent case is shown in Figure 10.2. I suspect this can be quite common and that many cases have been confused with dietary rickets. Presumably it is due to some enzyme inadequacy developing as part of the old age phenomenon.

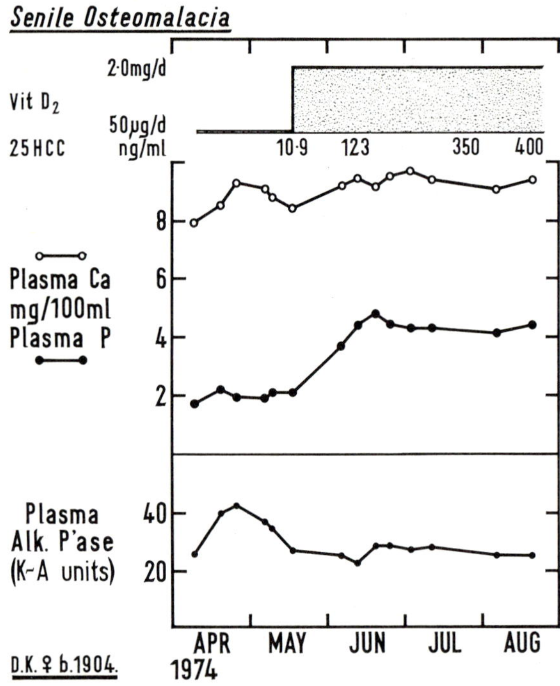

FIGURE 10.2 Mrs Krystos D. Senile osteomalacia. Biochemical findings and response to two dosage levels of vitamin D_2. Note that the low plasma P, usually the first abnormality to become normal on treatment of nutritional rickets, did not change on the smaller dose of D_2 given for 5 weeks although there was a rise in plasma Ca and a rise and fall ('phosphatase flare') in alkaline phosphates. We expect her eventual maintenance dose of vitamin D_2 to be about 0·25 mg daily.

Hypophosphataemic rickets accompanying neurofibromatosis and fibrous dysplasia

It has long been known that neurofibromatosis with bone changes is rarely associated with late presenting (around 30–50 years) hypophosphataemic osteomalcia (Albright and Reifenstein, 1948; Swan, 1954). We have also under follow-up a man now 28 years old with severe neurofibroma manifestations and who had hypophosphataemic rickets since infancy (Figure 10.3). Why should this be so? Could this be

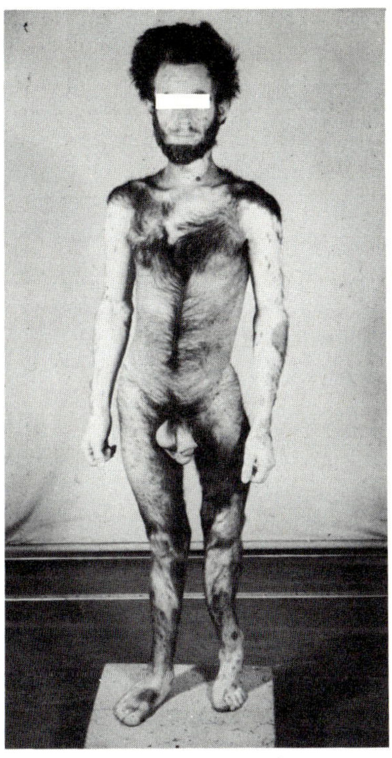

FIGURE 10.3 Paul R. at age 20 years. Neurofibromatosis and life-long hypophosphataemic rickets. He is grossly dwarfed (height 144·0 cm). as well as having rachitic deformities and asymmetry of bone growth.

another variant of tumour rickets? I recall that soon after Albright's description of 'Polyostotic fibrous dysplasia' there was a controversy with Thannhauser (1944) who claimed that the bone histology was really that of neurofibromatosis. I think most of us have supported the Albright view of two separate disease entities. However the problem needs reconsidering now in the light of the fact that rare patients are now being described, as in neurofibromatosis, with the combination of clear-cut fibrous dysplasia and hypophosphataemic rickets (reviewed by Ryan *et al.*, 1968). We have studied such a case recently in a young man of 22 years (Stephen F.) who had a history of bowing of the legs and repeated pathological fractures since the age of 4 years (Figures 10.4 and 10.5). He had a 'Coast of Maine' pigment patch on his right arm. During the last 3 years he had developed increasing pain, and orthopaedic measures to correct the leg deformities had failed owing to

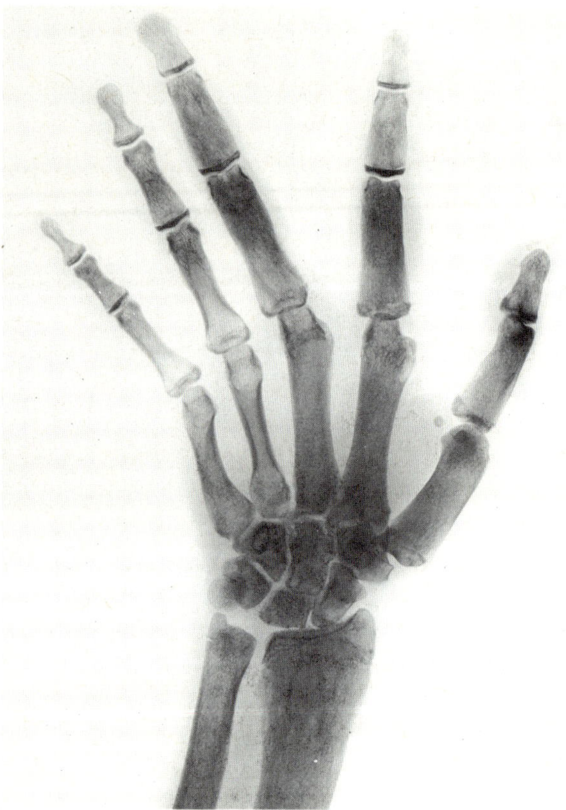

FIGURE 10.4 Stephen F. Fibrous dysplasia and recent osteomalacia. The hand shows typical X-ray changes.

lack of healing of the recent fractures. His plasma contained Ca, 9·8 mg; /100 ml; P, 2·3 mg/100 ml, with high alkaline phosphatase, high urinary total hydroxyproline and normal urinary phosphate. With vitamin D his pain has been relieved with the expected changes in calcium balance and urinary total hydroxyproline excretion. I think he had recently developed hypophosphataemic rickets to complicate the clinical picture.

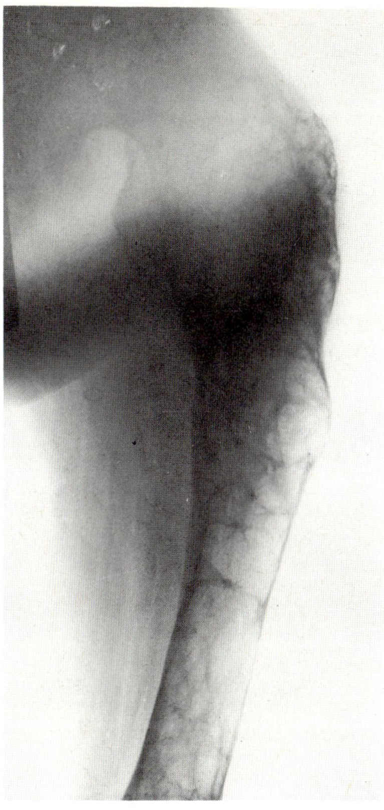

FIGURE 10.5 Stephen F. Fibrous dysplasia and recent osteomalacia. The femur shows gross cystic changes and the typical 'shepherd's crook' deformity.

This patient and the others already published makes it easier to clarify some other patients we have studied. Janet L. came to us aged 8 years with gross fibrous dysplasia of the mandible and jaw (Plate 10.6a). This had grown slowly since infancy producing grotesque facial deformity. A year before she had been noted to have hypophosphataemia and X-rays showed marked rickets (Figure 10.6b) which has since healed with high dosage vitamin D. She had no other features of Albright's fibrous dysplasia (pigmented patches of skin, precocious puberty) and there were no other bones affected by the cystic overgrowth. Another patient, William T., came to us in 1963 aged 52 years with a 2-year history of increasingly severe backache following lifelong fractures of long bones occurring through cystic areas. He had generalised fibrous dysplasia-type changes but they were symmetrical and

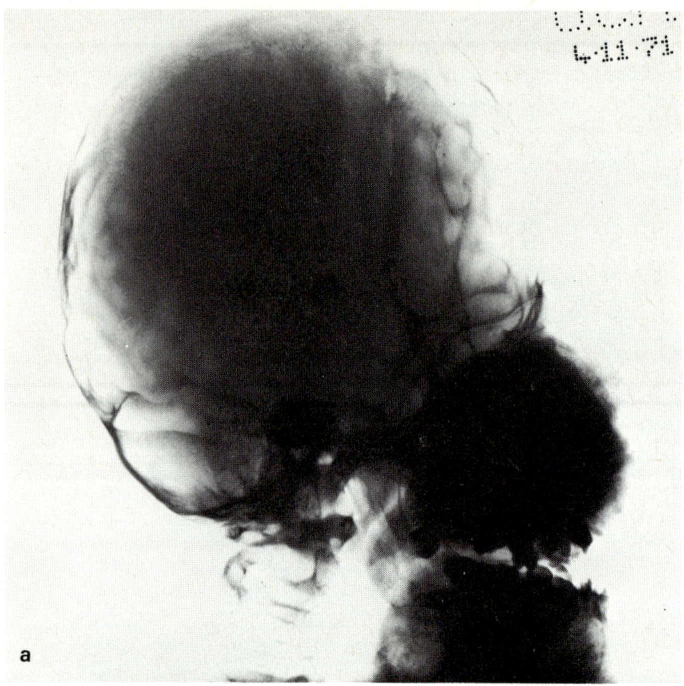

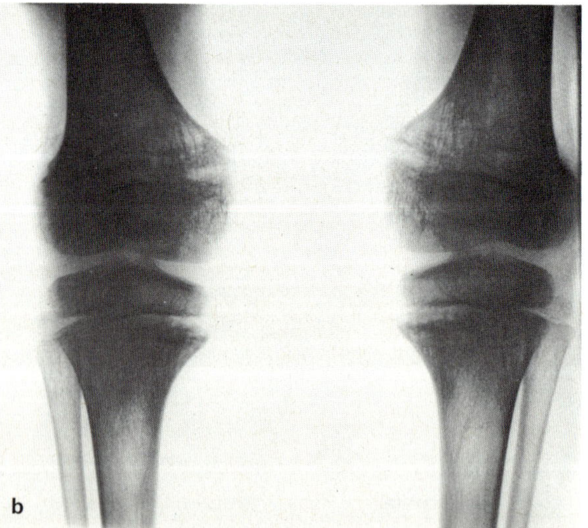

FIGURE 10.6 Janet L.(a) Fibrous dysplasia and hypophosphataemic rickets. Note gross changes in mandible and maxilla, not present elsewhere in skeleton. The skull vault shows 'copper beaten' appearances and upward growth from premature fusion of frontal suture. The father's skull shows this latter also, but he is otherwise normal. (b) The knees of 20 November 1970 show recently developed rickets.

associated with bizarre growth abnormalities as for instance in his metatarsal bones (Figures 10.7–10.9). He had no scoliosis, the vertebral bodies being rather biconcave. There were no pigmented patches or neurofibromata. He had marked hypophosphataemia (plasma P 2·0 mg/100 ml) and osteomalacic changes on bone biopsy. His osteomalacia responded well to treatment with vitamin D. He later became paraplegic from spinal cord compression due to bony overgrowth which required extensive laminectomy (he was Case 3 of Highman *et al.*, 1970). This latter complication we have also seen in sex-linked hypophosphataemic rickets (reviewed by Yoshikawa *et al.*, 1968; Highman *et al.*, 1970)

It is obvious that hypophosphataemic rickets is a complication of many other seemingly unrelated diseases and that Table 10.2 requires

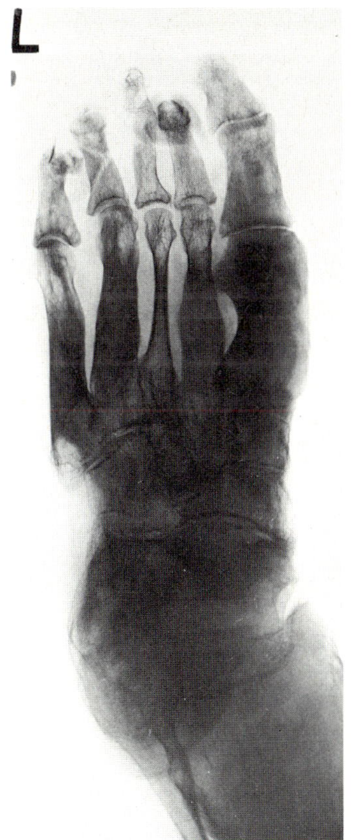

FIGURE 10.7 William T. Lifelong bone disease and recent hypophosphataemic osteomalacia. X-ray of left foot showing slender metatarsal and fibrous dysplasia elsewhere.

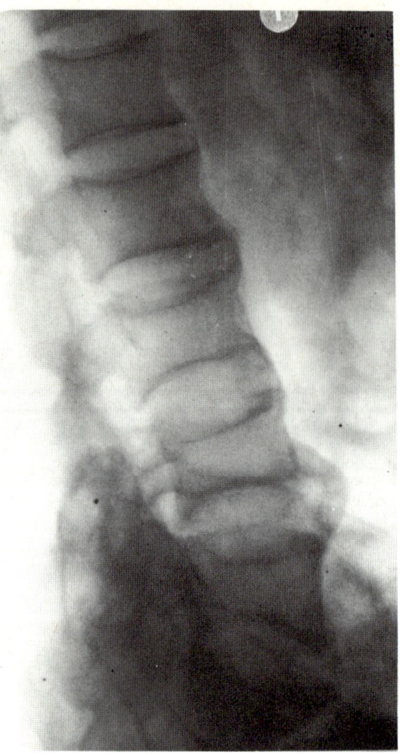

FIGURE 10.8 William T. Lifelong bone disease and recent hypophosphataemic osteomalacia. X-ray of spine shows some biconcavity of vertebral bodies and other degenerative changes.

considerable revision with the addition of the fibrous dysplasia group of diseases and I now think tumour rickets too. In all these cases there is a bone tumour or tumours. In the past it was usual to attribute hypophosphataemia to secondary hyperparathyroidism. The few assays that have been made, for instance in sex-linked rickets, have given contradictory results (Arnaud *et al.*, 1971; Lewy *et al.*, 1972; Reitz and Weinstein, 1973; Fanconi, 1974) and the whole matter needs reconsidering from the point of view of secondary vitamin D metabolic abnormality. It could be that terminal cancer patients with widespread bone metastases would provide readily available opportunities for study. They often manifest hypophosphataemia which I do not believe has been interpreted from this point of view, indeed it is usually ignored as being relatively unimportant in the circumstances. While radiologically visible hyperparathyroid bone disease is absent in all the types of hypophosphataemia,

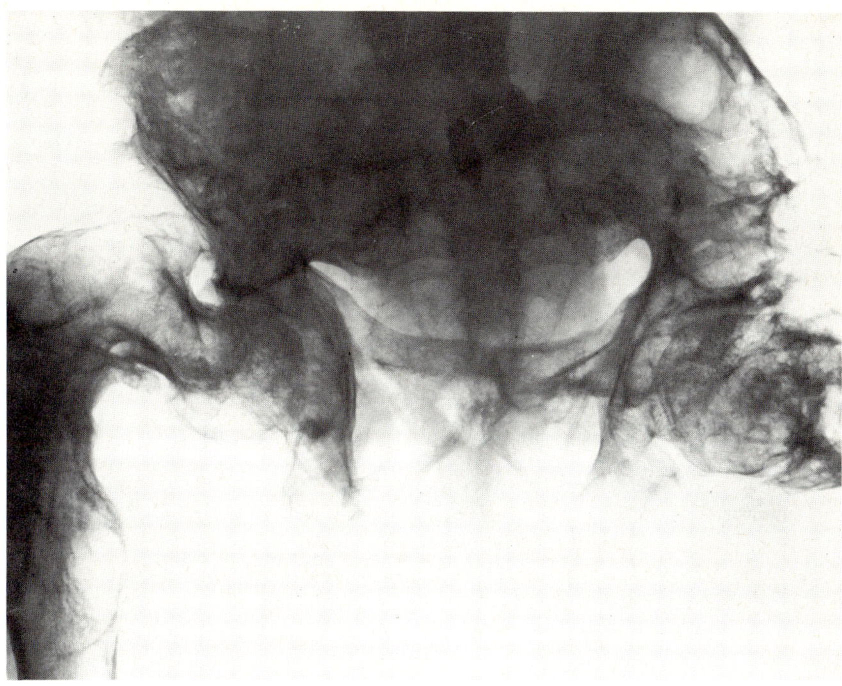

FIGURE 10.9 William T. Lifelong bone disease and recent hypophosphataemic osteomalacia. X-ray of pelvis and hips shows gross symmetrical cystic changes similar to those of fibrous dysplasia.

except in our one patient (above) with the steroid sensitive form, it must be pointed out that the development of autonomous ('tertiary') hyperparathyroidism has been described in two adult patients with the sex-linked form (Thomas and Fry, 1970; Hendrickse *et al.*, 1960) and we have another similar patient as yet unpublished. In these three patients it seems likely that a long period of secondary hyperparathyroidism must have preceded the growth of the autonomous adenoma.

Osteomalacia from overdosage with aluminium hydroxide

Our recent patient (Dent and Winter, 1974) fitted in well in all respects with the earlier described patients (Lotz *et al.*, 1964). Gross phosphate depletion thus induced produces unique biochemical accompaniments of the very overt osteomalacia, mainly a massive overabsorption of calcium from the diet and consequent gross hypercalcuria. The situation is that to be expected from an overproduction of calcium binding protein presumably from excessive local action of 1,25-dihydroxycholecalciferol. Although the clinical situation must be very rare it should be easy to mimic experimentally and thus give valuable further data as to vitamin D metabolite interactions with parathyroid hormone as well as of the physiology of calcium absorption from the diet.

I am also fascinated by the fact that simple phosphate depletion produces rickets while dietary calcium depletion produces osteoporosis. Presumably the key role of the parathyroid gland is relevant here in at any price maintaining normocalcaemia while not in any direct way being concerned in maintaining constant plasma phosphate levels.

Magnesium dependent rickets

The two children recently published (Reddy and Sivakumar, 1974) under this diagnostic label seemed to have the lifelong condition of magnesium dependent hypocalcaemia, which I believe is due to an isolated defect of magnesium absorption (Friedman *et al.*, 1967). The recently published children did not have tetany so no diagnosis was made nor treatment given till they were 2 and 5 years old when they presented with rickets and were then shown to have low plasma Ca and Mg. The usual treatment with extra oral Mg salts largely corrected the plasma abnormalities and cured the rickets which was not cured by large doses of vitamin D alone. Your lecturer remains speechless after reading about this since it does not seem to relate to any previously known rickets-producing mechanism. This is not an age related complication. Our original case (Friedman *et al.*, 1967) is now 9 years old and we still see him regularly. On his current 9 g of magnesium glycerophosphate daily he remains otherwise normal and has grown along a steady 25 percentile.

Diphosphonate osteodystrophy (in a case of myositis ossificans progressiva)

I cannot call this disease rickets owing to the inevitably more complicated nature of the actions of this important new type of drug. However there are aspects similar to those in rickets. Paul A. was 6 years old when he was started (28th July 1971) on 100 mg q.d.s. of disodium ethane-1-hydroxy-1,1-diphosphonate (EHDP) (kindly donated by Procter and

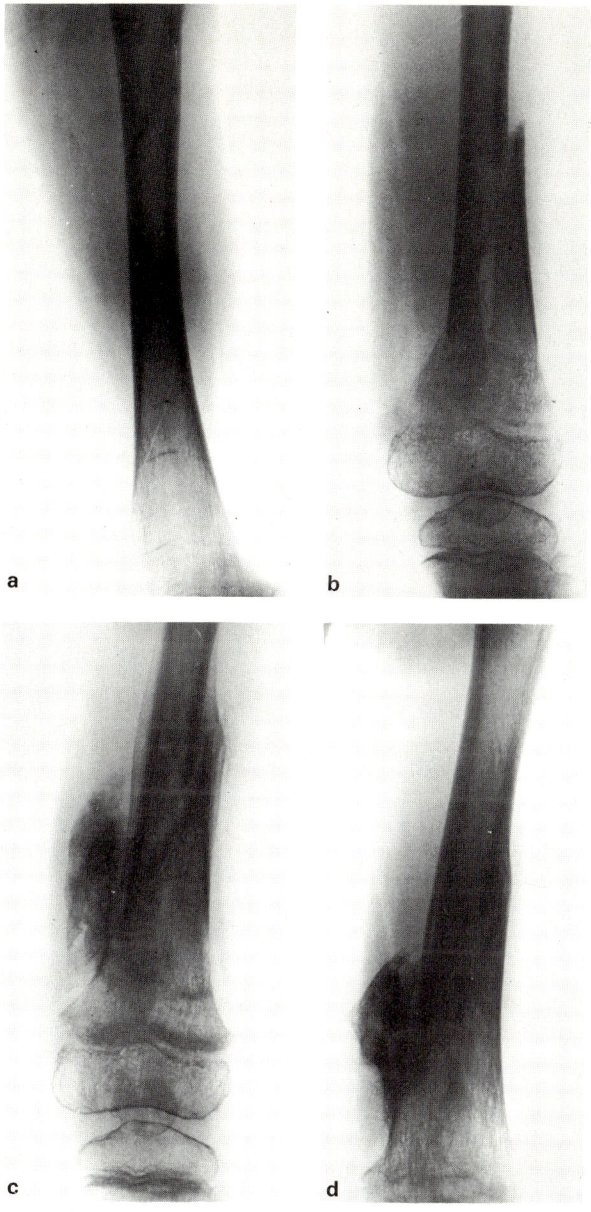

FIGURE 10.10 Paul A. Myositis ossificans progressive on and the after diphosphonate therapy: (a) X-ray (7th October 1971) of right femur after a fall. A spiral fracture is seen without displacement; (b) X-ray (14th January 1972) of right femur following further fall. The patient had been progressing well till then. The bone ends are now displaced. There has been no visible callus formation since the previous X-ray; (c) X-ray (28th February 1972). Gross callus has formed just over a month after stopping diphosphonate therapy; (d) X-ray (11th January 1973). Good union has now occurred.

Gamble). He had been increasingly incapacitated by the generalised ossification of his soft tissues and the taking of the drug was timed to coincide with surgical removal of a bony spur growing across his right antecubital fossa which had thus completely immobilised the elbow. During the next few months we noted on palpation recurrence of the spur and joint stiffness although no bone formation was visible there on X-ray. It was on 7th October 1971 that he stumbled and produced a fine spiral fracture in his right femur (Figure 10.10a) which it was decided to treat by immobilisation without splinting. The pain soon went and satisfactory healing was presumed, but on encouraging more activity he fell again, producing now a visible lump in the thigh. The X-ray (Figure 10.10b) of 15th January 1972 now showed movement of the broken ends of bone but there was no callus seen after over 3 months of having a fracture. EHPD was stopped on 20th January 1972 and the next X-ray (28th February 1972) just over a month later (Figure 10.10c) now showed gross callus formation, the bone finally healing well (Figure 10.10d). Clearly the drug had induced a defect of calcification just like that occurring in rickets as part of its action. The spur across his elbow also recalcified on stopping EHDP and now appears to be true bone on X-ray.

Rickets in congenital osteopetrosis

Most children with this very serious disease have fairly normal plasma Ca, P and phosphatase levels. Their long bone growth plates show very slow growth in a fairly normal manner. One of these children benefited greatly by severe dietary calcium depletion, the new bone growth showing much better structure on X-ray (Dent *et al.*, 1965). We have failed to repeat this result in a few further patients but fortunately Prof. June Lloyd has had a greater success with a child begun at 1 year of age on the regime and has allowed me to show you his X-rays (Figures 10.11a–10.11c) before and after 5 years of this regime.

The literature is confused on this topic but there are suggestions that some infants with the disease develop rickets-like changes on X-rays and abnormalities also in their relevant plasma levels. I now believe that the majority do this if they survive long enough and that these have a different disease which does not benefit so much by dietary calcium depletion.

Philip W. looked exactly like any other child with congenital osteo-

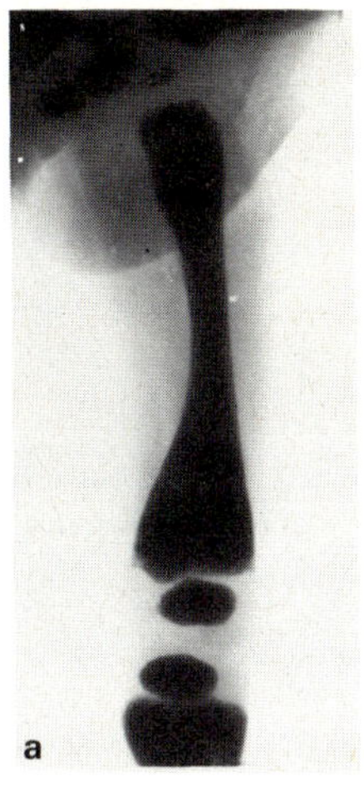

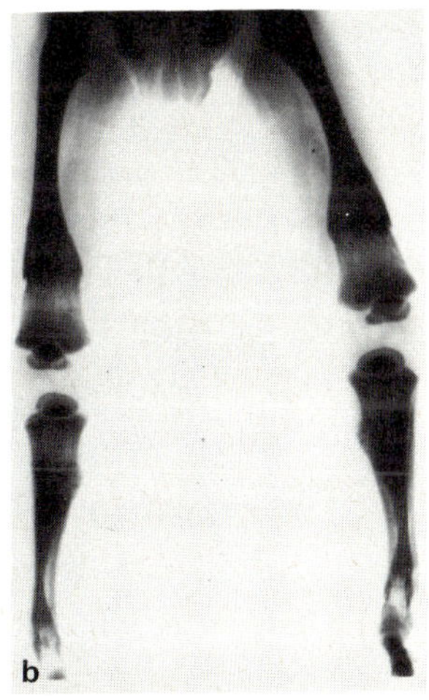

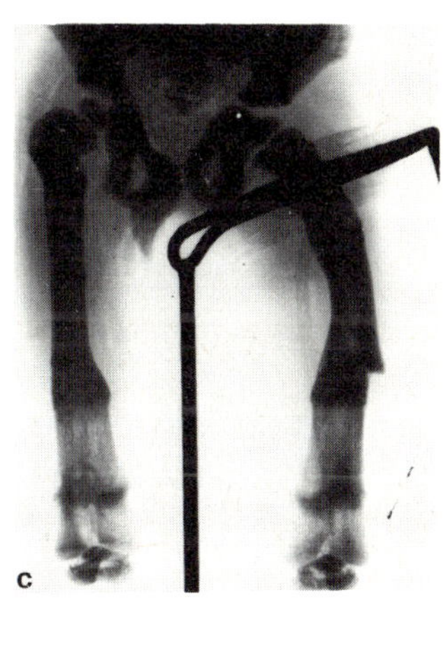

FIGURE 10.11 Matthew W. Born 9th September 1967. Congenital osteopetrosis. At age 1 year (a) he was begun on the low calcium intake regime. Bone growth since then (b and c) is seen as the additional much less radio-dense bone later grown. This new bone shows some trabecular structure, it also shows some normal modelling, and after giving radioactive Fe some concentration was detected over the new bone suggesting the formation of normal bone marrow there. The most recent X-rays show a marrow cavity forming in the shaft of the femur. (Dr June Lloyd's patient, with her kind permission.)

petrosis when he first came to us aged 1 year 8 months in May 1970. We treated him like our published case (above), with a little prednisolone to lessen his haemolysis, then splenectomy, and a low calcium diet and at first also cellulose phosphate. He still lives in moderate

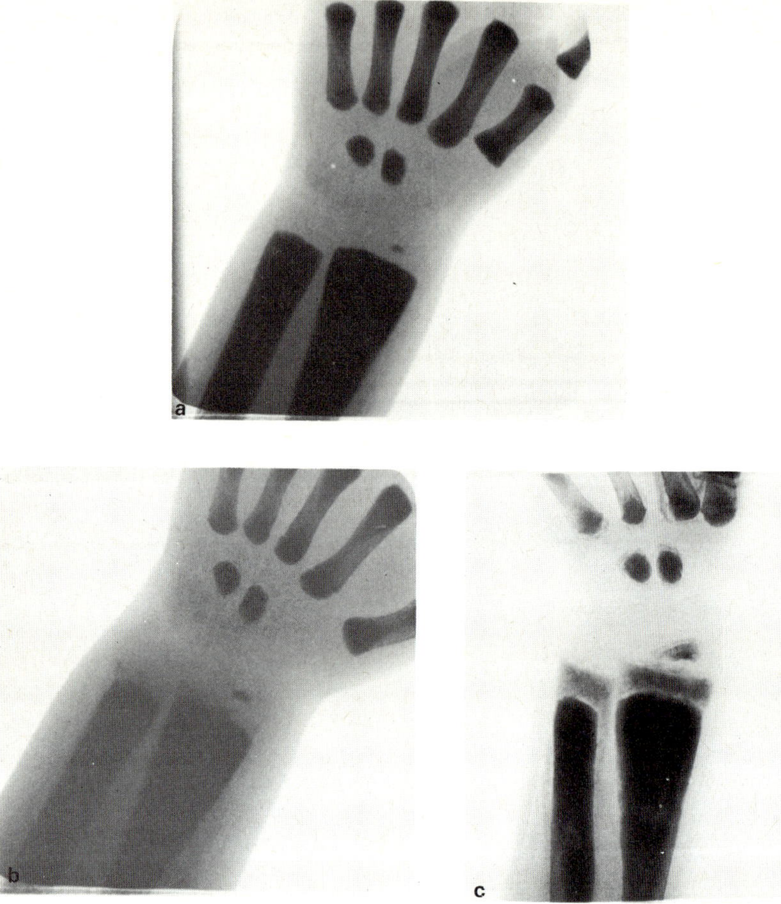

FIGURE 10.12 (a)–(c) Phillip W. Congenital osteopetrosis on essentially the same treatment as Matthew W. (above) (Figure 10.11): (a) X-ray (1st June 1970) of right knee. Low calcium diet was begun around this time; (b) X-ray (27th September 1971) of right knee. No growth of bone has occurred as with Matthew (Figure 10.11). The metaphysis now appears a little irregular and the biochemical signs of rickets are fully manifest; (c) X-ray (1st January 1974). There is still very little growth since 1970. A line of calcification in the widened growth plate suggests early healing of rickets. He has had enormous doses of various forms of vitamin D during this time.

general health today but during the time of observation he has hardly grown at all and his metaphyses have developed an irregular appearance with mottling in the widened growth plate, certainly rather like rickets (Figures 10.12a–10.12c). Treatment with vitamin D_2 up to 15 mg daily, or with DHT and 25-HCC all in enormous doses have caused only slight calcification of the growth plate. I think we must call this X-ray appearance rickets, modified in X-ray appearance by the lack of adequate growth. This interpretation is strongly supported by the biochemical findings. He has very low plasma Ca and P levels and a high alkaline phosphatase. He has gross aminoaciduria and a raised total hydroxyproline excretion. Other less well studied patients have resembled this one, convincing me of the reality of the two diseases which are so similar superficially in the early stages. This situation requires urgent and intensive study by modern methods. The rickets of osteopetrosis is the only form of rickets for which we have no treatment as well as such poor understanding. May I stress the apparent absurdity of this situation where defective calcification of the growth plate occurs at the same time as overcalcification of the bones elsewhere. Another curiosity is that most people consider the disease manifestation to be caused by inadequacy of osteoclastic action yet analysis of the urine showed high normal total hydroxyproline excretion, a finding that many of us associated with high bone turnover.

Rickets in cystinosis

The rickets can always be cured by a suitably large dose of vitamin D taken with the other routine measures (oral sodium and potassium salts). I have only recently noted that the dose of vitamin D_2 required may often be of the order of 1–2 mg daily but that if $25(OH)D_3$ is given a much smaller dose (20–40 μg daily) suffices. Either the equivalent strengths of these compounds is always very different from that usually stated or else there is something odd about vitamin D metabolism in cystinosis. I throw this out purely because we must exploit any new clue to unravel the pathogenesis of this disease of which we are totally ignorant in spite of intensive study in many centres. The defect in cystine metabolism is most striking, but the nature of the enzymopathy still remains unknown, as well as the reasons for the many secondary abnormalities, especially of the renal tubule. Could it be that there is a liver defect in 25-hydroxylation?

Rickets and vitamin D abnormalities in primary hyperparathyroidism

The clinical evidence is clear. When this disease occurs in childhood it may very rarely present in a form clinically indistinguishable from late-rickets (Wood *et al.*, 1958). More usually the children manifest osteitis fibrosa as the form of bone disease when present, and when the bones are normal on X-ray the disease is usually that of recurrent urinary stone formation. Adults are the same but the osteomalacia if present is more difficult to detect than is rickets in children. Nevertheless, we have complete data now from our over 430 cases of the adult disease to show us that some of these had typical osteomalacia as their main bone disease, which healed on removal of the parathyroid tumour. More had varying degrees of both osteomalacia and osteitis fibrosa as well as many with osteitis fibrosa only or, as is most common, with apparently normal bones.

These facts must be seen in relation to other work which suggests that something very much like vitamin D lack frequently occurs in these patients, especially in those with osteitis fibrosa. Relatively small doses of vitamin D given over a few months largely heal the bone disease (Woodham, Doyle and Joplin, 1971). These are most important findings which I am sure will be dealt with at this meeting by others more competent than me. It has very practical medical repercussions as well as important theoretical ones. Vitamin D lack can prevent the excess parathyroid hormone production from producing hypercalcaemia, thus greatly complicating the diagnosis. We currently give a small dose of vitamin D to patients suspected of having normocalcaemic primary hyperparathyroidism of this origin. If hypercalcaemia results which is then stable during our standard hydrocortisone schedule of administration we conclude that the diagnosis of parathyroid adenoma is confirmed (Dent *et al.*, 1975).

General comment and summing-up

I hope that by reviewing the whole picture and by stressing some of the details, I may have succeeded in making the main point of my discourse. This is that we have a mighty lot of work to do yet in unravelling all these huge problems, even when the scientific procedures seem at last to be available. May I stress this point with the summary in Table 10.4. where I have listed the approximate numbers of these diseases in a few aetiological categories. In adding them up I have counted all the causes of renal glomerular disease as one disease only. Likewise acquired Fanconi syndromes count as one only and also all the causes of acquired malabsorption syndromes. In other cases too I have counted as one disease what may well be two, for instance the child and adult presenting

Table 10.4 *Summary of aetiologies of the various forms of rickets and osteomalacia*

Acquired	17
Dominant gene	4
Recessive gene	11
Sex linked gene	2
Total	34 kinds

Table 10.5 *Some causes of rickets and osteomalacia*

1. Dietary (or solar) vitamin D lack
2. Senile osteomalacia
3. Gluten sensitive enteropathy
4. Other malabsorption syndromes
5. Partial or total gastrectomy
6. Hepatic diseases
7. Pancreatic insufficiency
8. Sex-linked hypophosphataemia
9. Autosomal hypophosphataemia
10. Vitamin D dependent (Pseudomangel)
11. Neurofibromatosis (child and adult)
12. Polyostotic fibrous dysplasia
13. Cystinosis with Fanconi syndrome
14. Glycogenosis with Fanconi syndrome
15. Child Fanconi without cystinosis
16. Fanconi with dominant inheritance
17. Adult presenting Fanconi
18. Occulocerebrorenal syndrome (Lowe)
19. Tyrosinaemia
20. Wilson's disease
21. Distal renal tubular acidosis
22. Glomerular renal failure (any origin)
23. Adult presenting hypophosphataemia
24. Hypercalcuric rickets
25. Acquired Fanconi syndromes
26. Ureterocolostomy
27. Neonatal rickets
28. Osteopetrosis
29. Tumour rickets
30. Anti-convulsant rickets
31. Primary hyperparathyroidism
32. Aluminium hydroxide overdosage
33. Corticosteroid sensitive
34. Magnesium dependent (? Autosomal recessive hypophosphataemia)

forms of rickets and osteomalacia occurring with neurofibromatosis. Even with these limitations I can count 34 different aetiologies which leads to a sizable number of sick people even bearing in mind that some of these causes are very rare (Table 10.5).

The diseases with recessive gene inheritance are clearly those in which we should expect enzyme abnormalities to occur and be most easily discovered, but I believe that so far only one has to date been elucidated, namely the inability to dihydroxylate vitamin D in vitamin D-dependent rickets (pseudomangelrachitis) (Fraser *et al.*, 1973). Even here there remain a few further facts to explain, for instance, how it is that these patients also respond well to high dosage vitamin D? The diseases with dominant gene inheritance should be more difficult according to our present day genetic philosophy. The mechanisms at fault here are more likely to concern complicated enzyme functions, such as membrane transport, regulation of rates of metabolic reactions and so on. Perhaps our techniques here are still inadequate. The acquired diseases concern a real rag-bag of causes from the fascinating bone tumour effect which so far only manifests itself if bone invasion is actually occurring, to complicated gammopathies and more simple-seeming things like heavy metal intoxications and obstructive uropathy.

I sincerely hope and believe that this conference will serve to highlight many of these problems and inspire and help us to work to their solution.

REFERENCES

ALBRIGHT, F., BUTLER, A. M. and BLOOMBERG, E. (1937). Rickets resistant to vitamin-D therapy. *Am. J. Dis. Child.*, **54**, 529

ALBRIGHT, F. and REIFENSTEIN, E. C. (1948). *The Parathyroid Glands and Metabolic Bone Disease.* (Baltimore : Williams and Wilkins)

ARNAUD. C., GLORIEUX, F. and SCRIVER, C. (1971). Serum parathyroid hormone in X-linked hypophosphataemia. *Science*, **173**, 845

CHICK, H., DALYELL, E. J., HUME, M., MACKAY, H. M. M. and SMITH, H. H. (1922). The aetiology of rickets in infants. *Lancet*, **iii**, 7

DENT, C. E. (1947). The aminoaciduria in Fanconi syndrome. *Biochem. J.*, **41**, 240

DENT, C. E. (1952). Rickets and osteomalacia from renal tubule defects. *J. Bone Jt. Surg. (Br.)*, **34B**, 266

DENT, C. E. (1969). Rickets (and osteomalacia), nutritional and metabolic (1919–1969). *Proc. R. Soc. Med.*, **63**, 401

DENT, C. E. (1971). Rickets and osteomalacia of various origins. *Birth Defects*, **7**, 79

DENT, C. E. and HARRIS, H. (1951). The genetics of 'cystinuria'. *Ann. Eugen. (Lond.)*, **16**, 60

DENT, C. E., SMELLIE, J. M. and WATSON, L. (1965). Studies in osteopetrosis. *Arch. Dis. Child.*, **40**, 7

DENT, C. E. and STOWERS, J. M. (1965). Adult Fanconi syndrome and cirrhosis. *Br. Med. J.*, **1**, 520

DENT, C. E. and WINTER, C. S. (1974). Osteomalacia due to phosphate depletion from excessive aluminium hydroxide ingestion. *Br. Med. J.*, **1**, 551

DENT, C. E., JONES, P. E. and MULLAN, D. P. (1975). *Lancet*, **i**, 1161

FANCONI, A., FISCHER, J. A. and PRADER, A. (1974). Serum parathyroid hormone concentrations in hypophosphataemic vitamin D resistant rickets. *Helv. Paediatr. Acta*, **29**, 187

FRASER, D., KOOH, S. W., KIND, H. P., HOLICK, M. F., TANAKA, Y. and DELUCA, H. F. (1973). Pathogenesis of hereditary vitamin D-dependent rickets. *N. Engl. J. Med.*, **289**, 817

FRIEDMAN, M., HATCHER, G. and WATSON, L. (1967). Primary hypomagnesaemia with secondary hypocalcaemia in an infant. *Lancet*, **i**, 703

HENDRICKSE, A., DECRAENE, P. and DE MOOR, P. (1960). Un cas d'hyperparathyroide associé a une osteomalacie pronuncée. *Ann. 'Endocrinol.*, **21**, 293

HIGHMAN, J. H., SANDERSON, P. H. and SUTCLIFFE, M. M. L. (1970). Vitamin D resistant osteomalacia as a cause of cord compression. *Quart. J. Med.*, **39**, 529

ILLIG., R. and PRADER, A. (1961). Primäre Tubulopathien 11. Ein Fall von idiopathischem Gluko-Amino-Phosphat-Diabetes. (DeToni-Debré-Fanconi Syndrome). *Helv. Pediatr. Acta*, **16**, 622

LEWY, J. E., CABANA, E. C., REPETTO, H. A., CANTERBURY, J. M. and REISS, E. (1972). Serum parathyroid hormone in hypophosphataemic vitamin-D-resistant rickets. *J. Pediatr.*, **81**, 294

LOWE, C. U., TERREY, M. and MACLAUCHLAN, E. A. (1952). Organic aciduria, decreased renal ammonia production, hydrophthalmos and mental retardation. *Am. J. Dis. Child.*, **83**, 164

LOTZ, M., NEY, R. and BARTTER, F. E. (1964). Osteomalacia resulting from phosphorus depletion. *Trans. Assoc. Am. Physicians*, **77**, 281

MCCANCE, R. A. (1947). Osteomalacia with Looser's zones due to raised resistance to vitamin D acquired about the age of 15 years. *Quart. J. Med.*, **16**, 33

MCCUNE, D. J., MASON, H. H. and CLARKE, H. T. (1943). Intractable hypophosphataemic rickets with renal glycosuria and acidosis (The Fanconi syndrome). *Am. J. Dis. Child.*, **65**, 81

Medical Research Council (1923). Studies of rickets in Vienna 1919–22. (Report to the Accessory Food Factors Committee appointed jointly by the M.R.C. and the Lister Institute). *Spec. Rep. Ser. Med. Res. Council* (*London*). *No.* 77 (London : H.M. Stationery Office)

MELLANBY, E. (1919). An experimental investigation on rickets. *Lancet*, **i**, 407

OMEN, G. S. (1971). Ectopic hormone syndromes associated with tumours in childhood. *Pediatrics*, **47**, 613

PRADER, A., ILLIG, R. and HEIERLI, G. (1961). Eine besondere Form der Primären vitamin-D-resistenten Rachitis mit Hypocalcämie und autosomal-dominantem Erbgang die hereditäre Pseudo-Mangelrachitis. *Helv. Paediatr. Acta*, **16**, 452

PRADER, A., ILLIG, R., UEHLINGER, E. and STALDER, G. (1959). Rachitis in folge Knochentumors. *Helv. Paediatr. Acta*, **14**, 544

REDDY, V. and SIVAKUMAR, B. (1974). Magnesium-dependent vitamin D-resistant rickets. *Lancet*, **i**, 963

REITZ, R. E. and WEINSTEIN, R. L. (1973). Parathyroid hormone secretion in familial vitamin D-resistant rickets. *N. Engl. J. Med.*, **289**, 941

RYAN, W. G., NIBBE, A. F., SCHWARTZ, T. B. and RAY, R. D. (1968). Fibrous dysplasia of bone with vitamin D-resistant rickets. A case study. *Metabolism*, **17**, 988

SALASSA, R. M., JOWSEY, J. and ARNAUD, C. D. (1970). Hypophosphataemic osteomalacia associated with 'non-endocrine' tumours. *N. Engl. J. Med.*, **283**, 65

SAVILLE, P. D., NASSIM, R., STEVENSON, F. H. MULLIGAN, L. and CAREY, M. (1955). The Fanconi Syndrome. Metabolic studies in treatment. *J. Bone Jt. Surg.* (*Br.*), **37B**, 529

STOWERS, J. M. and DENT, C. E. (1947). Studies of the mechanism of the Fanconi Syndrome. *Quart. J. Med.*, **26**, 275

SWAN, G. F. (1954). Pathogenesis of bone lesions in neurofibromatosis. *Br. J. Radiol.*, **27**, 623

THANNHAUSER, S. J. (1944). Neurofibromatosis (von Recklinghausen) and Osteitis Fibrosa Cystica Localisata et Disseminata (von Recklinghausen). *Medicine*, **23**, 105

THOMAS, W. C. and FRY, R. M. (1970). Parathyroid adenomas in chronic rickets. *Am. J. Med.*, **49**, 404

WOOD, B. S. B., GEORGE, W. H. and ROBINSON, A. W. (1958). Parathyroid adenoma in a child presenting as rickets. *Arch. Dis. Child.*, **33**, 46

WOODHOUSE, N. J. Y., DOYLE, F. H. and JOPLIN, G. F. (1971). Vitamin D deficiency and primary hyperparathyroidism. *Lancet*, **ii**, 283

YOSHIKAWA, S., SHIBA, M. and SUZUKI, A. (1968). Spinal cord compression in untreated adult cases of vitamin D-resistant rickets. *J. Bone Jt. Surg.* (*Am.*), **50A**, 743

II

X-linked hypophosphataemia and autosomal recessive vitamin D dependency: Models for the resolution of vitamin D refractory rickets

C. R. Scriver, F. H. Glorieux, Theresa M. Reade and Harriet S. Tenenhouse

Rickets was first reported as a formal clinical entity by English physicians in the mid-seventeenth century (cited by Park, 1923; and by Hunter, 1972). By the mid-nineteenth century, the epidemic nature of rachitic bone disease in industrial Europe was widely known (Loomis, 1970). Awareness of rickets provoked writing and reflection upon its cure, and physicians as exemplified by Theobald of eighteenth-century England, and West of nineteenth-century London, were moved to write prescriptions for its own cure, which are now, blessedly, out of date (Appendix I). The use of cod-liver oil as an effective cure of most cases of endemic rickets, was indeed known but largely ignored in the mid-nineteenth century (Appendix II). Only with the discovery (Mellanby, 1918; Park, 1923) of a substance eventually identified as vitamin D, and synthesised for therapeutic use, did the prevalence of rickets diminish dramatically.

As long as rachitic bone disease was endemic, and related to environmental mechanisms of vitamin D deficiency, it was unlikely that causes refractory to vitamin D therapy would gain attention. Only when the floods of deficiency rickets had abated could the monadnocks of vitamin D refractory rickets be observed in the landscape of metabolic bone disease. The fourth decade of the twentieth century marks the origins of our enlarged interest in these 'new' diseases (Albright *et al.*, 1937; McCance, 1947). Dent's superb classifications of metabolic bone disease (Dent, 1952; Dent and Harris, 1956; Dent, 1970) brought further insight to this difficult area of clinical medicine. An additional simple classification has been proposed recently according to whether the pathogenesis primarily affects the availability of phosphorus or calcium; to the former, we have given the term 'phosphopenic' rickets and to the latter, 'calciopenic' rickets (Scriver, 1974).

In the following paper we discuss two forms of hereditary metabolic bone disease refractory to vitamin D. The first, X-linked hypophosphataemia, is an example of phosphopenic rickets; the second, autosomal recessive vitamin D dependency, is an example of a calciopenic mechanism. Recognition of the primary pathogenesis permits the clinician to prescribe effective, rational therapy for these otherwise difficult clinical problems.

X-linked hypophosphataemia

EVIDENCE FOR A TRANSPORT DEFECT

We believe that X-linked hypophosphataemia (XLH) is a selective disorder in the trans-epithelial transport of orthophosphate (Scriver, 1974; Arnaud *et al.*, 1971; Glorieux and Scriver, 1972; Glorieux and Scriver, 1973). Net tubular reabsorption, or reclamation of orthophosphate (P_i), is impaired at the normal range of serum phosphate in affected patients. The maximum rate of tubular reabsorption of phosphate (T_{mPi}) is also depressed below normal (Glorieux and Scriver, 1972; 1973). Under the appropriate circumstances we have even observed *negative* reclamation ('secretion') of phosphate by the renal tubule in some XLH patients. However, in most, there is a small residual net reabsorption of phosphate by kidney; this retained function is insensitive to parathyroid hormone, but can be enhanced by calcium ion (Glorieux and Scriver, 1972; 1973).

Should the transport defect exist also in gut, XLH could be assigned to the class of inborn errors of membrane transport that affect epithelial transport tissues in general. The intestinal hypothesis found support with *in vivo* studies (Condon *et al.*, 1970) and from direct measurement of phosphate uptake in biopsied intestinal mucosa (Short *et al.*, 1973). However, other investigations (Gerbeaux-Balsan, 1965; Glorieux *et al.*, 1974) reveal that many XLH patients do not have abnormal intestinal transport of P_i. It is unclear at present, whether the discrepancies between reports reflect methodological variation or genetic heterogeneity among patients.

THE PTH-HYPERSENSITIVITY HYPOTHESIS

Even when elevated iPTH levels are not associated with further impairment of P_i reclamation by kidney (Arnaud *et al.*, 1971), serum immunoreactive PTH (iPTH) levels are essentially normal in untreated patients (Arnaud *et al.*, 1971; Lewy *et al.*, 1972; Reitz and Weinstein 1973; Fanconi, Fischer and Prader, 1974; Glorieux and Scriver, 1974). Nonetheless, investigators continue to examine the hypothesis that impaired reclamation of P_i in XLH, and other forms of vitamin D refractory rickets (Riggs *et al.*, 1969) may result from hypersensitivity of the renal tubule to circulating parathyroid hormone (PTH) (Arnstein and Hansen, 1969; Short *et al.*, 1974). The observations on serum

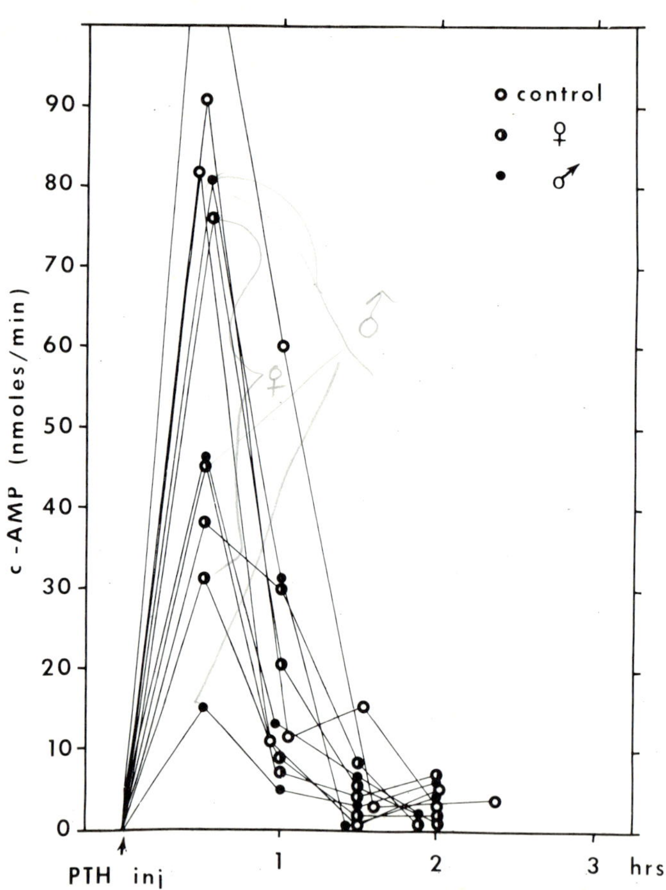

FIGURE 11.1 Urinary adenosine 3′,5′-monophosphate (cyclic AMP) excretion in patients with XLH. Basal levels (zero time) are normal. The 30-minute △ excretion response to bovine PTH infusion (200–400 units over 10 minutes intravenously) is within the normal range (cited by Chase, Melson and Aurbach, 1969). An appropriate fall in urinary calcium excretion accompanied the infusion of PTH (Glorieux and Scriver, 1972). (Cyclic AMP determinations were kindly performed by Dr Alan Tenenhouse.)

iPTH, if compatible with the 'hypersensitivity hypothesis', imply that the renal tubule is over-responsive, either to an unusual species of PTH synthesised by the XLH patient, or to normal amounts of normal hormone and its fragments. There is no evidence for or against the first proposal, and so far the weight of evidence is against the latter. For example, the XLH phenotype discreetly ignores solutes other than P_i; yet excess PTH provokes hyperaminoaciduria when acting normally on the tubule (Scriver, 1974). Moreover, the basal level of urinary adenosine 3′,5′-monophosphate (cAMP) is normal in XLH and not elevated as expected if the hypothesis is correct; following PTH infusion there is an appropriate rise in urinary cAMP (Figure 11.1) and urinary calcium excretion decreases appropriately by 50–70%.

The natural history of the XLH phenotype after parathyroidectomy provides another test of the hypersensitivity hypothesis, and we have had the opportunity to observe this situation in a patient with severe XLH who developed hyperparathyroidism as a complication of phosphate replacement therapy. Following seven-eighths parathyroidectomy, sufficient to permit sustained hypocalcaemia, there was no significant change in tubular reabsorption of phosphate (Table 11.1). We conclude

Table 11.1 *Response of renal tubular reclamation of phosphate following drastic subtotal parathyroidectomy for diffuse hyperplasma in XLH*

	Serum total calcium (mg/dl)	*Serum* P_i (mg/dl)	*Serum iPTH* (μEq/ml)[c]	*Tubular reabsorption of* P_i (% *of filtered* P_i)[d]
Before PTX[a]	9·4–10·9	1·5–2·6	270–490	34–80
Post PTX[b]	6·4–7·8*	1·6–3·4 (NS)	< 28*	28–62 (NS)

PTX = parathyroidectomy (7/8 of total mass).
a Range of values in month preceding PTX therapy; no P_i supplement; vitamin D_2, 1·25 mg/day.
b Range of values in two months following PTX.
c Normal value for age; < 40 mEq/ml (measured by Dr Claude Arnaud with GP-LM antiserum which detects C-terminal hormone).
d Normal value: > 80%, in range of serum P_i concentration experienced by patient.
* Difference from pre-PTX values is significant ($p < 0{\cdot}01$).
NS Difference from pre-PTX is not significant.

that the impairment of phosphate reclamation in this patient was not dependent on hyperresponsiveness of the renal tubule to PTH.

COMMENT

Phosphate, like calcium, may equilibrate with a mitochondrial compartment during transepithelial absorption (Borle, 1973). Since 'negative reabsorption' of P_i occurs in XLH kidney (Glorieux and Scriver, 1972), we believe the lesion in XLH could be a defect permitting back-flux of P_i from cytosol at the luminal membrane by

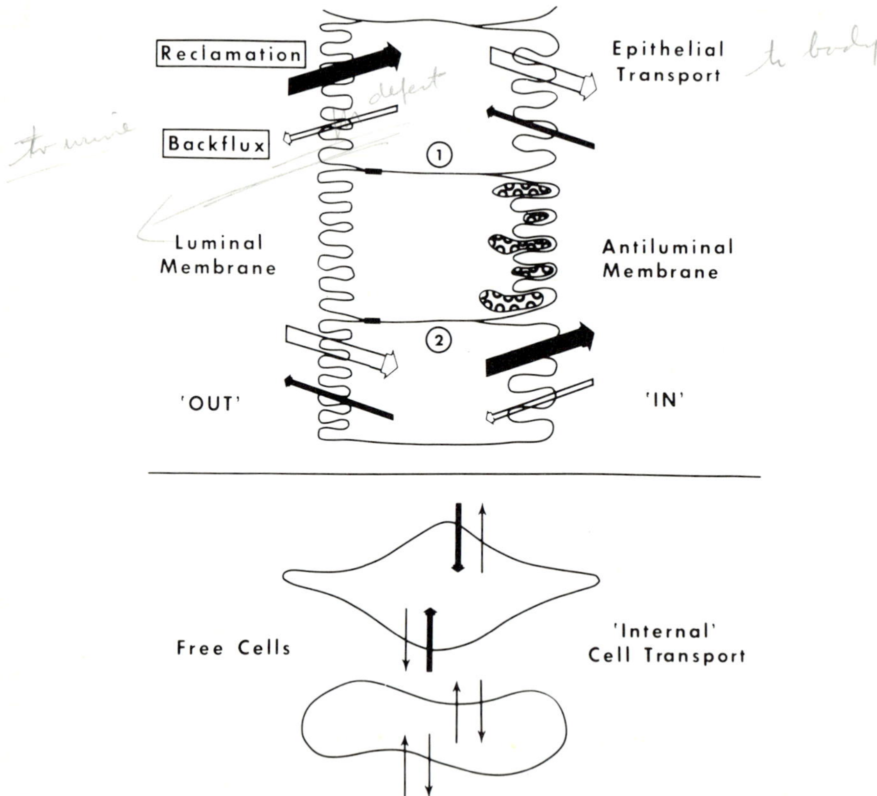

FIGURE 11.2 Topology of renal tubular reclamation of P_i compared to uptake of the same solute by 'internal' or free-floating, non-epithelial tissues (from Scriver and Bergeron, 1974). The net transepithelial reclamation involves flux equilibrium across two plasma membranes orientated in series; bidirectional fluxes occur from urine to blood and from blood to urine. Uptake by internal cells involves equilibrium across only one plasma membrane. Uptake of P_i is concentrative (against gradient) in kidney cortex, and is diffusional (down gradient) in the erythrocyte.

altering the normal Michaelis equilibrium (Scriver and Bergeron, 1974) that permits net reclamation at that surface of the epithelium before equilibration with mitochondria.

STUDIES IN THE XLH ERYTHROCYTE

The topology governing phosphate flux into an 'internal' cell, such as the erythrocyte, is quite different from that governing trans-epithelial absorption (Figure 11.2). We considered it advisable to compare phosphate transport in the erythrocyte with that in kidney. Furthermore, we wanted to know whether possible expression of the XLH allele in the erythrocyte membrane determines known changes in phosphate-dependent metabolism in XLH erythrocytes (Cartier *et al.*, 1970; Glorieux *et al.*, 1972). Whole-blood P_{50} values are low (Glorieux *et al.*, 1972) and the organic phosphate pool is diminished (Cartier *et al.*, 1970).

Phosphate entry into the normal erythrocyte was studied in the presence of iodoacetamide, an agent which permits little of the initial ^{32}P label to enter the organic phosphate pool (Figure 11.3). Phosphate slowly enters the intact, iodoacetamide-treated erythrocyte; down its concentration gradient (Tenenhouse and Scriver, 1975). The steady-state distribution ratio for P_i between erythrocyte water and plasma

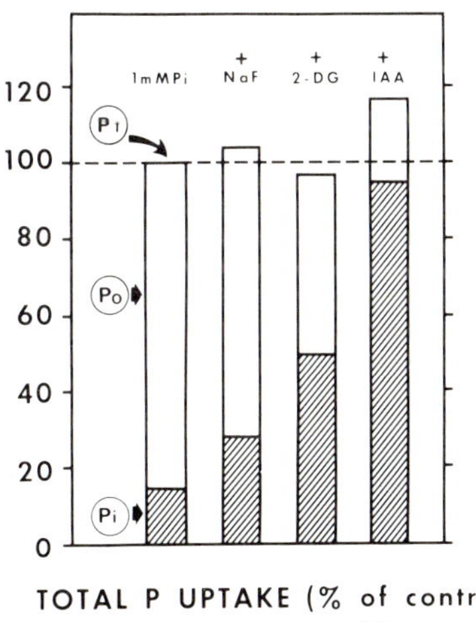

FIGURE 11.3 Effect of iodoacetamide and other agents (sodium fluoride and 2-deoxyglucose) on P_i entry into erythrocyte phosphate pools. Iodoacetamide, at pH 7·4 and 37 °C without preincubation inhibits 15-minute uptake of $(Po)_i$ into organic pools; about 88% of P_i entering cell is retained in the orthophosphate pool. With 5-minute preincubation in the presence of iodoacetamide, $<1\%$ of P_i enters the organic pools.

Table 11.2 *Comparison of P_i uptake by mammalian erythrocytes and kidney*

Characteristic	*RBC*	*Kidney cortex slice*[a]	*Tubular reabsorption*[b]
Uptake against gradient	No	Yes	Apparently
Steady-state distribution ratio[c]	0·6	10·0	—
Dependence on energy metabolism	No	Yes	Apparently
Evidence for specific carrier	Yes	Yes	Yes
Type of transport	Facilitated diffusion with symmetrical influx and efflux	Active transport inward	'Active' reclamation with T_m and back diffusion

a Preparation evaluates net uptake across basilar and lateral plasma membranes of tubular epithelium; luminal membrane not accessible.
b Net reabsorption (reclamation) across luminal membrane is measured.
c Distribution ratio refers to the *chemical* distribution ratio for P_i in intracellular water: P_i in extracellular water.

water is always less than 1·0 (Table 11.2) and a Donnan equilibrium readily accounts for the distribution of this anion across the erythrocyte membrane. By comparison, phosphate entry into kidney is rapid, and uptake of P_i by mammalian kidney cortex slices occurs against a concentration gradient (Glorieux *et al.*, 1974). Uptake across the luminal membrane *in vivo* must observe a similar gradient. Saturation of the P_i permeation process could not be demonstrated readily in the erythrocyte; by comparison, P_i reclamation by kidney *in vivo* manifests T_m, indicating saturation of the process; and *in vitro* uptake into slices is also saturable (Table 11.2). Rigorous tests of phosphate entry into the erythrocyte under conditions of equal influx and efflux reveal an anion carrier which interacts weakly with phosphate and arsenate. Movement on this anion carrier best fits the criteria for symmetrical exchange diffusion (Tenenhouse and Scriver, 1975). By comparison phosphate uptake by kidney observes active transport presumably on a different species of membrane carrier, and it is this mechanism that is affected by the XLH allele.

When we examined P_i entry into the XLH erythrocyte we could find no deviation from normal in either the rate of entry, the response to inhibitors, to temperature or to uptake at various phosphate concentrations (Tenenhouse and Scriver, 1975). Moreover, the P_i distribution ratio *in vivo*, across the erythrocyte membrane, at any concentration of serum phosphate in subject possessing the mutant allele, is not different from normal (Figure 11.4).

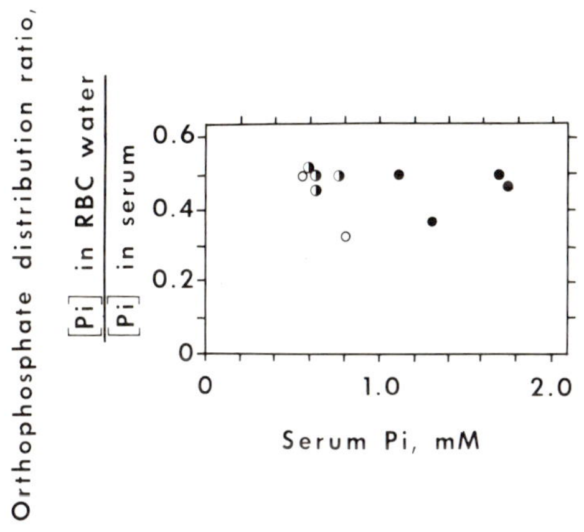

FIGURE 11.4 The distribution of P_i between erythrocyte water and plasma water in normal subject (filled circles) and heterozygous (half-filled circles) and hemizygous (open circles) XLH patients. The XLH mutation does not perturb the P_i distribution ratio *in vivo*. Phosphate anion species at pH 7·4 observe Donnan equilibrium *in vivo* (Tenenhouse and Scriver, 1975).

We deduce that the mutant allele is not expressed in the XLH erythrocyte membrane, or that the relevant gene product is not present even in the normal erythrocyte membrane. Earlier observations to the contrary (Cartier *et al.*, 1970) were probably an artefact of depleted erythrocyte P_i pools in XLH. Changes in phosphate-dependent metabolism in XLH erythrocytes can be attributed, quite simply, to the diminished concentration of phosphate in extracellular fluids which, in turn, is secondary to impaired tubular reclamation of phosphate in this disease.

TREATMENT OF X-LINKED HYPOPHOSPHATAEMIA

Use of phosphate

Treatment of XLH with vitamin D alone will heal the rickets, when the vitamin is given in large doses. However, the dose requirement is often close to the toxic range and the dwarfism is rarely corrected. The evidence for a phosphopenic mechanism in XLH rickets led us to emphasise phosphate replacement as a more effective way to neutralise the effect of the mutant allele (Glorieux *et al.*, 1972). We recognise moreover, that the diffusional mode of phosphate transport permits phosphate to enter cells even if the XLH allele impairs other mechanism of phosphate transport.

It has long been known that dietary phosphate will heal rachitic bone lesions in animals. Lilly, Peirce and Grant (1935) described this phenomenon, and reviewed the relevant literature as far back as 1872. In more recent times, Fraser and colleagues (Fraser *et al.*, 1957; Fraser *et al.*, 1958; Steendijk, 1961; and Scriver *et al.*, 1964) observed that intravenous infusion of phosphate promotes the healing of rickets in human hypophosphataemia states; and Gerbeaux-Balsan (1965) showed positive P_i and calcium balances after P_i supplementation by mouth in XLH. On the other hand, reports of 'failed-phosphate' treatment have not been lacking from the literature (e.g. Frame *et al.*, 1963; Stickler *et al.*, 1965). However, the latter seem to reflect more a failure to deliver the treatment effectively by mouth, and less a failure of the patient's ability to respond to phosphate.

It was Dent who taught us to appreciate that the blood response to pulsed phosphate loading is short-lived. For this reason, our phosphate treatment regimen is dependent on the administration of phosphate by mouth every 4 hours, up to five times a day (Glorieux *et al.*, 1972, Clow *et al.*, 1971). The supplemental phosphate mixture that we have used, and the method of administration, are described in Appendix III.

The serum P_i response

Early in the study of phosphate treatment we monitored six patients during 2725 days of home treatment. An acceptable serum P_i level was observed with the phosphate regimen (Table 11.3). The number of home visits required to support the favourable response to treatment should be noticed. Our experience now exceeds 20 000 treatment days

Table 11.3 *Serum P_i conc. and frequency of home visits during 12 month period in XLH patients*

Subject	*Age* (year)	*Sex*		*Serum P_i* (mg/dl) (*mean*, *SD*)		*Home visits per year* (*number*)
MC	10	F		3·7	1·1	30
SV	10	F		2·8	0·4	35
JB	8	M		3·2	0·6	*
EM	11	M		3·5	1·3	28
LA	11	M		5·1	1·4	24
OR	13	M		4·2	1·0	35
			Average	3·75	0·8	27·6

* Followed by telephone and through arrangement at local hospital 95 miles from Genetics Centre.

and we are convinced, more than ever, that constant support of patient and family is the key to successful therapy.

Healing of rickets

Regular treatment with orthophosphate supplementation by mouth in doses ranging from 1–4 g/day will heal the rickets of XLH. The mean radiographic density of bone, monitored by photodensitometry of a standard middle phalangeal X-ray image, in our cohort of patients, has always been normal when compared with age-matched control subjects.

Effect on linear growth

The average linear growth velocity in *untreated* XLH is only 63% of normal (Glorieux *et al.*, 1972). The same attenuation of growth rate is generally true of patients treated in the traditional manner with vitamin D alone. After the initiation of treatment of our patients with phosphate we observed a striking increase in the linear growth velocity in each subject. The average rate for the patient group on phosphate treatment was approximately two-fold greater than the corresponding pre-treatment rate. Moreover, the growth velocity during phosphate supplementation was 1·26 times the median rate for age-matched, normal subjects (Glorieux *et al.*, 1972). This acceleration of growth rate during phosphate treatment was apparent even in the lower segment which is the fastest growing portion of the body in childhood. Along with others (West, 1969; Harrison, Harrison, Lifeshitz *et al.*, 1966), we believe that phosphate therapy clearly permits true catch-up growth and will reduce the hazard of dwarfism in XLH.

Case history

We have had occasion to treat a male infant (YP) with phosphate, beginning at the third month of life. An affected male sibling (JP) had been treated with vitamin D_2 alone from 6 months until 30 months of age when his family moved to Montreal. Their mother is severely hypophosphataemic and dwarfed; she chose to feed her new offspring at the breast. Hypophosphataemia, in YP, was apparent in cord blood (4·2 mg/100 ml) and on the 1st day of life (3·4 mg/100 ml). The milk was low in phosphorus (54 mg/l, compared to normal human milk, 140–170 mg/l), and provided only 36–49 mg P_i/day (minimum requirement, 110 mg/day). A change to an evaporated milk formula, providing 990 mg P_i/l and delivering about 600 mg/day in the feedings, evinced a modest increase in serum P_i. But because the serum P_i level was still below normal and because early rachitic changes appeared in the long bones, we initiated dietary phosphate supplementation in the 5th month of life, to provide daily P_i intakes on the order of 0·9–1 g P_i/day. Serum P_i rose from previous values below 4·5 mg/100 ml to a level regularly above 4·5 mg/100 ml. The rachitic lesions healed rapidly. Linear growth which had slowed perceptibly returned to normal (Figure 11.5). At 20 months, the linear growth of YP is above the 10th percentile. By comparison, his sibling by the same age had experienced a marked failure of linear growth.

DIFFICULTIES WITH PHOSPHATE THERAPY

Delivery of treatment

The 'delivery system' is the most important aspect of the treatment of XLH. Because phosphate therapy is not easily accommodated by the patient or his family, we provide continuous support and reinforcement by means of home visits and demonstrations of progress under treatment (Clow *et al.*, 1971).

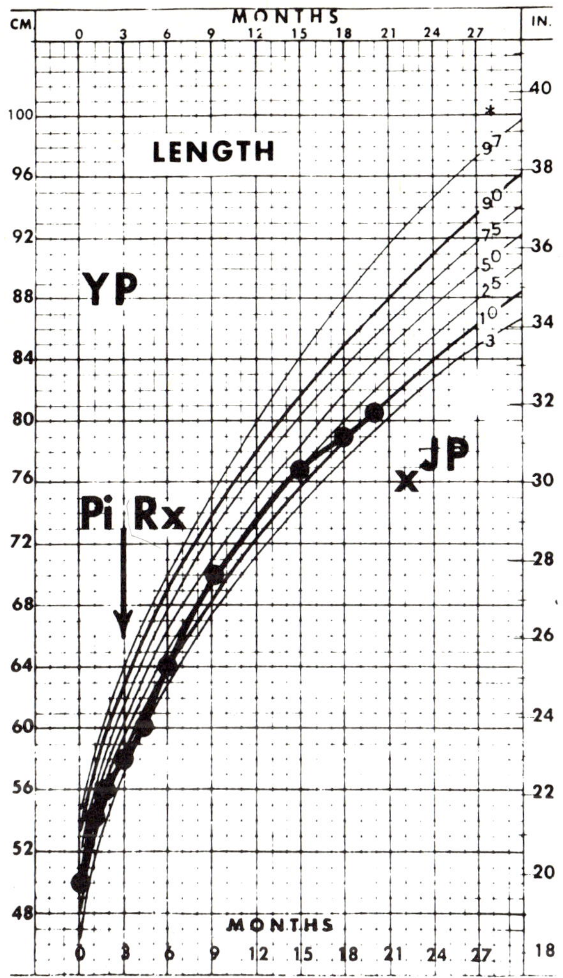

FIGURE 11.5 Linear growth of two sibs with XLH. JP was treated from 6 months of age with vitamin D_2 alone; YP was treated from 5 months of age with a dietary phosphate supplement and low doses of vitamin D_2. The beneficial effect of phosphate replacement on linear growth is apparent in YP. Healing of rickets at 20 months was also superior in YP.

We carry our message, even to the schools, so that patient-pupils can be helped to comply with their treatment regimen under challenging circumstances. We have not yet encountered a family, or a patient, who will not respond to these therapeutic manipulations, although some are less co-operative than others. It helps to have the support of the regional genetics programme sponsored by the Quebec Network of Genetic Medicine (Clow *et al.*, 1973).

Complications of treatment

Phosphate supplementation may cause transient diarrhoea; but persistence with the regimen will find the patient free of this symptom usually within 1 or 2 weeks.

The taste of the phosphate mixture is a problem, but an acidic preparation (Appendix III) has advantages over the neutral phosphate salt solution in this respect; the latter may be flavoured to the patient's choice, if it is preferred.

Sodium intake is high (up to 100mEq/day) particularly if the neutral phosphate salt mixture is used. We have not observed hypertension in our series of patients. There is a danger of an acid load with the acid phosphate mixture; we have not found this to be a complicating factor in patients with uncompromised acid-base metabolism.

Phosphate loading will lower ionised calcium and will raise the level of iPTH in serum (Reiss, Canterbury, Bercovitz and Kaplan, 1970). Characteristic hyperaminoaciduria with iminopeptiduria and bone changes will appear if there is sustained hyperparathyroidism; the latter occurred once in our series in our first patient. We use vitamin D_2 as an adjunct to phosphate therapy to avoid this complication. Our patients are given individualised doses of vitamin D_2 which vary from 0·1–1·2 mg/day depending on the dose of phosphate, and the particular need of the patient (Glorieux *et al.*, 1972). If transient hyperparathyroidism appears we intermit phosphate treatment and augment calcium repair (Glorieux *et al.*, 1972).

We have observed only four episodes of mild hypercalcaemia, due to Vitamin D_2 therapy, totalling about 60 days, in over 20 000 treatment days. No episode lasted more than 2 weeks, and serum calcium never exceeded 12·4 mg/100 ml. There has been no evidence of atopic tissue calcification as a complication of XLH therapy (Paunier *et al.*, 1968; Stickler, Jowsey and Bianco, 1971) or of urinary calculus formation in our patients; and glomerular filtration rate has remained normal in every instance.

Haemoglobin levels

We surveyed the relationship between whole blood haemoglobin and serum phosphorus in each of our patients looking for an exaggerated

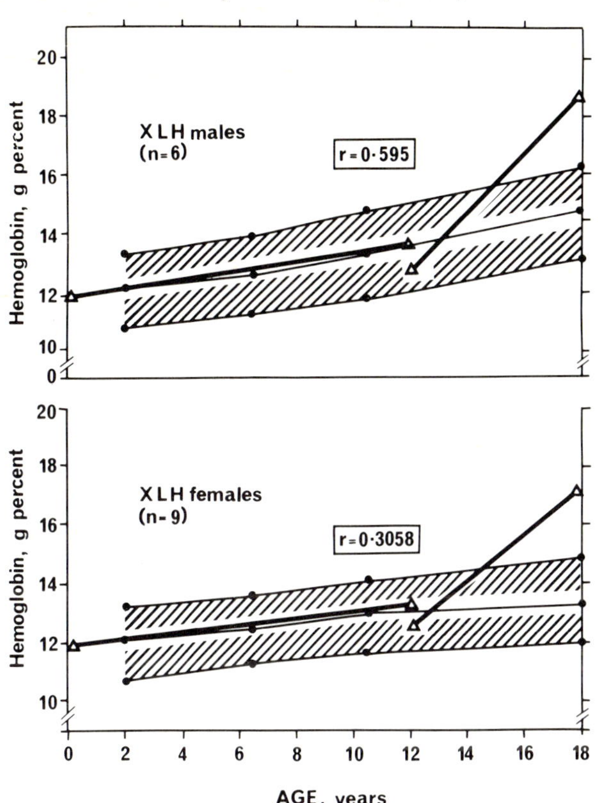

FIGURE 11.6 Age-dependent haemoglobin levels in a cohort of eight prepubertal XLH patients receiving P_i supplements. The values are in the normal range of Card *et al.* (1973). Two pubertal patients, in whom serum P_i values fell following poor treatment compliance, have experienced polycythaemia, accounting for the change in the regression line (r value given).

reciprocal relationship in accordance with current beliefs (Card) *et al.*, 1973). Dr James Popkin reviewed our patients' files and observed that haemoglobin values were normal throughout the period of treatment during childhood (Figure 11.6); P_i values in serum were also near normal. However, as patients enter puberty there has been a trend in some to develop erythrocytic polycythaemia. At present this observation is based on data from only two patients. Their polycythaemia is associated with a fall in serum phosphorus. The latter reflects, in part, the normal drop in serum P_i which accompanies puberty; but it is also the result of diminished compliance with treatment in these two patients. One of these patients has a severely affected mother; she also has mild polycythaemia with her persistant hypophosphataemia. None has elevated erythropoietin levels in urine or blood. The significance of these relationships and their interpretation is under investigation.

THE RESPONSE TO VITAMIN D HORMONE IN XLH

We have examined the effect of 1α,25-dihydroxycholecalciferol in XLH (Glorieux *et al.*, 1973). Rapid intravenous infusion of 1α,25$(OH)_2D_3$, at the 1 μg dose level, promotes, perhaps through its effect on calcium, a transient improvement of phosphate reclamation by the renal tubule; the phosphaturic response to bovine parathyroid hormone is also restored transiently. However, long-term treatment with 1α,25$(OH)_2D_3$ is not effective at physiological dose levels (1 μg/day) whether administered intravenously or by mouth. Serum phosphorus does not return to normal, and there is no healing of the rachitic process in our experience. We conclude that 1α,25$(OH)_2D_3$ is inadequate as a therapeutic agent in XLH and others appear to hold the same opinion. The finding is not surprising if our hypothesis is correct that XLH is a primary abnormality of trans-epithelial transport of phosphate.

Vitamin D dependency or 'pseudodeficiency' rickets

Autosomal-recessive, vitamin D dependency (ARVDD) (Fraser and Salter, 1958; Prader *et al.*, 1961; Fanconi and Prader, 1969; Arnaud *et al.*, 1970; Balsan *et al.*, 1972; Scriver, 1974) is associated with severe post-natal vitamin D deficiency, despite intakes of vitamin D_2, vitamin D_3 or 25-hydroxycholecalciferol that would normally prevent such manifestations. Resistant hypocalcaemia is accompanied by hypophosphataemia and generalised aminoaciduria; the two latter features reflect a renal tubulopathy associated with secondary hyperparathyroidism (Arnaud, *et al.*, 1970; Scriver, 1974). Elevated bone alkaline phosphatase activity, severe rachitic bone lesions and hypoplasia of dental enamel in teeth that form postnatally (Prader *et al.*, 1961; Arnaud *et al.*, 1970), indicate the severe disorder of mineralisation in this form of calciopenic rickets.

The basis for the calciopenia in ARVDD is a selective disturbance of calcium absorption by intestine (Hamilton *et al.*, 1970). The origin of the latter could be an impairment of biosynthesis, or of tissue responsiveness to the active hormone form of vitamin D (Scriver, 1970). Maintenance requirement for vitamin D prohormone (D_2, D_3 or 25$(OH)D_3$)

in ARVDD is in the pharmacological dose range, whereas the requirement for hormone, 1α-25$(OH)_2D_3$, is at dose levels in the microgram range, presumably equivalent to the physiological requirement (Fraser *et al.*, 1973). Although the enzyme defect has not yet been defined at the cellular level in any patient, the studies of Fraser and colleagues (1973), now corroborated by Balsan in France, by Prader and Fanconi in Switzerland (personal communications) and by ourselves, indicate that ARVDD, in all patients studied so far, is an inborn error of vitamin D hormone biosynthesis which affects the 1-hydroxylation step in kidney mitochondria. These observations do not obviate the possibility that future pedigrees will yield probands in whom there is defective responsiveness of target tissues to normal amounts of 1α,25$(OH)_2D_3$, or deficient conversion at other steps of biosynthesis.

An important question about the practical management of ARVDD remains open: notably whether therapy with the surrogate hormone 1α-hydroxycholecalciferol (1α$(OH)D_3$) would be more advantageous than treatment with 1α,25$(OH)_2D_3$. Chemical synthesis of 1α$(OH)D_3$ is more easily accomplished than that of 1α,25$(OH)_2D_3$ (Holick *et al.*, 1973). Moreover, 1α$(OH)D_3$ is likely to be a safe therapeutic agent which can be administered by mouth. In collaboration with Holick and DeLuca we have had the opportunity to examine the effect of the surrogate hormone on serum calcium homeostasis and bone mineralisation in ARVDD. The occasion also provided the first opportunity to estimate the 'physiological' requirement for this substance in man.

Patients

Four patients, between the ages of 17 months and 11½ years, have been investigated. Patients 1A and 1B are siblings (age 6 and 11½ years) who have been previously reported in detail (Arnaud *et al.*, 1970). Patient 2 was diagnosed at 18 months of age, and has been followed by us for the past 8 years. Patient 3 was recently diagnosed at 17 months of age at another hospital prior to the administration of maintenance therapy with vitamin D_2. Each patient has shown the characteristic chemical and biochemical features of ARVDD in the absence of maintenance therapy with vitamin D.

Requirement for vitamin D_2 in ARVDD

The requirement for vitamin D pro-hormone has been established in the first three patients: it lies between 0.6 mg and 1·5 mg/day. When related to body weight, the requirements are 41–55 μg/kg. This maintenance dose is 100 times normal; each patient has required it since the time of diagnosis.

Response to 25-hydroxycholecalciferol ($25(OH)D_3$

Patients 1B and 2 were given $25(OH)D_3$ by mouth in doses up to 40 μg per day; the normal maintenance requirement for this substance is approximately 3 μg/day (Fraser *et al.*, 1973). Neither patient exhibited a significant therapeutic response to $25(OH)D_3$ (Figure 11.4). Therefore the putative defect in vitamin D hormone biosynthesis lies beyond the 25-hydroxylation step, in the pathway for conversion of D_3 to $1\alpha,25(OH)_2D_3$.

Response to 1-hydroxylated forms of vitamin D in ARVDD

The effect of 1α-hydroxylated forms of vitamin D was investigated in patients A1, 1B and 2, after maintenance therapy had been withdrawn for a period of time sufficient for the natural phenotype of this hereditary trait to reappear. The response was also investigated in patient 3 prior to the administration of maintenance therapy with vitamin D prohormone.

Effect of $1\alpha(OH)D_3$

The substance was dissolved in propylene glycol and protected from oxidation by storage under nitrogen in the dark. It was administered daily by mouth in doses up to 3 μg/day. The response to $1\alpha(OH)D_3$ is shown in detail for patient 2 (Figures 11.7 and 11.8); the subject received the substance on three occasions; once at a dose level of 1 μg/day while in the normocalcaemia, hypophosphataemic stage of the vitamin D depletion syndrome; she also received the drug twice during the hypocalcaemia, hypophosphataemic state of depletion, at dose levels of 2 μg and 3 μg/day. Serum calcium rose on the first day of $1\alpha(OH)D_3$ treatment. A rise in serum phosphate followed slightly later, usually before the third day of treatment. The calcium $\times$ phosphorus product in serum also rises promptly under these conditions.

Patient 3 presented with florid rickets; after therapy with $1\alpha(OH)D_3$ (2 μg/day) her serum calcium rose, reaching a normal level within 7 days. Serum phosphate fell initially, rising only after the 4th week of treatment. Since this response was associated with rapid healing of rickets, the anomalous serum response may reflect vigorous bone remineralisation

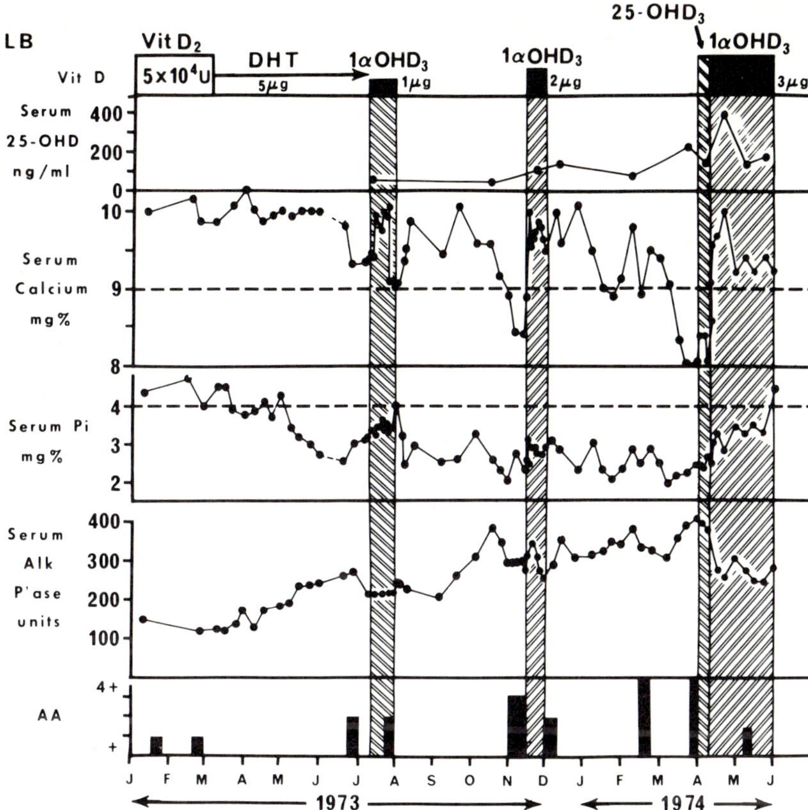

FIGURE 11.7 Time-course of response in Patient 2 with ARVDD after withdrawal of maintenance doses of vitamin D_2 (1·25 mg/day). Dihydrotachysterol at 'physiological' doses did not prevent evolution of the ARVDD phenotype. The surrogate hormone, 1α(OH) D_3, given by mouth at low doses (1–3 μg/day) offset the effects of the mutant allelle, with respect to serum levels of calcium and phosphorus, bone mineralisation and the tubulopathy, manifest as hyperaminoaciduria.

(Stearns and Boyd, 1931) permitted by replacement therapy with 1α(OH)D_3.

Bone response

All four subjects experienced an effect of 1α(OH)D_3 on bone. Alkaline phosphatase activity in serum fell immediately after initiation of treatment, and radiographic examination of bones revealed repair of the rachitic lesions. Patient 2 healed her rickets in 7 weeks with 1α(OH)D_3 therapy alone (3μg/day). Patient 3 was maintained on 1α(OH)D_3 (2 μg/day) during the primary healing process and achieved healing in 9 weeks of treatment.

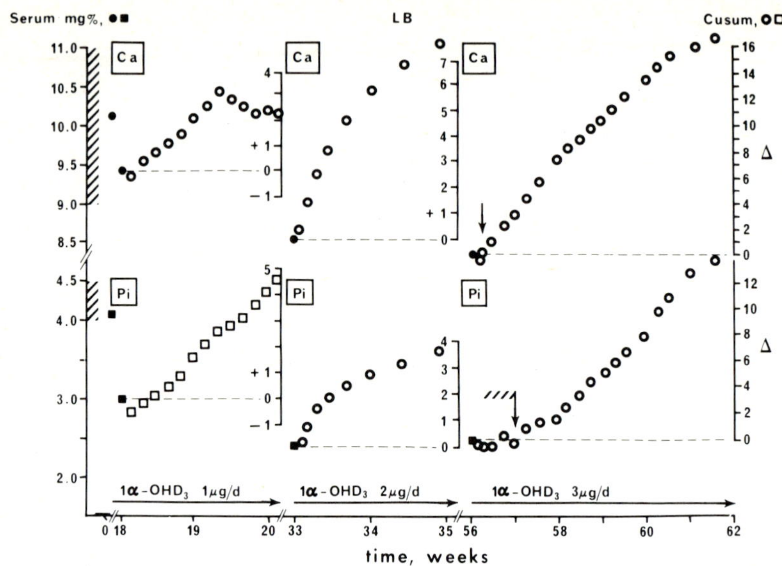

FIGURE 11.8 Cumulative sum (cusum) analysis (Healy, 1968) of the response to administration of 1α(OH)D_3 and following withdrawal of the surrogate hormone in patient 2. 1α(OH)D_3 acts within 1 day. After withdrawal, its effect persists for several days but the full vitamin D-depletion syndrome emerges within about 2 weeks. Thus the per-os dose requirement for 1α(OH)D_3 in men is of the order of 2 μg/day and its half life *in vivo* is of the order of 1 or 2 weeks.

Effect on the renal tubulopathy

Hyperaminoaciduria is a useful index of the tubulopathy, which is dependent on high levels of parathyroid hormone in serum (Arnaud *et al.*, 1970; Scriver, 1974). The presence of intracellular calcium depletion is an important determinant of PTH-dependent hyperaminoaciduria (McInnes and Scriver, 1974). Treatment of ARVDD with 1α(OH)D_3 was accompanied by a rapid decline in hyperaminoaciduria in each of our patients (Figure 11.7).

Response to withdrawal of 1α(OH)D_3

Serum calcium remains elevated for a short period, up to 2 weeks, before it falls after withdrawal of 1α(OH)D_3. Serum phosphorus falls within the first few days. Patient 2 exhibited this withdrawal response following termination of treatment at all dose levels of 1α(OH)D_3 (Figures 11.8).

Response to 1α,25(OH)$_2D_3$

The hormone was administered briefly at dose levels of 3 μg/day for

5 days *by mouth* to patient 1B when the ARVDD phenotype was fully manifest. An immediate rise in serum calcium was observed and serum inorganic phosphorus increased also. This response is similar to the observations of Fraser and colleagues (1973) who treated their patients with intravenous $1\alpha,25(OH)_2D_3$. Our observation suggests that the hormone is modestly effective by mouth as well.

Response to dihydrotachysterol (DHT)

There was no delay in the rate of appearance of the vitamin D depletion syndrome (Figure 11.7), when DHT was administered by mouth at low doses (5 μg/day) for the first 18 weeks after termination of maintenance therapy with vitamin D_2. The response to DHT was also examined in patient 1B during the hypocalcaemic, hypophosphataemic stage of vitamin D depletion. Dose levels of the synthetic metabolite up to 80 μg/day for 7 days had no therapeutic effect. The unresponsiveness to DHT is in marked contrast to the effect of $1\alpha(OH)D_3$, indicating that the ARVDD phenotype clearly distinguishes between the relative positions of the hydroxyl group in the A rings of the surrogate hormone and DHT.

Serum 25-hydroxyvitamin D in AVRDD

25-Hydroxyvitamin D levels in serum were measured in our patients by a competitive protein binding assay (Haddad and Chyn, 1971). Serum activity was 2·5–7 times greater than normal for age-matched, season-matched control subjects from our geographic region (Table 11.4); nonetheless, unequivocal manifestations of the vitamin D hormone depletion syndrome were present in all four patients. The high levels of 25-hydroxyvitamin D may reflect 'substrate' accumulation in the presence of the putative deficiency of 25-hydroxycholecalciferol-1-hydroxylase activity in ARVDD. On the other hand, these observations may reflect nothing more than an expanded pool of pro-hormone vitamin D metabolites in the presence of the previous high maintenance therapy with vitamin D_2. Even patient 3 did not escape exposure to vitamin D therapy; 5 weeks prior to diagnosis she had received vitamin D_2 (0·375 mg daily) in an attempt to initiate healing of her rickets. We report these observations to draw attention to the fact that high levels of 25-hydroxyvitamin D activity in serum in ARVDD are insufficient to maintain calcium homeostasis, and to prevent rickets.

Table 11.4 *Serum 25-hydroxycholecalciferol levels in ARVVD (ng/ml)*[a]

Subject	*Previous maintenance dose of vit.* D_2 (mg/day)	*Before treatment with* $1\alpha(OH)D_3$ *Last value*	*Range*[b]	*After treatment with* $1\alpha(OH)D_3$
1A	0·66	67	65–124	94–104
1B	1·475	167	87–167	141–167
2	1·25	217	56–217	141–194
3	(c)	153	–	50–158

a Measured by Dr Edgard Delvin with competitive protein binding assay of Haddad and Chyn (1971).

b Range of values obtained over 6 month period following withdrawal of maintenance dosage of vitamin D_2. Normal value = 29 ± 7 (Mean and 1 SD).

c Received vitamin D_2, 0·375 mg/day for 5 weeks just prior to diagnosis of ARVDD.

Comment and summary

We have reviewed in detail our experience with treatment regimes which offset the effects of two different mutant alleles, each causing hereditary forms of vitamin D refractory rickets. We have examined the hypothesis that familial, hypophosphataemic vitamin D resistant rickets, more accurately named X-linked hypophosphataemia (XLH), is a specific disorder of phosphate flux and reclamation across renal tubular epithelium. In the absence of any evidence for hyperparathyroidism, or for hypersensitivity of kidney to normal amounts of parathyroid hormone, there is no reason to consider this form of phosphopenic rickets other than potentially responsive to simple phosphate replacement. There are residual membrane carrier systems to permit phosphate anion entry into cells when the concentration of phosphate is sufficiently elevated in XLH. When inward movement of phosphorus is adequately restored, aberrations of intracellular, phosphate-dependent metabolism, and impairment of bone mineralisation, can be repaired. When this happens, normal growth rates can also be restored and dwarfism prevented. The role of vitamin D_2 therapy, in our approach to the treatment of XLH, is to prevent symptomatic hypocalcaemia during chronic phosphate loading. The rarity of significant complications during 70 patient-years of phosphate therapy is in sharp contrast to the oft-experienced complications of vitamin D therapy in XLH. We admit that phosphate treatment is not easy, but hopefully we have given enough information to indicate how it can be delivered to these patients with only modest perturbation of the quality of their lives.

By way of contrast, we have presented data on autosomal recessive, vitamin D dependency (ARVDD), a calciopenic form of rickets, refractory to vitamin D. It is likely that ARVDD was formerly confused with various forms of hypophosphataemic rickets associated with a generalised renal tubulopathy. The weight of evidence suggests that currently reported patients with ARVDD have a specific defect in the biosynthesis of $1\alpha,25(OH)_2D_3$. The putative enzyme impairment is 'leaky' since the patient can respond to pharmacological doses of prohormone, $25(OH)D_3$ and vitamin D_2. The message in our own studies is that rational interpretation of the mutant phenotype permits specific and highly effective treatment. At the present time, it would be difficult to entertain a life-long treatment protocol with intravenous $1\alpha,25(OH)_2D_3$. On the other hand, a relatively simple chemical synthesis yields a 'surrogate' hormone, $1\alpha(OH)D_3$, which can be given by mouth for treatment of affected probands. Although one cannot say, at present, whether $1\alpha(OH)D_3$ can be used reliably and with ease in a busy paediatric practice, there is every reason to believe that its use can be safely directed and monitored at the present time through the auspices of a regional medical genetics centre.

Acknowledgement

We are grateful to the following people for their help with this work, and in the preparation of the manuscript: To Dr Jessie Boyd Scriver, for many interesting, historical perspectives; to Dr Hector DeLuca, who provided us with various analogues of vitamin D; to Dr DeLuca again, and to Drs Arnaud, Dent, Fraser and Prader, for so many stimulating discussions about hereditary metabolic bone disease over many years; to Dr Edgard Delvin, for the competitive protein binding assay of 25-hydroxycholecalciferol in serum; to Dr James Popkin, for his assistance in the review of haemotological finding in X-linked hypophosphataemia; and finally to Mrs Carol Clow and Miss Susan Mackenzie, who with their colleague, Mrs Terry Reade, make the treatment of genetic disease a rewarding experience for everyone. We are also grateful to Lynne Prevost and Huguette Ishmael for assistance in the preparation of this manuscript and to Dr Roger Poirier for allowing us to study patient 3 with ARVDD.

APPENDIX I

EARLY TREATMENT OF RICKETS

Dr T. E. Cone Jr. of Harvard University brought to our attention the following annotation on rickets and its cure written by Dr J. Theobald in *The Young Wife's Guide to the Management of Her Children* (pp. 44–5) and printed by W. Griffen in London, 1764.

> 'This distemper most frequently affects children from nine months old, to two years and a half. The child at the beginning is seized with an aversion to motion, or exercise of any kind; the joints grow feeble and weak, and the flesh soft and flaccid; the head is over large, and the child's capacity exceeds its years. The belly is hard and very prominent; the bones of the arms and legs, grow crooked and are knotty at the joints; a cough comes on a difficulty of breathing; the pulse is low and languid, and an hectic fever carries off the child. Take of the best manna a drachm and and half, of dried raisins an handful, common ale a pint; infuse them together for twelve hours, and then strain them; let the child drink a draught of this frequently . . . Friction above everything must never be neglected especially on the back; and those parts which are apt to be the weakest; and the following ointment may be rubbed with advantage all over the back. Take the nerve ointment, and palm oil, each an ounce, oil of mace one drachms, spirits of sal armoniac (sic) forty drops, oil of amber twenty drops, mix them into a liniment, with which the parts affected may be anointed with a warm hand, two or three times in a day; the child may also take two grains of Ens Veneris in a spoonful of wine and water, every night . . .'

Dr Jessie Boyd Scriver shared her ancient copy of *Charles West's Lectures on the Diseases of Infancy and Childhood*, published by Lea in Philadelphia, 1874. On pp. 616 and 617 of that standard text for its age, is the following description which guided W. de Moulpied, M.D., the physician who cared for the mild deficiency rickets experienced in childhood by Walter de M. Scriver, the father of one of the authors of this paper.

'The *treatment* of rickets need not detain us long, for notwithstanding the importance of this disease, the principles to be borne in mind alike for its prevention and its cure are abundantly simple. Bad air and defective ventilation are its two great causes; and causes which among the poor it is often difficult, sometimes impossible, to remove. Even among the comparatively wealthy these causes of rickets are not infrequently met with. The nurseries are overcrowded; the infant is laid in a deep cot, wrapped up overwarmly in blankets, and left to breath for hours the atmosphere which is inclosed within the curtains or the sides of the cot; and which, moreover, is not seldom rendered still more impure by a want of the most sedulous attention to cleanliness on the part of the nurse. If to this be added the attempt to bring up the child entirely, or in great measure, on artificial food, we have at once the two conditions combined which are most certain to generate rickets.

Remove them; nourish the infant at the breast of a healthy nurse; place it in a large room, and in a cot which admits the air to pass freely over the child; let there be most careful attention to cleanliness; and improvement will become almost immediately apparent. If the disease is advanced, combine with all these precautions country or, still better, sea air, and even where marked deformity has already taken place, amendment will be sure to follow.

As the child grows older, and other food than the mother's or nurse's milk becomes necessary, let too exclusively farinaceous food be avoided. Beef tea at the age of eight or nine months; and a little underdone meat at fifteen or twenty months, are always desirable, while milk should always form an important part of the diet.

There is no specific for rickets—nothing which furnishes ready to hand, in a way in which it can be appropriated, the earthy matters in which the bones are deficient, and the notion that phosphate of lime supplied in large quantities to the child would directly promote its cure is but an unphysiological fallacy. Iron and cod liver oil* are the two great remedies on which, in this as well as in other cathectic diseases, we mainly rely. Their continuous employment, however, requires that attention be specially paid to the state of the digestive organs; but the simpler aperients, as rhubarb and magnesia, or caster oil, or syrup of senna, are to be preferred to the mercurial preparations which are so often employed without due occasion.'

* Charles West was evidently uncertain of the documented importance of cod liver oil in the cure of rickets.

APPENDIX II

A CURE FOR DEFICIENCY RICKETS

Appendix I reveals that Professor West in London knew of cod liver oil for the cure of rickets. But are we certain that he was truly convinced of its efficacy? He appears to be similar to many other physicians of his generation, who may have heard the message but did not yield to it with conviction. An English translation of an article, first published in the *Gazette Med. de Paris*, appeared in the *British Association Journal of Medicine* (Vol. IV) in 1848–9 entitled '*The History of Fish Liver Oil.*' The article clearly states that 'fish liver oil is without exception the best remedy for rickets in all its stages'. Professor Hanner of Munich described, in 1855, his success with the treatment of 200 cases of rickets; he prescribed 3–4 desert spoonfulls of cod liver oil. All his patients were cured of their rickets. Professor Vogel of Vienna reiterated the theme in 1884. Rickets remained endemic in the society in which these fine men lived and taught. Melanby identified a deficiency state as the cause of rickets in 1918; but the curative factor in cod liver oil, and known to be influenced by sunlight, was still referred to as substance X in the 1923 review of Parks.

Further perspectives of historical interest will be found in the articles by Loomis (1970) and Park (1923). The closing in Park's review might be found in today's Whole Earth Catalogue: 'Rickets is indeed a price paid by man for his abandonment of a life out-of-doors and a natural diet for life in houses and a diet of denatured food stuffs; it is a sign of the operation of the immutable law of nature that nothing out of accord with her shall flourish.' Park did not know about the hereditary forms of rickets.

APPENDIX III

The use of phosphate mixture in the treatment of X-linked hypophosphataemia

We have shifted from the use of a neutral phosphate mixture (pH 7·4) to an acidic phosphate mixture in the majority of our patients.

Acidic (Joulie's) phosphate solution

(1)	Dibasic sodium phosphate anhydrous, or $Na_2HPO_4 \cdot 12\ H_2O$	136 g
(2)	Phosphoric acid (NF 85%)	58·8 g
(3)	Make up with distilled water to	1000 ml

The solution is easily made by dissolving the phosphate salt in warm water to which is added the phosphoric acid followed by the addition of water up to 1 l, keep at room temperature.

The solution contains 483 mg inorganic phosphate /10 ml if made with the anhydrous salt, and 304 mg/10 ml when made with the dodecahydrate; the pH of the former solution is 5·9 and of the latter 4·3.

Treatment protocol

Phosphate supplementation is given five times daily and provides 1–4 grams of inorganic phosphorus per day. To begin treatment we administer 5 ml t.i.d. on the 1st day; 10 ml t.i.d. on the 2nd day; 10 ml q.i.d. on the 3rd day; 10 ml q.4.h. five times a day on the 4th day; and if necessary, 15 ml q.4.h. five times a day thereafter. The parents are warned to expect loose bowel movements initially but this is rarely a problem after treatment has been established.

Joulie's solution is taken with meals where possible; and when given between meals is followed by a drink of the patient's choice (3–4 oz).

The object of treatment is to obtain serum phosphorus levels in children of about 4 mg /100 ml. Frequent home visits, demonstration of serum response, measurement of linear growth and demonstration of catch-up growth and X-ray evidence of healing rickets provides positive encouragement to the patient and family regarding the benefits of treatment.

We have found that the night dose of phosphorus is important hence the reinforcement of the benefits of therapy, since this is a difficult treatment dose to give.

We recommend that the consumption rate of the phosphorus solution be monitored to assure that the maintenance dose is being followed.

REFERENCES

ALBRIGHT, F., BUTLER, A. H. and BLOOMBERG, E. (1937). Rickets resistant to vitamin D therapy. *A. J. Dis. Child.*, **54**, 529

ARNAUD, C., GLORIEUX, F. and SCRIVER, C. R. (1971). Serum parathyroid hormone in X-linked hypophosphataemia. *Science*, **173**, 145

ARNAUD, C., MAIJER, R., READE, T., SCRIVER, C. R. and WHELAN, D. T. (1970). Vitamin D dependency: An inherited postnatal syndrome with secondary hyperparathyroidism. *Pediatrics*, **46**, 871

ARNSTEIN, A. R. and HANSEN, C. A. (1969). Nature of renal phosphate leak. *N. Engl. J. Med.*, **281**, 1427

BALSAN, S., GARABEDIAN, M. and LEBOUADEC, L. (1972). Le rachitisme vitamino-resistant pseudocarentiel hypocalcémique. *Arch. Fr. Pediatr.*, **29**, 287

BORLE, A. B. (1973). Calcium metabolism at the cellular level. *Fed. Proc.*, **32**, 1944

CARD, R. T., BRAIN, M. C., LOTT, D. E. and MCNAMARA, M. A. (1973). The 'Anemia' of childhood, evidence for a physiological response to hyperphosphatemia. *N. Engl. J. Med.*, **288**, 388

CARTIER, P., LEROUX, J. P., BALSAN, S. and ROYER, P. (1970), Etude de la glycolyse et de la perméabilite des erythrocytes aux ions orthophosphates dans le rachitisme vitamino-résistant hypophosphatémique héréditaire. *Clin. Chim. Acta.*, **29**, 261

CHASE, L. R., MELSON, G. L., and AURBACH, G. D. (1969). Pseudo-hypoparathyroidism defective excretion of 3′, 5′-AMP in response to parathyroid hormone. *J. Clin. Invest.*, **48**, 1832

CLOW, C. L., FRASER, F. C., LABERGE, C. and SCRIVER, C. R. (1973), On the application of knowledge to the patient with genetic disease. *Prog. Med. Genet.*, **9**, 159

CLOW, C. L., READE, T. and SCRIVER, C. R. (1971). Management of hereditary metabolic disease. The role of allied health personnel. *N. Engl. J. Med.*, **284**, 1292

CONDEN, J. R., NASSIM, J. R. and RUTTER, A. (1970). Defective intestinal phosphate absorption in familial and non-familial hypophosphatemia. *Br. Med. J.*, **3**, 138

DENT, C. E. (1952). Rickets and osteomalacia from renal tubule defects. *J. Bone and Joint Surg. (Br).*, **34B**, 266

DENT, C. E. (1970). Rickets (and osteomalacia), nutritional and metabolic (1919–69). *Proc. R. Soc. Med.*, **63**, 401

DENT, C. E. and HARRIS, H. (1956). Hereditary forms of rickets and osteomalacia. *J. Bone and Joint Surg. (Br).*, **38B**, 204

FANCONI, A., FISCHER, J. A. and PRADER, A. (1974). Serum parathyroid hormone concentrations in hypophosphatemic vitamin D resistant rickets. *Helv. Paediatr. Acta*, **29**, 187

FANCONI, A. and PRADER, A. (1969). Die hereditäre pseudomangel rachitis. *Helv. Paediatr. Acta*, **24**, 423

FRAME, B., SMITH, R. W. Jr., FLEMING, J. L. and MANSON, G. (1963). Oral phosphates in vitamin D-refractory rickets and osteomalacia. *Am. J. Dis. Child.*, **106**, 147

FRASER, D., JACO, N. T., YENDT, E. R., MILNE, J. D. and LIN, E. (1957). The induction of *in vito* and *in vivo* calcification in bones of children suffering from vitamin D-resistant rickets without recourse to large doses of vitamin D. *Am. J. Dis. Child.*, **93**, 84

FRASER, D., GEIGER, D. W., MUNN, J. D., SLATER, P. E., JAHN, R. and LIN, E. (1958). Calcification studies in clinical vitamin D deficiency and in hypophosphatemic vitamin-D refractory rickets. The induction of calcium deposition in rachitic cartilage without administration of vitamin D. *Am. J. Dis. Child.*, **96**, 460

FRASER, D., KOOH, S. W., KIND, H. P., HOLICK, M. F., TANAKA, Y. and DELUCA, H. F. (1973). Pathogenesis of hereditary vitamin D-dependent rickets. An inborn error of vitamin D metabolism involving defective conversion of 25-hydroxy vitamin D to 1α,25-dihydroxyvitamin D. *N. Engl. J. Med.*, **289**, 817

FRASER, D. and SALTER, R. B. (1958). The diagnosis and management of the various types of rickets. *Pediatr. Clin. N. Am.*, **5**, 417

GERBEAUX-BALSAN, S. (1965). L'Absorption intestinale du phosphore dans le rachitisme vitamino-résistant hypophosphatémique héréditaire. Effects de fortes surcharges de phosphore et dès régimes très pauvres en calcium. *Rev. Fr. Etudes Clin. Biol.*, **10**, 65

GLORIEUX, F. H. and SCRIVER, C. R. (1972). X-linked hypophosphatemia: Loss of a PTH-sensitive component of phosphate transport. *Science*, **175**, 997

Glorieux, F. H. and Scriver, C. R. (1973). Transport, metabolism and clinical use of inorganic phosphate in X-linked hypophosphatemia. In B. Frame, A. M. Parfitt, and H. Duncan (eds), *The Clinical Aspects of Metabolic Bone Disease*, p. 421. (Amsterdam: Excepta Medica)

Glorieux, F. H. and Scriver, C. R. (1974). Parathyroid hormone secretion in X-linked hypophosphatemia. *N. Engl. J. Med.*, **290**, 1329

Glorieux, F. H., Scriver, C. R., Eicher, E. M., Southard, J. L. and Travers, R. (1974). X-linked hypophosphatemia in *Hyp/Y* mouse (abstract). *Pediatr. Res.*, **8**, 389

Glorieux, F. H., Scriver, C. R., Holick, M. F. and DeLuca, H. F. (1973). X-linked hypophosphatemic rickets: Inadequate therapeutic response to 1,25-dihydroxycholecalciferol. *Lancet*, **ii**, 287

Glorieux, F. H., Scriver, C. R., Reade, T. M., Goldman, H. and Rosenborough, A. (1972). Use of phosphate and vitamin D to prevent dwarfism and rickets in X-linked hypophosphatemia. *N. Engl. J. Med.*, **287**, 481

Glorieux, F. H., Travers, R., Delvin, E. E., Morin, C. L. and Poirier, R. (1974). Intestinal phosphate transport in familial hypophosphatemia (abstract). *Pediatr. Res.*, **8**, 381

Haddad, J. G. Jr., and Chyn, J. C. (1971). Competitive protein-binding radioassay for 25-hydroxycholecalciferol. *J. Clin. Endocrinol.*, **33**, 992

Hamilton, J. R., Harrison, J., Fraser, D., Radde, I., Morecki, R. and Paunier, L. (1970). The small intestine in vitamin D dependent rickets. *Pediatrics*, **45**, 364

Healy, M. J. R. (1968). The disciplining of medical data. *Br. Med. Bull.*, **24**, 210

Holick, M. F., Semmler, E. J., Schnoes, H. K. and DeLuca, H. F. (1973). 1α-hydroxy derivative of vitamin D_3: A highly potent analogue of 1α,25-dihydroxyvitamin D_3. *Science*, **180**. 190

Hunter, R. (1972). Rickets, Rinckets, Rekets or Rackets. *Lancet*, **i**, 1176

Lewy, J. E. Cabara, E. C., Repetto, H. A., Canterbury, J. M. and Reiss, E. (1972). Serum parathyroid hormone in hypophosphatemic vitamin D-ressitant rickets. *J. Pediatr.*, **81**, 294

Lilly, C. A., Peirce, C. B. and Grant, R. L. (1935). The effects of phosphates on the bones of rachitic rats. *J. Nutr.*, **9**, 25

Loomis, W. F., (1970). Rickets. *Sci. Am.*, **223**(**6**), 77

McCance, R. A. (1947). Osteomalacia with Looser's nodes (Mulliman's syndrome) due to a raised resistance to vitamin D acquired about the age of 15 years. *Quart. J. Med.*, **16**, 33

McInnes, R. R. and Scriver, C. R. (1974). Mechanism of amino-aciduria produced by calciotropic hormones and dibutyryl cAMP. *Clin. Res.*, **22**, 538A

Mellanby, E. (1919). An experimental investigation on rickets. *Lancet*, **i**, 407

Park, E. A. (1923). The etiology of rickets. *Physiol. Rev.*, **3**, 106

Paunier, L., Kooh, S. W., Conen, P. E., Gibson, A. A. M. and Fraser, D. (1968). Renal function and histology after long-term vitamin D therapy of vitamin D refractory rickets. *J. Pediatr.*, **73**, 833

Prader, Von A., Illig, R., and Heierli, E. (1961). Eine besondere Form der primären vitamin-D resistenten Rachitis mit Hypocalcämie und autosomal-dominantem Erbgang: die hereditäre Pseudo-Mangelrachitis. *Helv. Paediatr. Acta.*, **16**, 452

Reiss, E., Canterbury, J. M., Bercowitz, M. A. and Kaplan, E. L. (1970). The role of phosphate in the secretion of parathyroid hormone in man. *J. Clin. Invest.*, **49**, 2146

Reitz, R. E. qnd Weinstein, R. L. (1973). Parathyroid hormone secretion in familial vitamin D resistant rickets. *N. Eng.l J. Med.*, **289**, 941

Riggs, B. L., Sprague, R. G., Jowsey, J. and Maher, F. T. (1969). Adult-onset vitamin -D-resistant hypophosphatemic osteomalacia. Effect of total parathyroidectomy. *N. Engl. J. Med.*, **281**, 762

Scriver, C. R. (1970). Vitamin D dependency. *Pediatrics*, **45**, 361

Scriver, C. R. (1974). Rickets and the pathogenesis of impaired tubular transport of phosphate and other solutes. *Am. J. Med.*, **57**, 43

Scriver, C. R. and Bergeron, M. (1974). Amino acid transport in kidney. The use of mutation to dissect membrane and transepithelial transport. In W. L. Nyhan (ed.), *Hereditable disorders of Amino Acid Metabolism*, p. 155. (New York: Wiley)

Scriver, C. R., Goldbloom, R. B. and Roy, C. C. (1964). Hypophosphatemic rickets with renal hyperglycinuria, renal glucosuria, and glycylprolinuria. A syndrome with evidence for renal tubular secretion of phosphorus. *Pediatrics*, **34**, 357

Short, E. M., Binder, H. J. and Rosenberg, L. E. (1973) Familial hypophosphatemic rickets: defective transport of inorganic phosphate by intestinal mucosa. *Science*, **179**, 700

SHORT, E., SEBASTIAN, A., SPENCER, M. and MORRIS, R. C. Jr. (1974). Hyper-responsiveness of the phosphaturic effect of parathyroid hormone in X-linked hypophosphatemic vitamin-D-resistant rickets (FHR) (Abst. 282) *J. Clin. Invest.*, **53**, 75a

STEARNS, G. and BOYD, J. D. (1931). The healing of rickets coincident with low serum inorganic phosphorus. *J. Clin. Invest.*, **10**, 591

STEENDIJK, R. (1961). The effect of a continuous intravenous infusion of inorganic phosphate on the rachitic lesions in cystinosis. *Arch. Dis. Child.*, **36**, 321

STICKLER, G. B., HAYLES, A. B. and ROSEVEAR, J. W. (1965). Familial hypophosphatemic vitamin D-resistant rickets. *Am. J. Dis. Child.*, **110**, 664

STICKLER, G. B., JOWSEY, J. and BIANCO, A. J. (1971). Possible detrimental effect of large doses of vitamin D in familial hypophosphatemic vitamin D resistant rickets. *J. Pediatr.* **79**, 68

TENENHOUSE, H. S. and SCRIVER, C. R. (1975). Orthophosphate transport in the erythrocyte of normal subjects and of patients with X-linked hypophosphatemia. *J. Clin. Invest.*, **55**, 644

12

1α–hydroxyvitamin D : A comparative study in children

S. Balsan, M. Garabedian, R. Sorgniard, M. F. Holick and H. F. DeLuca

In 1972 Omdahl *et al.* described a method for the production of biosynthetic 1,25-dihydroxycholecalciferol (1,25$(OH)_2D_3$). This technique has been utilised in our laboratory for the past 2 years for the production of the hormonal form of cholecalciferol. The 1,25$(OH)_2D_3$ prepared was given orally to children with different types of D-resistant rickets. Preliminary results indicated that patients with 'pseudo-deficiency' rickets, an inherited disorder described by Prader *et al.* (1961), were sensitive to small doses of 1,25$(OH)_2D_3$, i.e. 2 μg/day, contrasting with their requirements for large doses of 25-hydroxycholecalciferol (25$(OH)D_3$), i.e. 265 μg/day. This observation and the fact that the doses of 1,25$(OH)_2D_3$ used were considered in the physiological range for humans led us (Balsan *et al.*, 1974) to suggest the hypothesis that this disorder may be related to a defect in the kidney enzyme 25-hydroxycholecalciferol 1α-hydroxylase. Similar results were observed by Fraser *et al.* (1973) who reached the same conclusion. In the absence of more direct evidences for a deficit of this kidney enzyme in patients with 'pseudo-deficiency' rickets we decided to test the validity of this hypothesis by investigating the minimal curative dose of 1,25$(OH)_2D_3$ for children with nutritional rickets and children with 'pseudo-deficiency' rickets. The assumption was that if both groups were in fact 1,25$(OH)_2$ D_3-deficiency rickets they would respond similarly to the same minimal active dose of the drug. But, amounts of 1,25$(OH)_2D_3$ sufficient for long-term clinical trials were not easily available. Therefore, the study was done with a synthetic analogue of 1,25$(OH)_2D_3$: 1α-hydroxyvitamin D_3 (1α$(OH)D_3$), (Holick *et al.*, 1973). First, the biologic effects of short-term oral administration of 1α$(OH)D_3$ were studied in patients belonging to the same diagnostic groups that had previously been studied with 1,25$(OH)_2D_3$. Once it was verified that 1α$(OH)D_3$ could be considered a valuable substitute to the hormonal form of cholecalciferol, the therapeutic effects of 1α(OH)D_3 were compared in a child with simple nutritional rickets and one with 'pseudo-deficiency' rickets.

Comparative effects of short-term oral administration of 1,25$(OH)_2D_3$ and 1α(OH)D_3

Investigations were carried out in 20 subjects* including one normal control aged 14 years 6 months, four children with D-deficiency rickets, four patients with 'pseudo-deficiency' D resistant rickets (PDR), two with hereditary hypophosphataemic D-resistant rickets (VDRR), one adolescent with late acquired D-resistant rickets as described by McCance (1947), and who had been in spontaneous recovery for 18 months, one patient with chronic idiopathic hypoparathyroidism, four children with terminal stage chronic renal failure and two children with cystinosis. In these different diagnostic groups the effects of short-term administration of 1,25$(OH)_2D_3$ were studied with some patients whereas 1,α(OH)D_3 was given to the others. The two children with cystinosis had severe impairment of their glomerular functions, i.e. creatinine clearances respectively of 6 and 40 ml/min/1·73 m^2, both received 1,25$(OH)_2D_3$. The effects of 1,25$(OH)_2D_3$ and of 1α(OH)D_3 were analysed in the same patient with chronic idiopathic hypoparathyroidism. All children with VDRR or with PDR, the adolescent with late acquired D-resistant rickets and the one with chronic idiopathic hypoparathyroidism had been previously treated with vitamin D or 25(OH)D_3. Therapy had been stopped for 2–16 months when the present study was started. None of the other subjects had received any vitamin D.

The 1,25$(OH)_2D_3$ used was biosynthetically prepared in the Laboratoire des Tissues Calcifies, Paris, from synthetic 25(OH)D_3 (Laboratoire Roussel, Paris, France) and D-deficient chick kidney homogenate according to the technique described by Omdahl *et al.* (1972). 1α(OH) D_3 was synthetised in the department of Biochemistry, University of Wisconsin Madison, Wis., USA by M. F. Holick and H. F. DeLuca. The drugs were administered orally as propylene glycol solution. Doses used were 2 μg/d/5 d for 1,25$(OH)_2D_3$ and 1 μg/d/5 d for 1α(OH) D_3 in all cases studied, except for the patient with chronic idiopathic

* Informed consent was obtained from the parents and when appropriate from the child.

hypoparathyroidism who was given 2 μg/d/5 d of 1,α(OH)D_3 then, after an interval of 7 days, 2 μg/d/5 d for 1,25$(OH)_2D_3$.

Results with 1,25$(OH)_2D_3$.

This compound had no effect on any of the biochemical parameters studied in the two children with cystinosis. For all other patients oral administration of 2 μg/d for 5 days of the active metabolite of vitamin D promoted a clear-cut rise in serum calcium concentrations (Figure 12.1). An increase in serum phosphorus concentrations was observed in the child with D-deficiency rickets, three patients with 'pseudo-deficiency' rickets and the child with VDRR (Figure 12.2). In this last patient a transient rise in TRP, i.e. 61% during therapy versus 36% during the control period, occurred. Serum phosphorus decreased slightly then increased sharply in the two children with severe chronic renal failure. In contrast, in the adolescent with chronic idiopathic pypoparathyroidism 1,25$(OH)_2D_3$ administration promoted a fall in serum phosphorus concentration, this effect persisted one week after cessation of therapy. No changes of endogenous creatinine clearance were observed during this investigation. The effects of 1,25$(OH)_2D_3$ on serum citrate as on the other parameters studied, were variable from case to case.

Results with 1α$(OH)D_3$

Figure 12.3 illustrates the maximal variations in serum calcium concentrations. A rise was observed in all subjects studied. This augmentation occurred either during 1α$(OH)D_3$ administration or during the post-treatment period. The most important variation from base-line level (+ 1·4 mg/100 ml) was found in a D-deficient severely hypocalcaemic child who had been given i.v. calcium gluconate infusion 12 hours prior to 1α$(OH)D_3$ therapy. Serum phosphorus concentration (Figure 12.4) decreased in the patient with chronic idiopathic hypoparathyroidism; in all other subjects, except one child with chronic renal failure receiving anticonvulsant therapy, serum phosphorus concentration rose. An augmentation in serum citrate concentration was found in seven out of eight subjects studied. A transient rise in TRP occurred during therapy in the child with VDRR. 1α$(OH)D_3$ did not modify endogenous creatinine clearance and urinary excretion of calcium; the effects on serum alkaline phosphatase and urinary excretion of cAMP were variable.

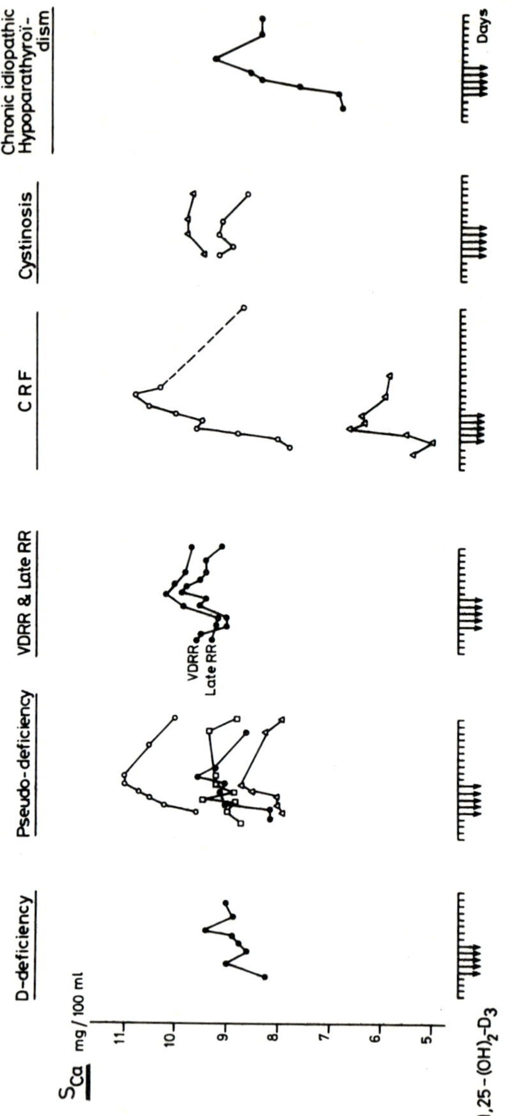

FIGURE 12.1 Serum calcium concentrations (SCa) during short-term protocol with 1,25(OH)$_2$D$_3$. The arrows on the horizontal axis represent days of oral 1,25(OH)$_2$D$_3$ administration. VDRR = hereditary hypophosphataemic rickets; late RR = Late acquired D-resistant rickets; CRF = Chronic renal failure.

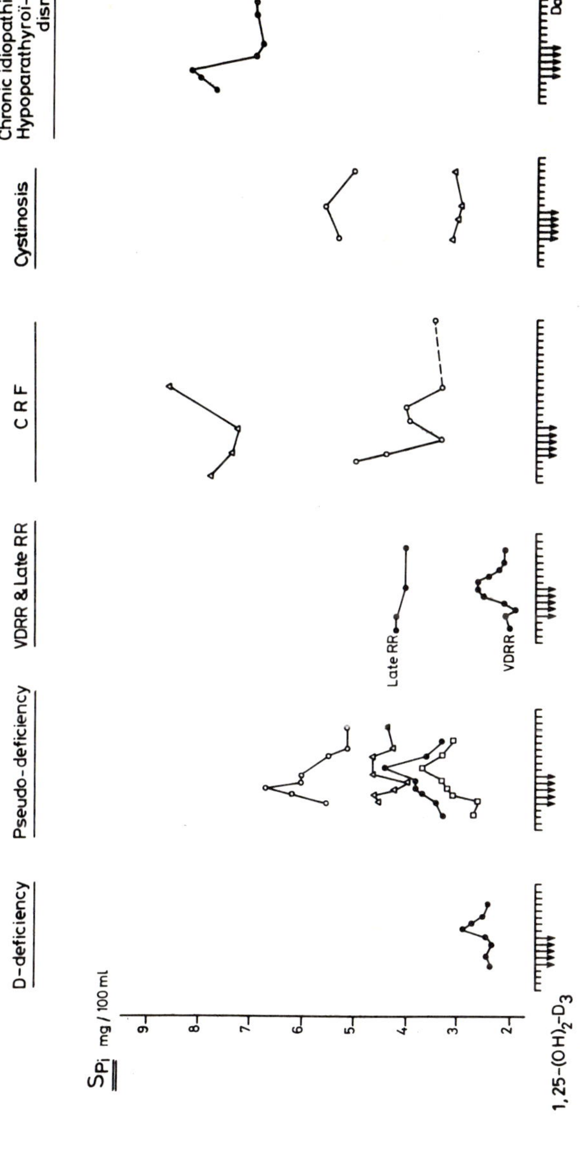

FIGURE 12.2 Serum phosphorus concentrations (SP_i) during short-term protocol with 1,25$(OH)_2D_3$. Same symbols and abbreviations as in Figure 12.1.

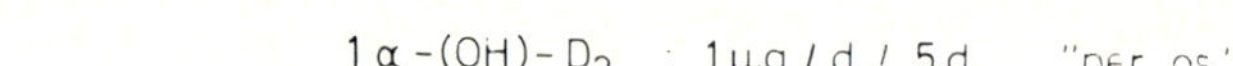

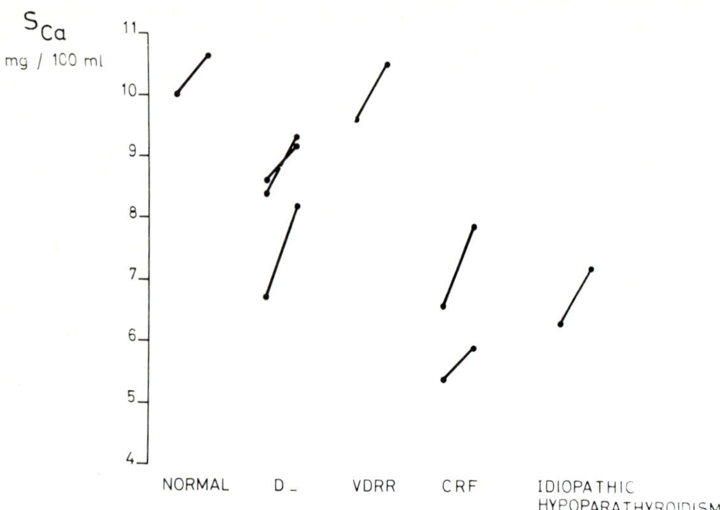

FIGURE 12.3 Serum calcium concentrations. Maximal variations (mg/100 ml) observed during short-term protocol with $1\alpha(OH)D_3$.

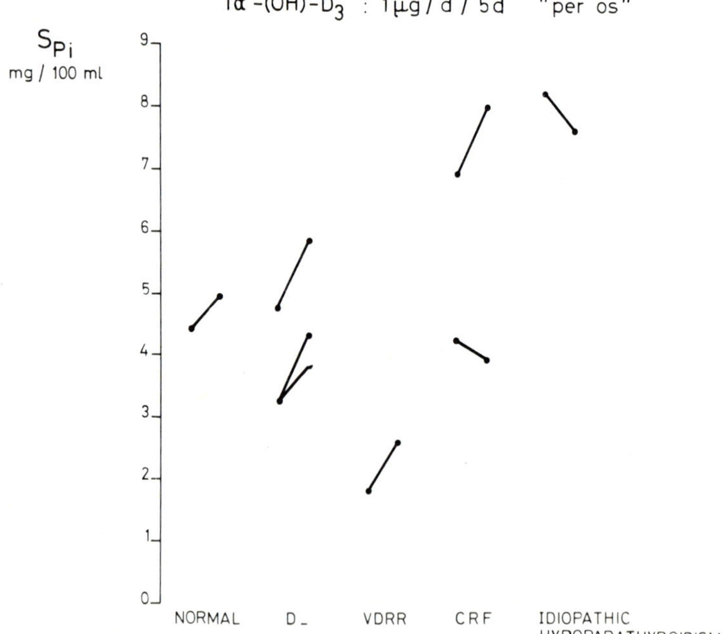

FIGURE 12.4 Serum phosphorus concentrations. Maximal variations (mg/100 ml) observed during short-term protocol with $1\alpha(OH)D_3$.

Comparative effects of long-term oral administration of 1α(OH)D_3 in a child with nutritional rickets and one patient with PDR

The effects of long-term administration of 1α(OH)D_3 were investigated with two patients : a 16-month-old child with D-deficiency rickets and one patient with 'pseudo-deficiency' rickets who had been previously treated with 1,25$(OH)_2D_3$. For the child with D-deficiency, treatment was restarted with 1α(OH)D_3 5 days after the end of the short-term protocol. At that time, his blood chemistry was as follows: serum calcium 9·1 mg/100ml; serum phosphorus 4·1 mg/100 ml; serum alkaline phosphatase 29 Bodansky units (Figure 12.5). Serum

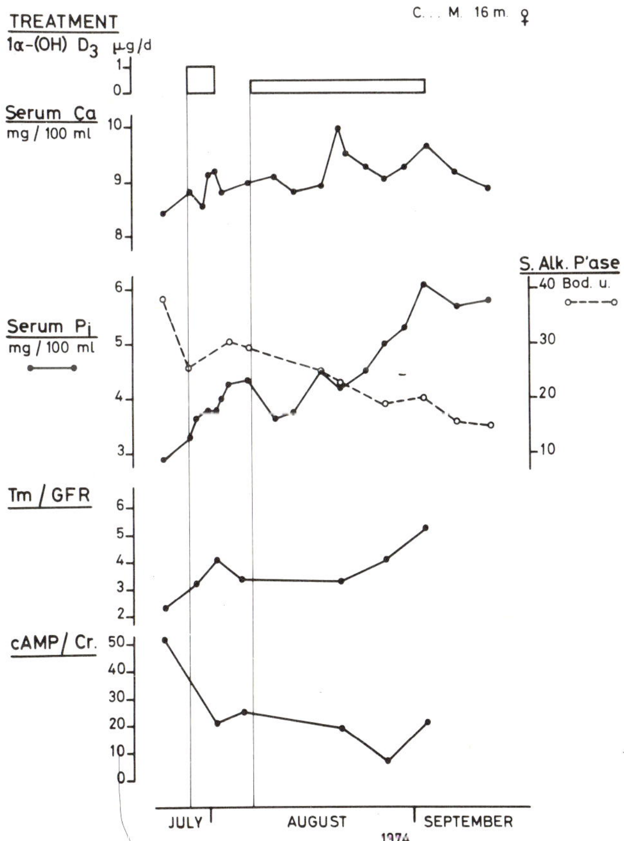

FIGURE 12.5 Effects of short-term and long-term administration of biosynthetic 1,25$(OH)_2D_3$ on two sibs with 'pseudo-deficiency' rickets. The arrows indicate the days and the doses of 1,25$(OH)_2D_3$ therapy.

citrate was normal at 2·3 mg/100 ml. The urinary cAMP/creatinine ratio was elevated, i.e. 25 and phosphorus Tm/GFR was 3·44. On treatment with 0·5 μg/d for 28 days serum calcium and citrate remained in the normal range, serum phosphorus concentration increased progressively and reached 6·1 mg/100 ml on the 28th day and serum alkaline phosphatase activity became normal. Tm/GFR reached 5·19, while urinary cAMP/creatinine ratio fell to 7·2 on the 21st day. Comparison of radiographs obtained at the start and at end of the 1α(OH)D_3 therapy demonstrated initiation of healing of the bone lesions. One week after cessation of treatment serum calcium had decreased from 9·7 to 8·9 mg/100 ml with serum phosphorus still at a high normal concentration (5·8 mg/100 ml).

The effects of 1α(OH)D_3 therapy were evaluated at two dose-levels, i.e. 5 μg/d/25 d then 1 μg/d/20 d on a 7-year-old patient with PDR. This child and her brother aged 5 years had been previously treated with biosynthetic 1,25$(OH)_2D_3$, i.e. 1 μg/d/28 d. As reported elsewhere (Balsan *et al.*, 1974) this treatment promoted in both children normalisation of serum chemistry (Figure 12.6) and initiated healing of skeletal lesions. When the present investigations was started (Figure 12.7) the patient was in biochemical relapse; X-ray examination demonstrated

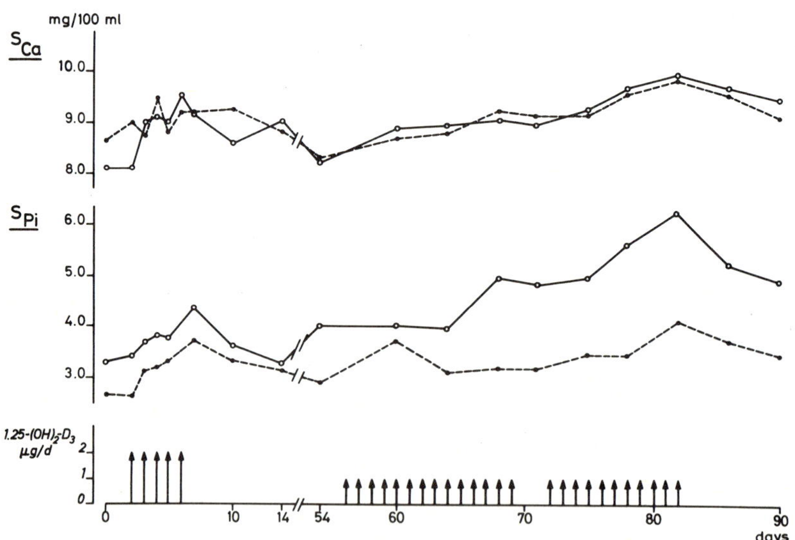

FIGURE 12.6 Effects of short-term and long-term administration of 1α(OH)D_3 on a D-deficient child aged 16 months. cAMP/cr = urinary cAMP (μmol) to creatinine (g), ratios.

the reappearance of bone lesions and balance studies showed a negative calcium balance with a poorly positive phosphorus balance (Figure 12.8).

On long-term treatment with 0·5 g/d/25 d (Figure 12.7), serum calcium concentration augmented progressively and reached 7·9 mg/100 ml. Serum phosphorus concentrations, after an initial rise to 4·2 mg/100 ml,

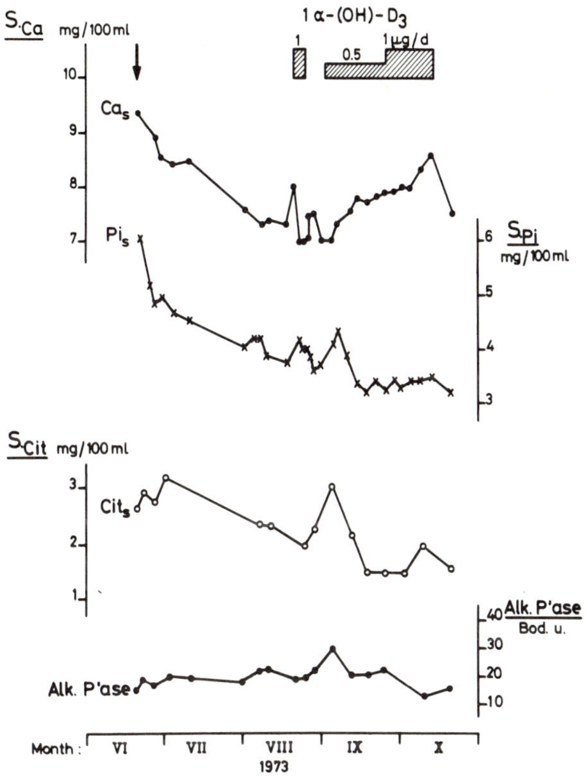

FIGURE 12.7 Long-term therapy with $1\alpha(OH)_2D_3$ of one of the sibs with PDR. The arrow indicates the end of $1,25(OH)_2D_3$ treatment shown on Figure 12.5. S_{cit} = serum citrate concentrations.

fell and remained stabilised around 3·2 mg/100 ml, likewise serum citrate concentration increased from 2·2 mg to 3·0 mg/100 ml on the 5th day, then decreased to 1·4 mg/100 ml. The results obtained in the first period of the balance studies during long-term indicated a positive balance for calcium (+114 mg/d) and for phosphorus (1+ 253 mg/d); during the subsequent periods calcium balances were at equilibrium and phosphorus balances were only slightly positive. When the daily

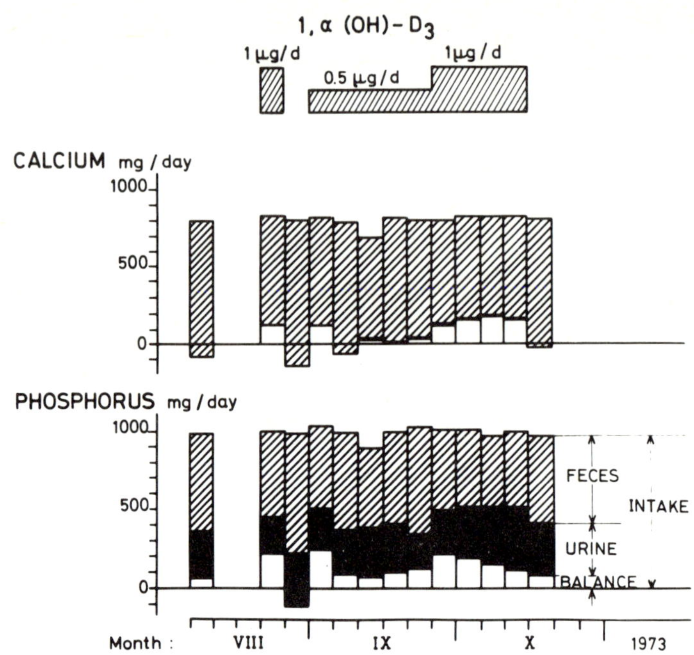

FIGURE 12.8 Stable calcium and phosphorus balance studies of the child with PDR, before, during and after 1α(OH)D_3 therapy. Each column represents a 5-day period. Carmine was used as a faecal marker.

oral dose of 1α(OH)D_3 was doubled, the calcium balance of this patient became positive again (+ 112 mg/d) and remained so throughout the study. A further elevation of serum calcium concentration occurred; serum calcium reached 8·6 mg/100 ml after 3 weeks of therapy. Serum alkaline phosphatase fell from 22·3 to 11·4 Bodansky units. In contrast, no significant changes in serum phosphorus concentration were observed. Net intestinal absorption of phosphorus increased, as shown by a diminution of faecal phosphorus excretion (Figure 12.8). However, this improvement in intestinal absorption was followed, after 10 days of treatment with 1 μg/d of 1α(OH) D_3, by an increased urinary output and a decreased phosphorus Tm/GFR (calculated according to the normogram of Bijvoet, Morgan and Fourman, 1969). As a consequence the phosphorus balances became less and less positive during the last two periods of 1α(OH)D_3 therapy. Five days after 1α(OH) D_3 treatment was stopped, serum calcium concentration fell to 7·5 mg/100 ml, and once again net intestinal calcium absorption decreased leading to a negative calcium balance. For this patient, the radiologic examinations done at the end of 1α(OH)D_3 therapy at each dose level, showed the persistence of rachitic lesions. When these X-rays were compared to the pretreatment radiographs, neither healing nor deterioration could be detected.

Summary

This investigation confirms the high biological activity and the similarity of the effects of small doses of 1,25$(OH)_2D_3$ and of its analogue 1α(OH)D_3 on children with nutritional rickets, 'pseudo-deficiency' rickets (PDR), hereditary hypophosphataemia, chronic idiopathic hypoparathyroidism and chronic renal failure. It also shows that cystinotic patients may develop at the end-stage of the disease a certain degree of resistance to 1,25$(OH)_2D_3$.

The comparison of the therapeutic effects of long-term oral administration of 1α(OH)D_3 to a D-deficient child and one patient with PDR demonstrates differences in sensitivity. In the patient with nutritional rickets 0·5 μg/d of 1α(OH)D_3 corrects the biochemical abnormalities and initiates healing of skeletal lesions in 28 days. In contrast, it appears clearly that this dose, followed by a double dose for another 20-day period, is only partly active in PDR.

These observations indicate that the hypothesis of a deficit in 25-hydroxycholecalciferol 1α-hydroxylase in patients with PDR must await for confirmation more direct evidence, and that such a deficit, even if proven, may not account for all the biochemical and skeletal alterations seen in patients with this inherited disorder.

Acknowledgement

This investigation was supported in part by grants from the Centre National de la Recherche Scientifique (ATP No. 5305) and the Délégation Générale pour la Recherche Scientifique et Technique (DGRST No. 72 7 0026).

REFERENCES

Balsan, S., Garabedian, M., Pavlovitch, H. and Sorgniard, R. (1974). 1,25-dihydroxycholecalciferol: biological and therapeutic effects in children. In S. Taylor (ed.), *Endocrinology* 1973, p. 379. Proceedings of the IVth international symposium (London : Heinemann).

Bijvoet, O. L. M., Morgan, D. B. and Fourman, P. (1969). The assessment of phosphate reabsorption. *Clin. Chim. Acta*, **26**, 15

Fraser, D., Kooh, S. W., Kind, H. P., Holick, M. F., Tanaka, Y. and DeLuca, H. F. (1900). Pathogenesis of hereditary vitamin D dependent rickets. An inborn error of vitamin D metabolism involving defective conversion of 25-hydroxycholecalciferol to 1α,25-dihydroxyvitamin D. *N. Engl. J. Med.*, **289**, 817

Holick, M. F., Semmler, E. J., Schnoes, H. and DeLuca, H. F. (1973). 1α-hydroxy derivative of vitamin D_3 : A highly potent analog of 1α,25-dihydroxyvitamin D_3. *Science*, **180**, 190

McCance, R. A. (1947). Osteomalacia with Looser's nodes (Milkman's syndrome) due to a raised resistance to vitamin D acquired about the age of 15 years. *Quart. J. Med.*, **61**, 33

Omdahl, J. L., Gray, R. W., Boyle, I. T., Knutson, J., DeLuca, H. F. (1972). Regulation of metabolism of 25-hydroxycholecalciferol by kidney tissue *in vitro* by dietary calcium. *Nature*, **237**, 63

Prader, A., Illig, R. and Heierli, E. (1961). Eine besondere Form der primären vitamin-D resistenten Rachitis mit Hypocalcämie und autosomal-dominantem Erbgang : die hereditäre Pseudo-mangelrachitis. *Helv. Pediatr. Acta*, **16**, 452

13

Tubular Fanconi Syndromes with bone involvement

J. Brodehl

The DeToni-Debré-Fanconi Syndrome (DDFS) is characterised by functional disturbances of the tubular cells in the kidney. The physiological role of these tubules is to reabsorb most of those many substances filtered through the glomerular basement membrane into the tubular lumen, in order to maintain the homeostasis of body fluids. Gross impairment of these reabsorptive processes lead to changes in the acid-base and electrolyte content of the body fluids which may affect normal growth and functioning of many organs including the skeletal system. Dwarfism, therefore, and rickets, are predominant features of the renal Fanconi Syndrome.

Historical remarks

A special tubular type of renal rickets was first postulated by DeToni, who in 1933 at the London International Congress of Paediatrics presented a case of a 5-year-old girl who showed severe renal rickets which was accompanied by hypophosphataemia and renal glucosuria. A similar case was observed by Debré *et al.* and published one year later. Debré's case was an 11-year-old girl who in addition to glucosuria and rickets exhibited an excessive urinary loss of organic acids bound to fixed bases and ammonia.

In 1936 Fanconi described three additional cases of the 'nephrotic–glucosuric dwarfism with hypophosphataemic rickets', including one who had already been mentioned by him in 1931. Fanconi was able to show that one of his cases had an excessive loss of organic acids also, which he reasoned could possibly be amino acids. This was proved in 1943 by McCune *et al.*, who demonstrated that 82% of organic acids excreted in a case with Fanconi Syndrome were indeed free amino acids. Dent, using paper chromatography, finally demonstrated the renal origin and the generalised type of hyperaminoaciduria in this syndrome.

Definition

I will not go further into the intricate history of this syndrome, but rather try to define it as it is understood today: the DeToni-Debré-Fanconi Syndrome, which is often just referred to as the renal Fanconi Syndrome, is a syndrome of generalised dysfunction of the proximal renal tubules leading to excessive loss of amino acids, glucose, phosphate, bicarbonate and some other substances while the glomerular filtration is not primarily affected. The metabolic consequences are acidosis, hypophosphataemia and dehydrations which provoke rickets, osteoporosis and growth retardation. This syndrome may be congenital or acquired, idiopathic or symptomatic.

In the following I shall first discuss the pathophysiology of the Fanconi Syndrome, with emphasis on the pathomechanisms of those essentials of the syndrome., i.e. the hyperaminoaciduria, glucosuria and phosphate diabetes including the bone involvement. Then I will try to give a certain classification of the different types of the Fanconi Syndrome and finally present some additional aspects of typical cases.

Hyperaminoaciduria

The first symptom to be discussed in hyperaminoaciduria. In the DDF-syndrome, the amounts of free amino acids found in the urine are greatly increased. In Figure 13.1 the urinary excretion rates of free amino acids in a child with Fanconi Syndrome and glycogenosis are compared with the excretion rates of normal children. All amino acids are involved in this hyperaminoaciduria, the individual amino acids to a very variable degree.

The hyperaminoaciduria is of renal origin and is not due to increased plasma levels of amino acids. The rates of tubular reabsorption are reduced in this syndrome as shown for alanine in Figure 13.2, where the reabsorption rates in 34 normal children are compared with those of six patients with the Fanconi Syndrome, of whom two had glycogenosis and the other four cystinosis. The endogenous tubular load calculated from the glomerular filtration rate, measured by inulin, and the plasma concentration of alanine is plotted against the net tubular reabsorption (T_{Ala}). The values for the normal children are just below the line of identity of load and reabsorption regardless of the height of the endogen-

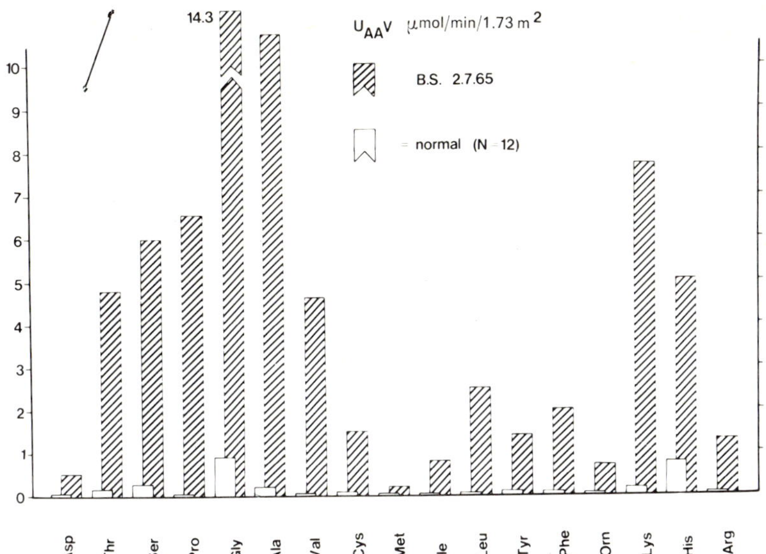

FIGURE 13.1 Endogenous urinary excretion rates of free amino acids in a boy with glycogenosis and Fanconi Syndrome (B.S., hatched columns) in comparison with normal excretion rates (from Brodehl and Gellissen, 1968).

ous load. This means, that in normal states alanine is reabsorbed by the tubules almost completely. In contrast patients with the Fanconi Syndrome show variable rates of reabsorption at given loads. The vertical distance from the symbol up to the line of identity represents the net amount of alanine excreted in the urine, while the vertical line down to the abscissa represents the net amount of reabsorption. Both rates are rather variable, even in the same patient, and the percentage of alanine which is reabsorbed is obviously independent of the total amount filtered by the glomeruli. The percentage tubular reabsorption (%TAA) is, therefore, the best parameter to assess the tubular handling of amino acids.

In Figure 13.3 the rates of percentage tubular reabsorption are given for 17 amino acids as they were found in seven children with the Fanconi Syndrome, of whom three had cystinosis, two had glycogenosis, and one each had galactosaemia and nephropathy due to outdated tetracycline. There are some amino acids which are highly excreted, and others exhibiting only slight decreases in the percentage reabsorption. A certain pattern seems to evolve which will be recognised much more easily when the mean values are calculated for each individual amino acid.

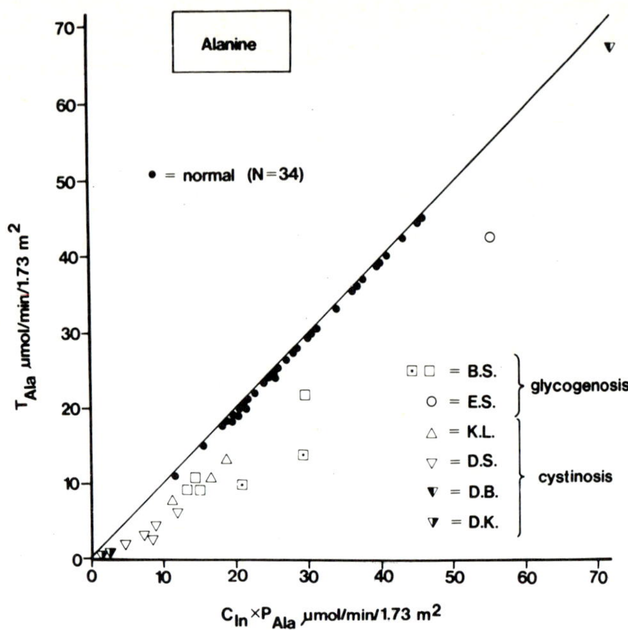

FIGURE 13.2 The tubular reabsorption of alanine (T_{Ala}) in 34 normal children (black circles) and six children with Fanconi Syndrome. T_{Ala} is plotted against tubular load ($C_{In} \times P_{Ala}$).

In Figure 13.4 those mean values of the same patients are compared with the normal values of percentage tubular reabsorption (see Brodehl and Gellissen, 1968). The distinct pattern of generalised hyperamino-aciduria becomes quite obvious: those amino acids which physiologic-ally show the lowest reabsorption rates, namely glycine and histidine, have also the lowest percentage rates in the Fanconi Syndrome, while those amino acids which normally show almost complete reabsorption, such as proline, valine, isoleucine, ornithine, and arginine preserve high reabsorption rates in the Fanconi Syndrome also. Thus, the hyper-aminoaciduria of the Fanconi syndrome shows a generalised pattern which is an exaggeration of the pattern found normally.

The mechanism by which generalised hyperaminoaciduria is pro-duced is not thoroughly understood. It usually is explained by a defective tubular reabsorption. Some experimental studies, however, indicate that increased leakage from the tubular cells could also be responsible for the hyperaminoaciduria. Rosenberg and Segal (1964) found in experi-mental maleic acid intoxication that the efflux of amino acids from the tubular cells was indeed increased. More recently Bergeron and Vadebonceour (1971) showed by micropuncture studies in the rat that maleic acid did not reduce the tubular reabsorption of arginine and leucine but produced an increase in the leakage from the peritubular space into the tubular lumen, which could be responsible for the increased amount of amino acid in the urine. These findings still have to be confirmed. If they are confirmed it would change drastically our understanding about the mechanism of hyperaminoaciduria.

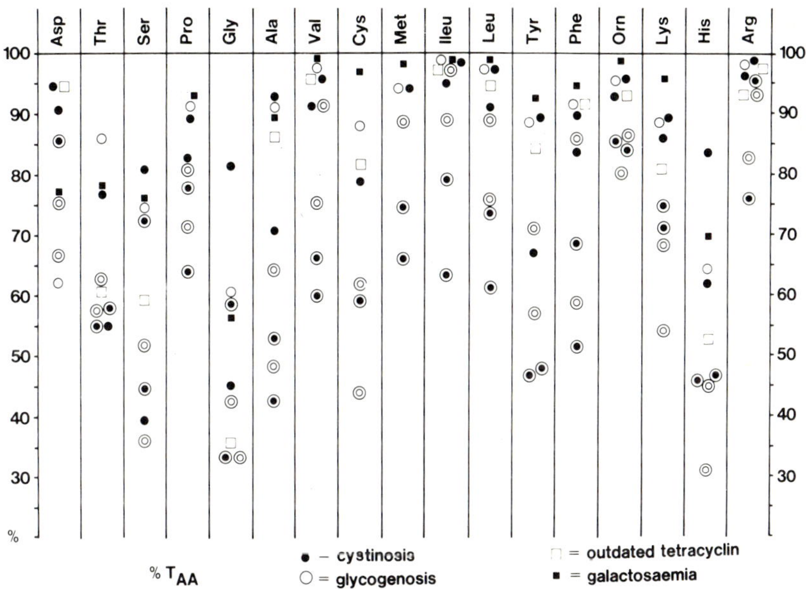

FIGURE 13.3 The percentage tubular amino acid reabsorption (%T_{AA}) in seven children with Fanconi Syndrome (three cystinosis, two glycogenosis, one galactosemia, one outdated tetracycline).

Glucosuria

Glucosuria is the second cardinal symptom of the Fanconi syndrome. It is also of renal origin as already described by DeToni in his first report. The amount of glucose excreted is very variable which allows us to differentiate different types of this syndrome as will be shown later.

Normally the tubular reabsorption of glucose is almost complete until the blood glucose level reaches the renal threshold which is about 180 mg/100 ml. This behaviour is indicated by the solid line on Figure 13.5, in which the tubular reabsorption (T_G) is plotted against tubular

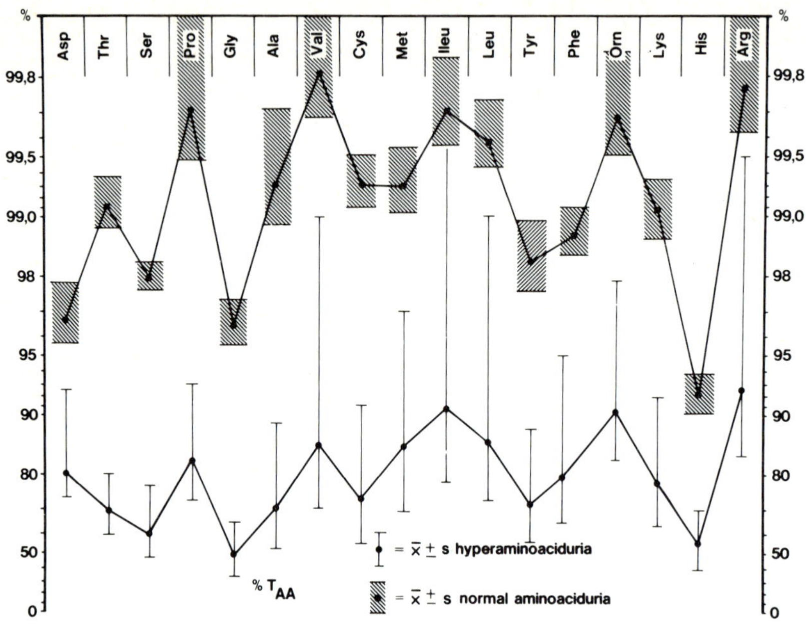

FIGURE 13.4 The mean values of percentage tubular amino acid reabsorption (%TAA) in 12 normal children (from Brodehl and Gellissen, 1968) compared with means values values of seven children with Fanconi Syndrome (see Figure 13.3).

load ($C_{In} \times P_G$). Two patients with the Fanconi syndrome due to cystinosis, show T_G values only slightly below the line of identity. They have therefore only slight to moderate glucosuria in normoglycaemia in contrast to the boy with the glycogenosis (B.S.) who exhibits a highly disturbed tubular reabsorption of glucose even under normo- or hypoglycaemia. The renal threshold for glucose, which can be calculated by T_G/C_{In} seems to be extremely low in this case, leading to excessive urinary loss of glucose.

Glucose loading tests to determine maximal glucose reabsorption may be dangerous in some types of the Fanconi Syndrome. Therefore, only a few data on Tm_G are available. In Figure 13.6 the Tm_G values, divided by C_{In}, are plotted against the glucose load, calculated from C_{In} and the plasma glucose level. The normal values derived from 16 children (Brodehl *et al.*, 1972) are shown by the shadowed area. As can be seen in a low range of glucose load, between 300 and 600 mg/min, there was a marked lowering of Tm_G/C_{In}, as measured in three cases with Fanconi Syndrome. In one case however the continued glucose

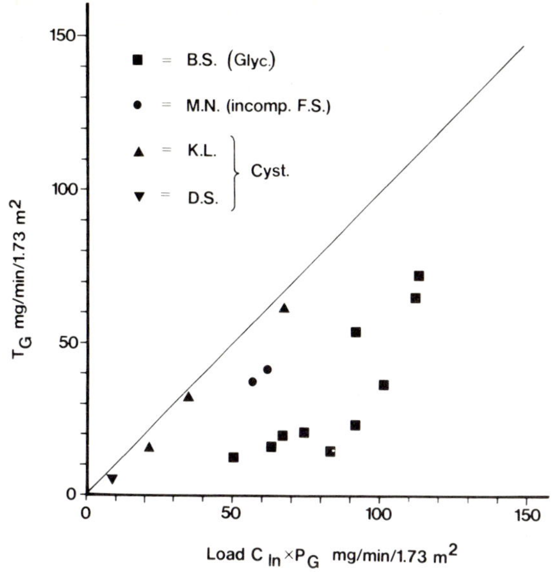

FIGURE 13.5 The tubular reabsorption of glucose (T_G) in relation to tubular load ($C_{In} \times P_G$) in four children with Fanconi Syndrome. The diagonal line of identity represents complete reabsorption as normally found.

loading led to an unexpected elevation of glucose load up to 1200 mg/min which then was accompanied by normal values of T_{mG}/C_{In}. The same phenomenon has been described by Bauer (1968) in a case with glycogenosis. Whether this would be true in all cases with Fanconi Syndrome remains a completely open question.

Glucosuria in the Fanconi Syndrome, therefore, is of variable degree and is the result of both a lowered renal threshold for glucose and a lowered maximal capacity of tubular glucose reabsorption. Both could be explained by a highly increased functional or morphological heterogeneity of the nephron population. Clinically the massive glucosuria may produce hypoglycaemias especially in those cases with glycogenosis.

Phosphate diabetes

Phosphate diabetes is considered to be the most critical symptom of the Fanconi Syndrome. It is closely related to the changes in mineralisation of the skeletal system.

In Figure 13.7 the urinary excretion rates of phosphate in four children with the Fanconi Syndrome are compared with those of normal

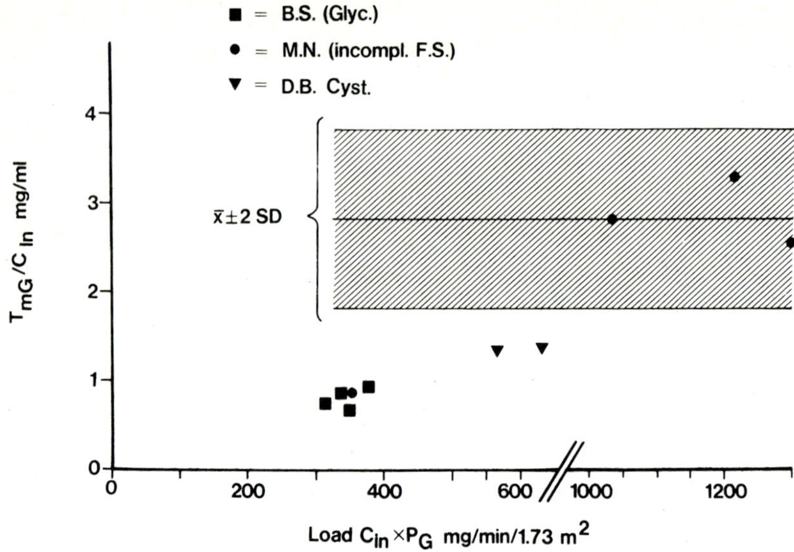

FIGURE 13.6 The maximal tubular reabsorption of glucose corrected for glomerular filtration rate (T_{mG}/C_{In}) in three children with Fanconi Syndrome compared with normal values (from Brodehl *et al.*, 1972). T_{mG}/C_{In} is plotted against tubular load ($C_{In} \times P_G$)

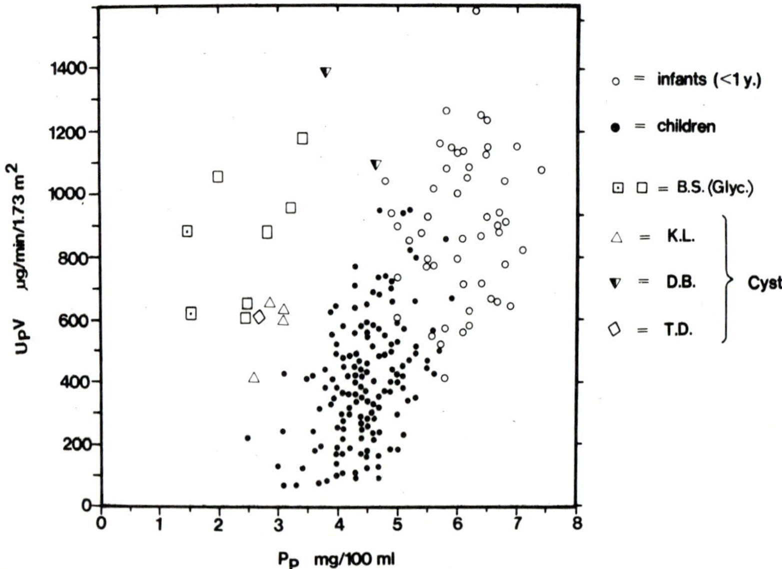

FIGURE 13.7 The urinary phosphate excretion (U_PV) in normal infants ($n = 31$) and children ($n = 143$) compared with those of four children with the Fanconi Syndrome. U_PV is plotted against plasma phosphate concentration (P_P).

infants and children. The urinary phosphate excretion U_pV is plotted against the plasma level of phosphate P_p. All values were obtained by clearance studies. As can easily be recognised the rates of urinary phosphate excretion are not significantly higher in patients with the Fanconi Syndrome than in normals, they are, however, accompanied by significantly lower values of plasma phosphate. Hypophosphataemia, therefore, is the main pathophysiological parameter of phosphate diabetes, and not hyperphosphaturia *per se*.

Hypophosphataemia is produced by a decrease in tubular phosphate reabsorption. The most determining factor for plasma phosphate is the fractional phosphate reabsorption which can be calculated as T_p/C_{In}. This is significantly lowered in all cases of Fanconi Syndrome, as shown on Figure 13.8. The only exception seemed to be one infant with

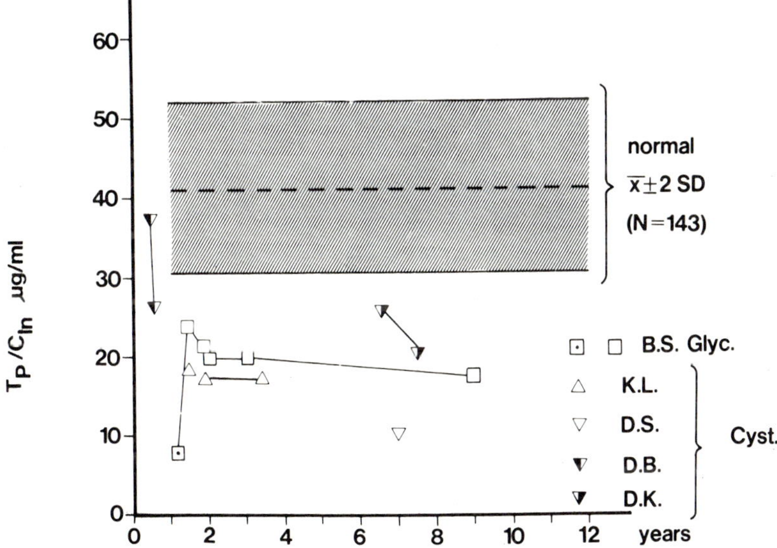

FIGURE 13.8 Fractional phosphate reabsorption (T_p/C_{In}) in five children with Fanconi Syndrome compared to normal values (hatched area). T_p/C_{In}) is plotted against age, the lines connect identical cases examined at various ages.

cystinosis (D.B.), who was 6 months old when first examined. The second investigation however, performed only 2 weeks later, did already reveal the decrease in T_p/C_{In}. He, obviously, was just at the point of developing phosphate diabetes.

Phosphate loading does not increase the tubular rates of phosphate reabsorption as is shown in a few cases with Fanconi Syndrome in

Figure 13.9. The endogenous rates are shown on the left, the rates after intravenous phosphate loading on the right. In normal children too there is no increase of T_p/C_{In} after loading, as indicated by the shadowed area.

Thus, hypophosphataemia is a constant finding in the Fanconi Syndrome. The low plasma phosphate levels are the result of a decrease in the fractional tubular phosphate reabsorption and are the most important factor in the impaired mineralisation of skeletal system.

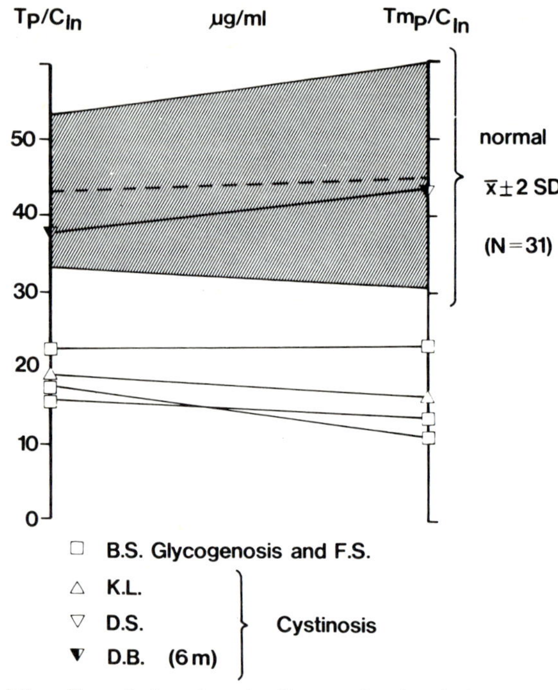

FIGURE 13.9 The effect of phosphate loading on fractional phosphate reabsorption (T_p/C_{In}) in four children with Fanconi Syndrome compared with normal children ($n = 31$). T_p/C_{In} represent endogenous values, Tm_p/C_{In} values obtained after acute phosphate loading, demonstrating no significant changes.

There is much evidence, that the tubular defect in phosphate transport is a cellular one, and not just mediated by hyperparathyroidism, as has occasionally been postulated.

There are more additional signs of tubular impairment in the DDF syndrome which include the decreased threshold for bicarbonate, the increased clearances of potassium and urate, the defective urinary concentrating ability, the organic aciduria and a certain type of tubular proteinuria. These symptoms, which will not be discussed further may be responsible for acidosis, hypokalaemia, hypouricaemia and polyuria with polydipsia and dehydration. All these signs are as variable as the tubular defects and depend on the rate of glomerular filtration which may be impaired secondarily.

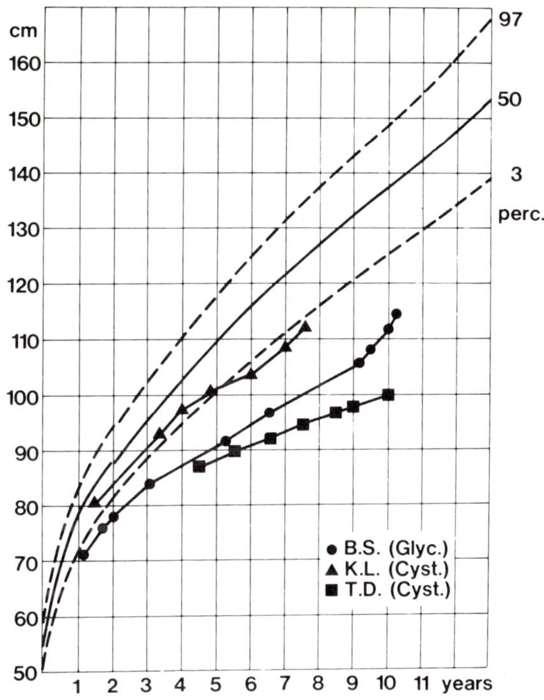

FIGURE 13.10 The growth curves in three children with Fanconi Syndrome.

Bone involvement

The bone involvement is the most prominent clinical finding in the Fanconi Syndrome. It shows a wide spectrum which includes defective mineralisation and demineralisation, rickets or osteomalacia, osteoporosis and in advanced cases with glomerular insufficiency osteodystrophy. These changes will produce growth retardation, fractures and pseudofractures, and crippling deformities of the bones.

Growth is retarded in most cases of Fanconi Syndrome. The growth rates of three children with Fanconi Syndrome are depicted in Figure 13.10. Two of them suffered from cystinosis, one from glycogenosis. All three are below the 3rd percentile for height although there are great individual differences, irrespective of the type of Fanconi Syndrome as demonstrated by the two children with cystinosis. The patient K.L. was treated continuously from the age of 1 year with vitamin D and alkali, while the other one could not receive such consistent treatment, which may partly explain the differences.

On X-ray examinations the bones are demineralised and show signs of rickets especially on the epiphyseal lines of the long bones. In advanced cases of cystinosis there will be overt signs of hyperparathyroidism which accompanies the glomerular insufficiency.

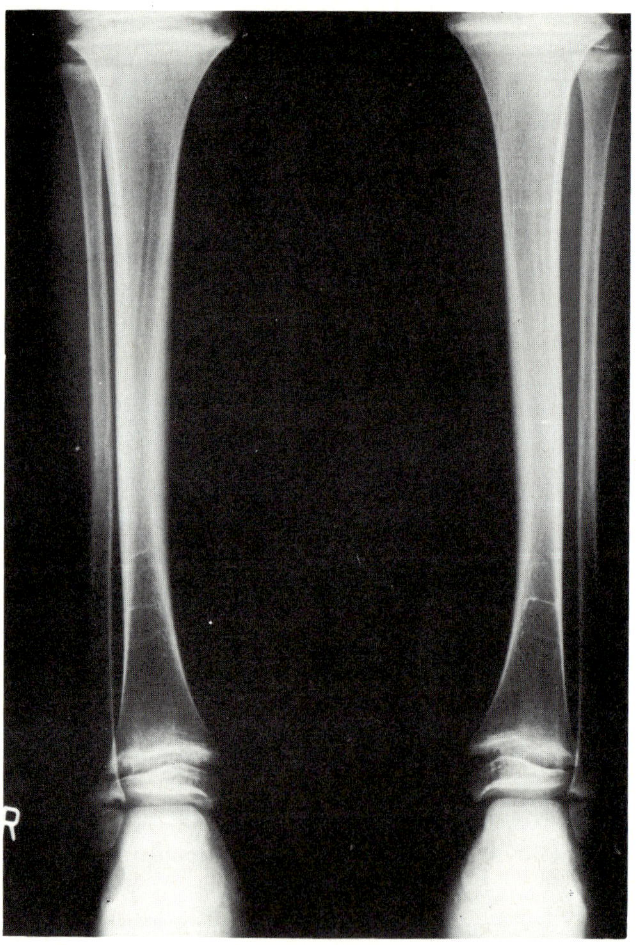

FIGURE 13.11 X-ray of leg in boy with glycogenosis (B.S.) demonstration severe osteoporosis.

In the Fanconi Syndrome with glycogenosis the most prominent sign on X-rays is osteoporosis (Figure 13.11), which is not found in cystinosis, while the signs of rickets very much depend on treatment and often are not found in treated cases. There is no sign of hyperparathyroidism in this type of Fanconi Syndrome which has completely normal glomerular filtration rates at all times.

The bone histology confirms the X-ray findings. The biopsies of our patients were obtained from the iliac crest by the technique of Burckhardt, and processed by Dr Vykoupil of the Pathological Institute of the Medical School, Hanover. The biopsy from a cystinotic patient demonstrates seams and patches of unmineralised osteoid (Figure 13.12). The normal lamellar structure of the bone is still preserved, there are, however, signs of increased activity of osteoblasts with lacunar erosions as signs of secondary hyperparathyroidism.

The biopsy of the boy with glycogenosis is quite different (Figure 13.13). Here the most prominent finding is extreme osteoporosis as can easily be recognised in comparison with Figure 13.12, which shows identical regions of the bone. The osteoid however, when present, is normally mineralised and no signs of hyperparathyroidism are visible.

The skeletal changes depend on the homeostasis of calcium and phos-

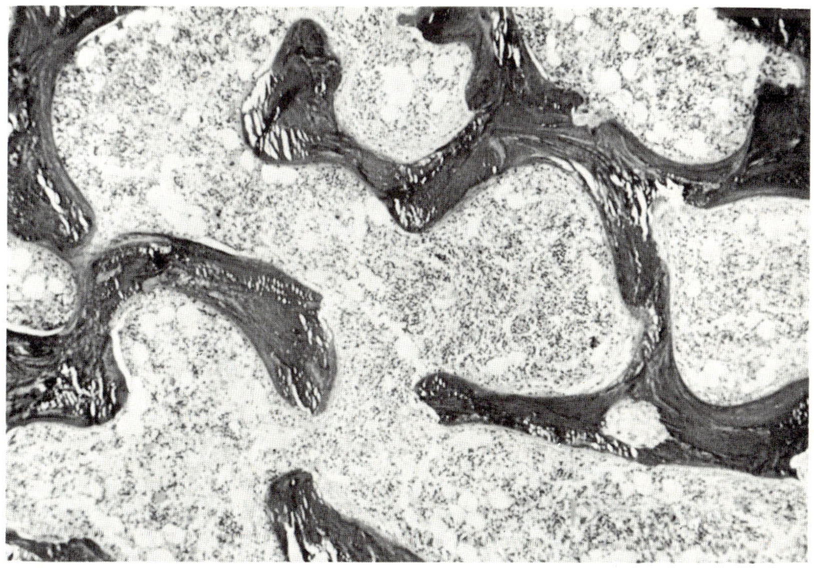

FIGURE 13.12 Bone biopsy from iliac crest of patient with cystinosis. By courtesy of Dr Vykoupil, Pathological Institute of Hanover Medical School (Prof. Georgii).

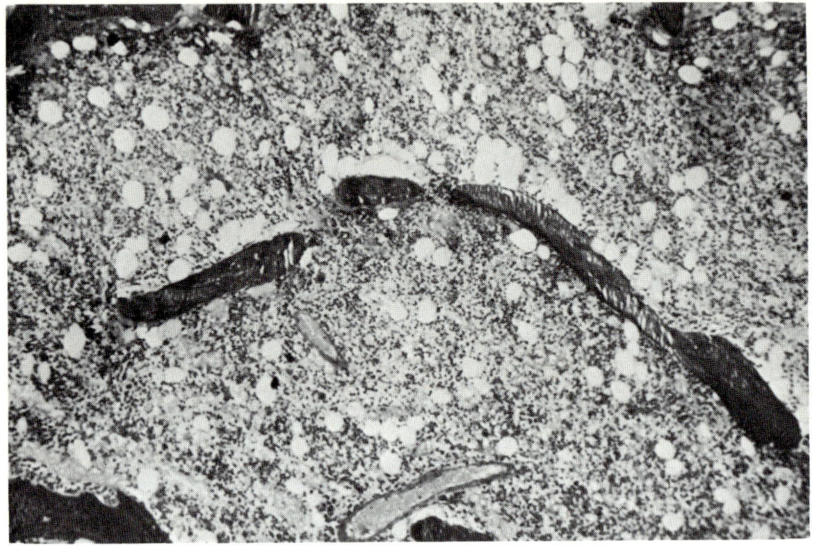

FIGURE 13.13 Bone biopsy from iliac crest of patient with glycogenosis and Fanconi Syndrome (B.S.) By courtesy of Dr Vykoupil, Pathological Institute of Hanover Medical School (Prof. Georgii).

phorus in the extracellular fluid, on endocrine control and glomerular function, and on the presence and activation of vitamin D. The bone histology thus reflects many parameters which have to be considered in the individual case, in order to find more effective ways of treatment to prevent severe bone changes, deformities, and growth retardation.

Classification

Variability is found in the severity of tubular defects, as already pointed out, and in the extent to which the various transport systems are involved in individual cases. The DDF-syndrome is obviously not a nosological entity, but is characterised by a variety of aetiologies, phenomenologies and clinical courses. These have to be differentiated by thorough clinical examinations of the whole patient and quantitative analysis of the disturbed metabolism and function.

In Table 13.1 a classification is attempted according to the underlying pathogenetic mechanisms leading to the syndrome. One may differentiate between the renal DDF-syndrome, in which the primary defect is located within the tubular cells, and the prerenally caused DDF-syndrome, in which toxic metabolites outside the kidney lead to toxic changes in the tubular function.

The renal type can be pure, which means that no other primary metabolic derangements are found, and this type is then called 'idiopathic', or the renal type can be associated with an extra-renal metabolic disorder, in such a way that both the tubular and the extra-renal cells are submitted to the same metabolic block. This type which is really a mixed renal and prerenal one, is found in cystinosis, and may also exist in glycogenosis and in Lowe's Syndrome.

Table 13.1 *Classification of DeToni–Debré–Fanconi Syndrome* (DDFS)

I Renal DDFS
- (a) 'Idiopathic' (pure renal)
- (b) Renal with associated pre renal metabolic disorder
  - (1) Cystinosis
  - (2) Glycogenosis
  - (3) Lowe's Syndrome

II Pre Renal DDFS ('Symptomatic')
- (a) Inborn errors:
  Galactosaemia, fructose intolerance, tyrosinaemia, ornithinaemia, Wilson's disease
- (b) Acquired:
  Multiple myeloma, nephrotic syndrome, transplanted kidney
- (c) Intoxications:
  Heavy metals, maleic acid, lysol, degraded tetracycline

There was much debate whether the tubular defect in cystinosis is just produced by an overloading with cystine or whether the tubular cells are directly disturbed by the same metabolic defect found in the whole organism. Recent clinical trials with renal transplantations in patients with cystinosis, however, showed clearly that the Fanconi Syndrome does not return in spite of the fact that cystine was again found to accumulate in the transplanted kidney (Briggs *et al.*, 1972; Hambridge *et al.*, 1969; Lucas *et al.*, 1969; Mahoney *et al.*, 1970). This indicates that a primary *renal* cause of the DDF syndrome must exist in cystinosis. Whether the same pathogenetic mechanism operates in glycogenosis and in Lowe's Syndrome must remain questionable, as long as the underlying metabolic defect in these syndromes is not recognised.

The symptomatic or prerenal types of the DDF syndrome can either be produced by inborn errors of metabolism, such as galactosaemia, fructose intolerance, tyrosinaemia and others, or by acquired diseases like multiple myeloma or the nephrotic syndrome, or by intoxications with heavy metals, organic substances or drugs such as outdated tetracycline. These prerenal types are usually reversible as long as the underlying cause can be eliminated.

Some types of the DDF syndromes exhibit rather distinct patterns of functional involvement. They may, therefore, be differentiated by exact quantitative measurements of the defective tubular functions, as will be illustrated with a few clinical observations.

IDIOPATHIC FANCONI SYNDROME

The first case (C.H.) is a girl of 7 years, who suffered from an idiopathic type of the DDF syndrome. Her main complaint had been muscular weakness and bone pain prior to admission. She had a bilateral congenital cataract which was operated on at 4 years of age. Enzymatic tests for uridyltransferase and galactokinase activities were normal. She was still of normal height for her age while her weight was 5 kg below the 3rd percentile.

The values of kidney function tests in this patient are given in Table 13.2. Her glomerular filtration rate was completely normal, while the *p*-amino hippurate clearance (C_{PAH}) was severely impaired indicating a defect in tubular PAH secretion.

The endogenous phosphate clearance was greatly increased, the fractional tubular phosphate reabsorption T_P/C_{In} being correspondingly very low. The amino acid clearance was also greatly increased, the type of hyperaminoaciduria being generalised. The glucose reabsorption was only moderately impaired, with a glucose clearance of 27 ml and a glucose threshold T_G/C_{In} of 57 mg/100 ml.

Thus, this idiopathic type is characterised by a severe defect in phosphate and amino acid reabsorption and PAH secretion while the glucose reabsorption is only moderately impaired.

The renal biopsy, which was kindly made available to us by Dr Zobl (Pathological Institute of the Medical School, Hanover) showed dilatations of the tubuli on light microscopy. The diameters of the tubules

Table 13.2 *Renal function in the idiopathic Fanconi Syndrome* (*C.H.*)

C_{In}	= 149 ml/min/1·73 m² (117 ± 17)
C_{PAH}	= 194 ml/min/1·73 m² (534 ± 104)
FF	= 0·77 (21·8 ± 2·1)
C_p	= 56·1 ml/min/1·73 m² (8·8 ± 4·1)
T_p/C_{In}	= 7·1 μg/ml (41 ± 5·4)
C_{AA}	= 20·0 ml/min/1·73 m² (1·7)
$\%T_{AA}$	= 86·4% (98·6)
C_G	= 26·5 ml/min/1·73 m² (0·0)
C_G/C_{In}	= 0·18
T_G/C_{In}	= 57 mg/100 ml

Normal values in brackets (mean ± S.D. own laboratory).

measured up to 300 μm, which means that they were sometimes as wide as Bowman's capsule.

The proximal tubular cells (Figure 13.14) were partly swollen and contained a fine granular material, while other parts looked completely normal. The electronmicroscopic examination, performed by Dr v.

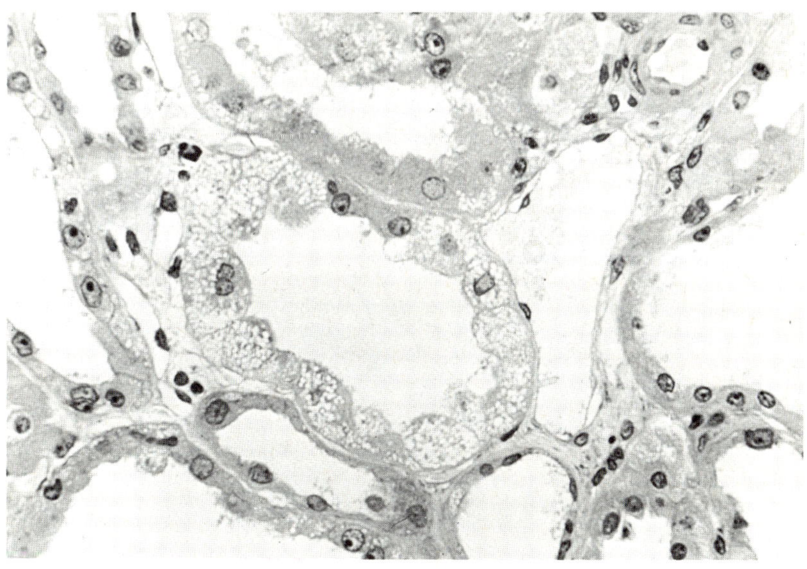

FIGURE 13.14 Kidney biopsy in patient with idiopathic Fanconi syndrome (C.H.). By courtesy of Dr Zobl, Pathological Institute of Hanover Medical School (Prof. Georgii).

Bassewitz, Münster, showed grossly enlarged mitochondria located around the nucleus of the tubular cell (Figure 13.15).

These giant mitochondria show triple-layered cristae which are dislocated laterally or even marginally and occasionally contain electron-dense material.

Some tubular cells also contain dark granules in the cytoplasm

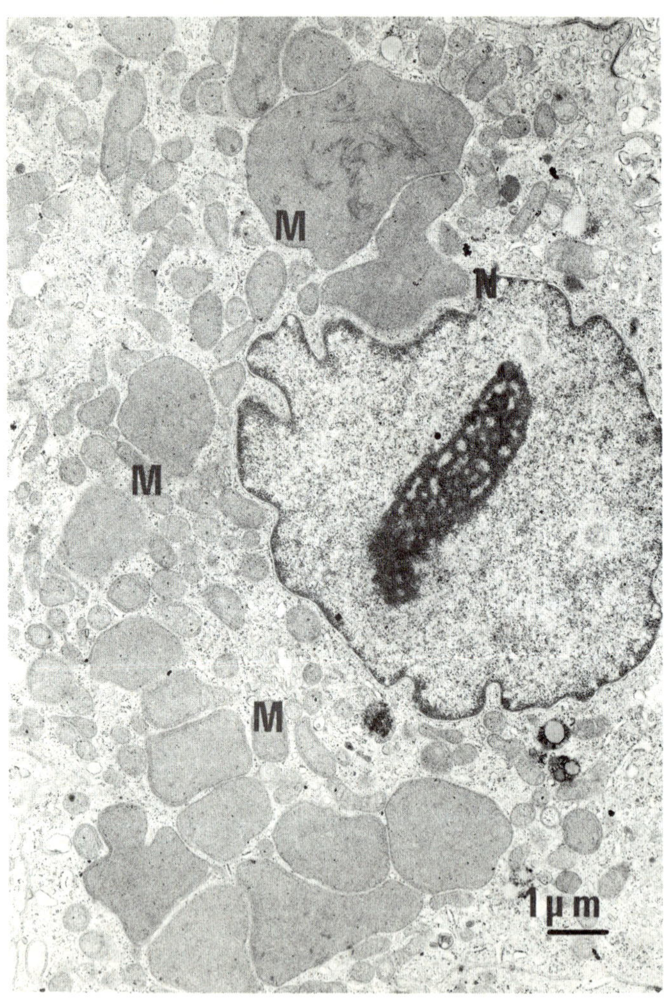

FIGURE 13.15 Electron microscopy of kidney biopsy in idiopathic Fanconi Syndrome (C.H.), demonstrating giant mitachondria. By courtesy of Dr v. Bassewitz, Institute of Medical Cytobiology, University of Münster. (Prof. Themann). M = Giant mitochondria, N = nucleus, magnification 8000 ×.

which probably represent glycogen. The main histological finding therefore consists of the giant mitochondria which may indicate that the energy supplying or transferring apparatus of the cells are somehow involved in this syndrome.

GLYCOGENOSIS WITH FANCONI SYNDROME

The second case (B.S.) is a DDF syndrome associated with glycogenosis of the liver. This type was first described by Fanconi and Bickel (1949). Since then only a few more cases have been published (see Table 13.3).

Table 13.3 *Maximal urinary glucose excretion in glycogenosis with DDF Syndrome (renal glucose losing syndrome)*

Author	*Age*	*Max.* U_G (g/100 ml)	U_GV (g/day)	U_GV (g/day/1·73 m^2)
Fanconi and Bickel 1949	4 years	6·0	64	240
Rotthauwe *et al.*, 1963	4 years	5·8	55	206
Odievre 1966 R. L.	2 years	?	50	210
B. B.	6 years	?	21 (Av.)	74
Lampert and Mayer, 1967	4 years	8·0	73	230
Bauer, 1968	5 years	?	53	178
Brodehl *et al.*, 1969	1 year	5·4	43	200

Our patient was 1 year old when he was first seen by us. He had suffered from fever, thirst and malnutrition, had typical signs of rickets and showed an enlarged abdomen with hepatomegaly. His parents are consanguineous. An older sister had died at the age of 5 months with unexplained high fever.

The laboratory findings revealed a severe hypophosphataemia (0·6 mmol/l). Serum bicarbonate was low, as was the fasting glucose level. Serum lactate stayed in the normal range.

The glycogen content of the liver, kindly determined by Prof. Hers, Louvain, amounted up to 9 g/net weight. The activities of the glycogenolytic enzyme in the liver and in the muscles were within the normal range. Thus a clear cut enzymatic defect could not be established in this boy nor in other identical cases described in the literature.

The kidney function in B.S. is shown on Table 13.4. There was a severe decrease in the fractional phosphate reabsorption and a massive generalised hyperaminoaciduria (see Figure 13.1). The most remarkable defect, however, was seen in glucose reabsorption. In normoglycaemia a glucose clearance of C_G of 89 ml was measured and the ratio of glucose clearance to inulin clearance C_G/C_{In} was 0·7. This means, that 70% of the glucose filtered through the glomeruli is excreted in the urine, or only 30% is reabsorbed respectively. This could repeatedly be measured in this boy and stayed constant over a 9-year period of observation.

Table 13.4 *Renal function in glycogenosis with Fanconi Syndrome (BS)*

C_{In}	= 128 ml/min/1·73 m^2
C_{PAH}	= 434 ml/min/1·73 m^2
FF	= 0·23 ml/min/1·73 m^2
C_p	= 59 ml/min/1·73 m^2
T_p/C_{In}	= 8·0 μg/ml
C_{AA}	= 47·4 ml/min/1·73 m^2
$\%T_{AA}$	= 63%
C_G	= 89 ml/min/1·73 m^2
C_G/C_{In}	= 0·70
T_G/C_{In}	= 23 mg/100 ml

See Table 13.2 for normal values.

The glucosuria in all these cases with glycogenosis and DDF syndrome is indeed remarkably severe (Table 13.3). Almost all cases reported in the literature show maximal daily urinary glucose excretion rates of 200 g/1·73 m^2 or more. One has to realise that this is occurring continuously in these patients, in spite of the fact that they are normo— or even hypo-glycaemic.

This is much more than in other cases with the DDF syndrome. It therefore was proposed by Fellers, Piedrahita and Galan (1967) to call this syndrome 'pseudo-phlorizin-diabetes' while we preferred to call it 'renal glucose losing syndrome' (Brodehl *et al.*, 1969).

The clinical course of the glycogenosis type of DDF syndrome is favourable. The patient is now 10 years old, active and doing well. His height however, is far below the 3rd percentile (see Figure 13.10).

CYSTINOSIS WITH FANCONI SYNDROME

In cystinosis, finally, there is a secondary impairment of the glomerular filtration rate which shows a steady decline leading to renal insufficiency. In Figure 13.16 the inulin clearance rates in two boys with cystinosis are plotted against age. The closed symbols represent values corrected to the surface area of adults, while the open symbols represent the actual rates measured. There is a progressive decline of the GFR per 1·73 m², while the actual rates seem to be comparatively stable. One could speculate that after the early severe kidney injury caused by the metabolic defect, there is actually no more growth of the nephrons along with somatic growth, or that a certain population of nephrons could be resistant to the metabolic defect, and the slow deterioration would be explained by interstitial infiltrations and fibrosis of the kidney.

The tubular defects in cystinosis are not as severe as in glycogenosis, as was shown earlier. There is, however, a very early and severe impairment in the tubular PAH secretion. In Figure 13.17 the values of

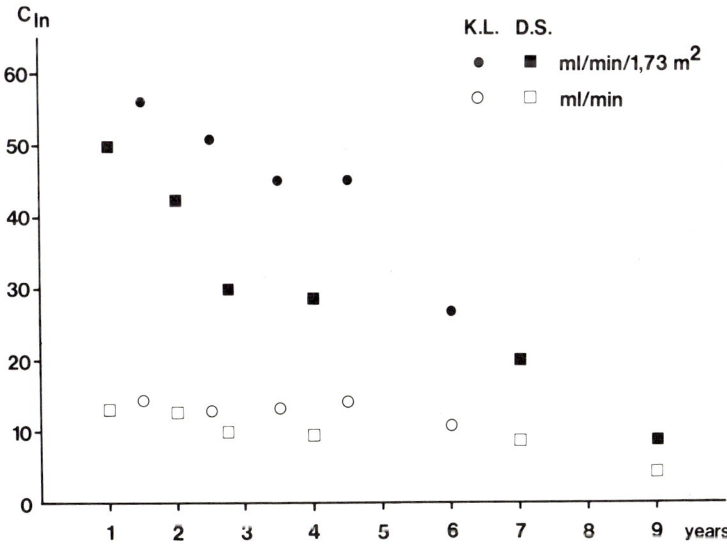

FIGURE 13.16 The development of glomerular filtration rate (C_{In}) in two boys with cystinosis. The actual values measured and the same values corrected for surface area adults are given

maximal tubular PAH secretion (Tm_{PAH}), in a boy with cystinosis are compared with normal values. There is strong inhibition of PAH-secretion, which is not simply due to decline of glomerular filtration rate, as the ratio of Tm_{PAH}/C_{In} shows the same decrease.

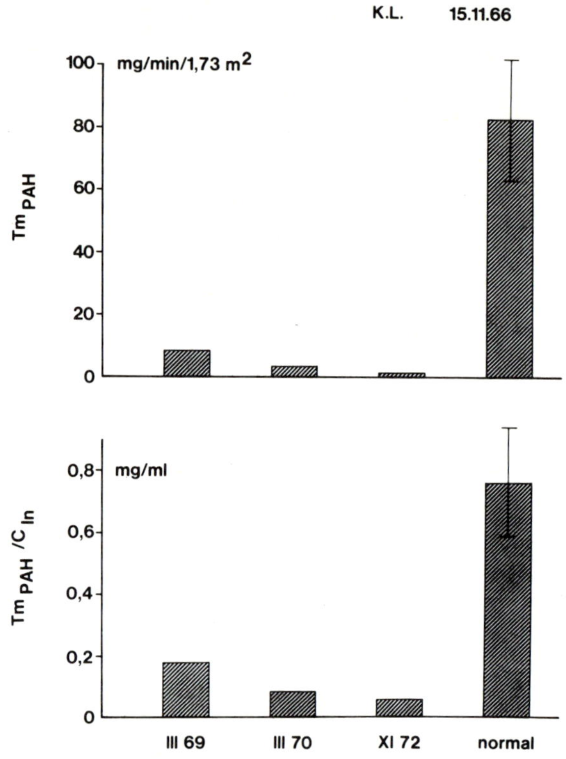

FIGURE 13.17 The maximal tubular secretion of p-amino hippurate (PAH) in a boy with cystinosis in comparison to normal values.

Summary

The DeToni–Debré–Fanconi Syndrome is a complex dysfunction of the tubular cells, which may be caused by various aetiological factors, which can be differentiated according to the severity and extent of the tubular defects and which are accompanied by variable changes in the skeletal system including rickets, osteoporosis and growth retardation. The clinical course and the response to therapy depend on the type of the DDF syndrome.

REFERENCES

Bauer, B. (1968). Debré-DeToni–Fanconi Syndrom mit Glykogenese der Leber. *Klin. Wochenschr.*, **46**, 317

Bergeron, M. and Vadeboncoeur, M. (1971). Microinjections of L-Leucine into tubules and peritubular capillaries of the rat. II. The maleic acid model. *Nephron*, **8**, 367

Briggs, W. A., Kominami, N., Merrill, J. P. and Wilson, R. E. (1972). Kidney transplantation in Fanconi Syndrome. *N. Engl. J. Med.*, **286**, 25

Brodehl, J. and Gellissen, K. (1968). Endogenous renal transport of free amino acids in infancy and childhood. *Pediatrics*, **42**, 395

Brodehl, J., Gellissen, K. and Hagge, W. (1969). The Fanconi syndrome in hepato renal glycogen storage disease. In G. G. Peters and F. Roch-Ramel, (eds.), *Progress in Nephrology*, p. 241. (Berlin-Heidelberg–New York : Springer-Verlag)

Brodehl, J., Franken, A. and Gellissen, K. (1972). Maximal tubular reabsorption of glucose in infants and children. *Acta Paediatr. Scand.*, **61**, 413

Debré, R., Marie, J., Clerét and Messimy, R. (1934). Rachitisme tardif coexistant avec une néphrite chronique et une glycosurie. *Arch. Med. Enfants*, **37**, 597

Dent, C. E. (1947). The amino-aciduria in Fanconi syndrome. A study making extensive use of techniques based on paper partition chromatography. *Biochem. J.*, **41**, 240

DeToni, G. (1933). Remarks on the relations between renal rickets (renal dwarfism) and renal diabetes. *Acta Paediatr.*, **16**, 479

Fanconi, G. (1931). Die nicht diabetischen Glykosurien und Hyperglykämien des älteren Kindes. *Jahrb. Kinderh.*, **133**, 257

Fanconi, G. (1936). Der frühinfantile nephrotisch-glykosurischer Zwergwuchs mit hypophosphatämischer Rachitis. *Jehrb. Kinderh.*, **147**, 299

Fanconi, G. and Bickel, K. (1949). Die chronische Aminoaciduria (Aminosäurendiabetes oder nephrotisch-glukosurischer Zwegwuchs) bei der Glykogenose und der Cystinkrankheit. *Helv. Paediatr. Acta.*, **4**, 359

Fellers, F. X., Piedrahita, V. and Galan, E. M., (1967). Pseudo-phlorizin-diabetes. (Abstract) *Paediatr. Res.*, **1**, 304

Hambridge, K. M. *et al.*, (1969). Accumulation of cystine following renal homotransplantation for cystinosis. *Pediatr, Res.*, **3**, 364

Lampert, F. and Mayer, H. (1967). Glykogenose der Leber mit Galaktoseverwertungsstörung und schwerem Fanconi-Syndrom. *Zeitschr. Kinderh.*, **98**, 133

Lucas, Z. J., Kempson, R. L., Palmer, J. Korn, D. and Cohn, R. B. (1969). Renal allotransplantation in man. II. Transplantation in cystinosis, a metabolic disease. *Am. J. Surg.*, **118**, 159

Mahoney, C. P., Striker, G. E., Hickman, R. O., Manning, G. B. and Marchioro, Th. L. (1970). Renal transplantation for childhood cystinosis. *N. Engl. J. Med.*, **283**, 397

McCune, D. J., Mason, H. H. and Clarke, H. T. (1943). Intractable hypophosphatemic rickets with renal glycosuria and acidosis. The Fanconi-Syndrome. *Am. J. Dis. Child.* **65**, 81

Odievre, M. (1966). Glycogénose hépato-rénale avec tubulopathie complex. *Rev. Int. Hepatologie* **16**, 1

Rosenberg, L. E. and Segal, S. (1964). Maleic acid-induced inhibition of amino acid transport in rat kidney. *Biochem. J.* **92**, 345

Rotthauwe, H. W., Fichsel, H., Heldt, H. W., Kirsten, E., Reim, M., Schmidt, E., Schmidt, F. W. and Weseman, W. (1963). Glykogenose der Leber mit Aminoacidurie und Glukosurie. *Klin. Wochenschr.* **41**, 818

14

Diseases of bone in search of an inborn error

C. O. Carter

Introduction

Paraphrasing Dr J. O'Brien (1969), who discovered the hexominidase A deficiency in Tay-Sachs disease, the stages in the discovery of an inborn error are:

(a) the clinical delineation of the disease or syndrome;
(b) the demonstration of its mode of inheritance—usually autosomal or X-linked recessive;
(c) the discovery of chemical abnormality in urine, plasma or cultural cells;
(d) the discovery of the precise enzyme (or structural protein) defect.

Steps (a) and (b) are the task of the paediatrician and clinical geneticist, steps (c) and (d) the task of the biochemist and particularly the enzyme chemist.

In the field of skeletal disorders this sequence has been nicely illustrated by the history of the mucopolysaccharidoses (McKusick, 1972). The initial recognition of a disease, or as we now know a group of diseases, came with Hunter's paper in 1917 and Hurler's in 1919. The realisation that there could be X-linked inheritance as well as the more usual autosomal recessive inheritance came in the 1940s, because of the excess of male patients and individually clearly X-linked pedigrees, such as that of Njå reported in 1946. Njå also first proposed the clinical distinction between the X-linked Hunter and the autosomal recessive Hurler. The recognition of excess mucopolysaccharide excretion and intracellular accumulation of mucopolysaccharide came in the 1950s and the recognition that Morquio's disease, recognised clinically since 1929, belonged to the mucopolysaccharidoses came at the same time. In the 1960s came the recognition of the Sanfilippo and Scheie forms. Later in the 1960s came the demonstration that those forms, for example the Hurler and Scheie, which had related biochemical defects, did not correct each other's deficiency in mixed fibroblast culture. In 1972 came the first clear delineation of specific enzyme defects α-L-iduronidase in Hurler's and heparan sulphate sulphatase in Sanfilippo A and *N*-acetyl-α-D-glucosaminidase in Sanfilippo B. The recognition of the two genetically distinct forms of Sanfilippo disease is purely biochemical since no clinical differences have been shown between these two forms and the two enzyme deficiencies affect adjacent steps in biochemical degradation.

Most osteochondrodystrophies are still at stage (b) of O'Brien's scheme and I will mention some of those whose inheritance is probably autosomal or X-linked recessive and which therefore are presumably inborn errors of metabolism in the sense of being specific enzyme defects. Dominant conditions will be mentioned only incidentally, though these must also depend essentially on biochemical error since the function of genes is to produce biologically active peptides. But, since in these the mutant gene by definition produces significant abnormality in the heterozygote, it is reasonable to suppose, as McKusick has suggested, that the gene product is part of a structural protein rather than an enzyme. For example the bone collagen in osteogenesis imperfecta appears to contain an excess of hydroxylysine.

Until the biochemical defect is known the classification of these osteochondrodystrophies must be largely anatomical, according to whether the metaphyses, the epiphyses, the spine and the epiphyses, or the diaphyses are most affected. The evidence on the genetics of these conditions has recently been summarised by Carter and Fairbank (1974) and the radiological features by Spranger *et al.* (1974).

Metaphyseal conditions

It is now clear that two forms of what was thought to be severe achondroplasia, lethal in the neonatal period, are quite distinct from classical achondroplasia. The commoner of the two is *thanatophoric dwarfism*, this probably includes more than one entity. Almost all cases have occurred sporadically and the condition is most likely to be dominant. This condition has a higher frequency at birth than true achondroplasia and than the next condition I will be mentioning, achondrogenesis. The radiological features are surprisingly like those for the homozygous form of true achondroplasia; but the latter is genetically quite distinct since both parents must have true achondroplasia, while with thanatophoric dwarfism both are normal.

Achondrogenesis

This rare severe lethal form of osteochondrodystrophy, described first by Parenti in 1936 and well delineated by Maroteaux and his colleagues in 1968, is probably autosomal recessive. Scott (1972) reports personal communication from Silverman, from Saldino and from Houston of families with two or more patients in a sibship born to normal parents. The pedigree of a family reported by Laxova, O'Hara and Ridler (1973) is shown in Figure 14.1. Three of five girls were affected and stillborn;

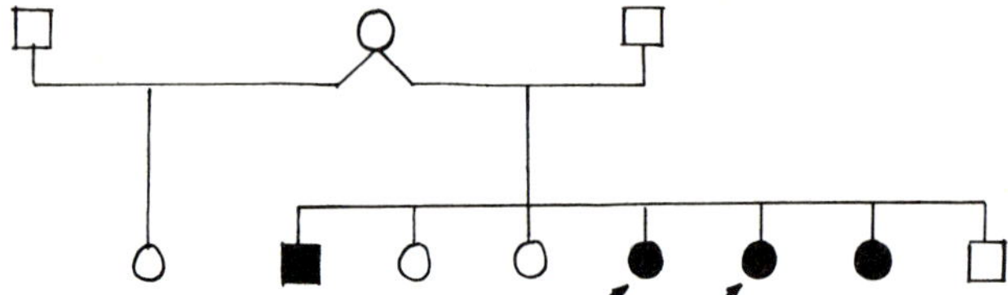

FIGURE 14.1 Achondrogenesis: recessive.

the parents were first cousins. The limbs are even shorter than in thanatophoric dwarfism, the trunk is also shorter, but the thorax not so narrow. Radiologically the whole skeleton is poorly calcified, especially the vertebral bodies and the sacrum. The metaphyseal ends of the long bones are much enlarged. In contrast to the thanatophoric dwarfs the femora are not bowed, and the metaphyses are more cupped. Histologically resting cartilage is hypercellular consisting of large hollowed chondrocytes with little intercellular matrix. There is no cellular formation and endochondral ossification is completely disorganised. There is an indication that this is a storage disease of cartilage since Laxova *et al.* (1973) reported the presence of lipid-like granules in cells from fibroblast cultures from two of these still born infants, but this needs confirmation.

Asphyxiating thoracic dystrophy

This usually, but not always, lethal condition was first recognised as a familial condition by Jeune in 1958 and is almost certainly autosomal recessive. In Jeune's family two brothers and a sister born to normal parents were all affected. A dozen or so further examples of affected sibs born to normal parents have been reported since. In one instance minor signs of the anomaly were present in the mother, possibly an example of clinical manifestation in the heterozygote. The long narrow chest wall is almost completely immobile in infancy and death usually occurs from respiratory insufficiency. Radiologically the ribs are short and horizontally placed, the thorax narrow, long and cylindrical. The iliac wings are short and square. The medial part of the acetabular roof projects downwards like a hook. The clavicles are high. The long bones show epiphyseal enlargement, they may be short but are usually of normal length. Some patients have ulnar polydactyly and this appears to be genetically distinct since affected sibs resemble each other in the presence of polydactyly. Radiological features resemble those of the Ellis–van Creveld Syndrome, but the ectodermal and cardiac anomalies of the latter syndrome are absent. The histological findings are said to be non-specific.

Metaphyseal chondroplasia

There are several conditions generically called just metaphyseal dysplasia. The rare severe Jansen form is probably dominant and the common Schmid form is certainly dominant. The Spahr form is probably recessive but only one family has been reported. But the form with pancreatic inficiency and neutropenia, Schwachman's syndrome, is almost certainly recessive. The skeletal features and short stature have probably been missed in many patients reported to have just pancreatic insufficiency and neutropenia. The dysplasia affects especially the hips, but may also affect knees, wrists and vertebrae. Radiologically zones of rarification and condensation are seen in both femoral necks and remodelling of these leads to bilateral coxa vara.

Epiphyseal conditions

The common mainly epiphyseal lesion, multiple epiphyseal dysplasia, is in most families dominant. So probably are the Conradi–Hunerman varieties of chondrodysplasia punctata. In contrast the severe rhizomelic form of chondrodysplasia punctata is autosomal recessive. A number of examples of two or more sibs born to normal parents have been reported and at least two instances of parental consanguinity are known. As the name implies the limbs are strikingly short, the face is flat and the bridge of the nose very depressed. There is congenital cataract. Patches of cicotricial alopecia develop in the skin. Most patients are mentally retarded. Radiologically epiphyseal centres are stippled and the centres of calcification may extend into the soft tissues. The metaphyses are splayed, cupped and show disturbed ossification. Histologically endochondral bone formation is grossly abnormal with deficient columnar arrangement, little calcification of the matrix and diminished vascularity.

Spondyloepiphyseal conditions

There are several varieties of spondyloepiphyseal dysplasia including dominant, autosomal recessive and X-linked forms.

X-linked forms of spondyloepiphyseal dysplasia

This form is well defined. The appearance is suggestive of Morquio's disease though of later onset and lesser severity. A typically X-linked pedigree was reported by Milsonne as early as 1927 and an extensive one by Jacobson in 1937 which has since been updated (Bannerman 1969). Carter and Sutcliffe (1970) reported a family (shown in Figure 14.2)

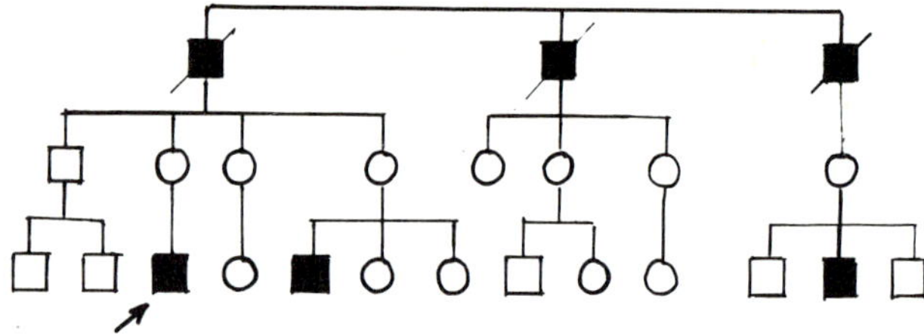

FIGURE 14.2 X-linked spondyloepiphyseal dysplasia tarda.

where three affected brothers had four affected grandsons through their necessarily carrier daughters. The vertebrae and articular cartilages of the long bones are affected, but not the growth cartilage. Radiologically there is a characteristic humpbacked mound of dense bone seen at the back of the upper and lower plates of the flattened vertebrae.

Diastrophic dwarfism

A well-defined autosomal recessive form of spondylepiphyseal dysplasia is diastrophic dwarfism, first fully described by Lamy and Maroteaux in 1960. Some dozen instances of affected sibs born to normal parents have been reported and parental consanguity noted on several occasions. The main clinical features are short limbs with bilateral talipes equinovarus. Later severe scoliosis may develop. Cleft palate is not uncommon. In infancy cystic swellings develop in the ear which later give the appearance of the professional boxer's cauliflower ear. Both hips may dislocate and this is probably not congenital. There is some neonatal mortality from respiratory insufficiency. Radiologically the long bones are short and the epiphyses are flattened and distorted. The metatarsals and metacarpals are short and this is particularly true of the first metacarpal which is oval or even triangular. Histologically there is a reduction in the number of chondrocytes in the resting, proliferative and columnar zones and the chondrocytes have larger, clearer and rounder nuclei than normal.

Pseudoachondroplastic spondyloepimetaphyseal dysplasia

Until Maroteaux and Lamy defined this condition in 1959 these children were called achondroplastics. The distinction, however, is clear. There is no involvement of the growth plates which are not associated with articular cartilage, so the skull, the pelvis, the ribs and the pedicles of the spine are not involved. The dwarfism in childhood is more severe than in achondroplasia, but unlike achondroplasia the condition is not usually recognised at birth. The most severe variant of the condition is recessive. Two sibs born to normal parents have been reported and one instance of parental consanguinity. The pedigree of a remarkable family with four sibs affected is illustrated (Dennis and Renton, 1975) in Figure 14.3. Radiologically the epiphyses appears more irregular than in achondroplasia, the vertebrae are flat and show an anterior projection; in contrast the skull is normal, the sacrosciatic

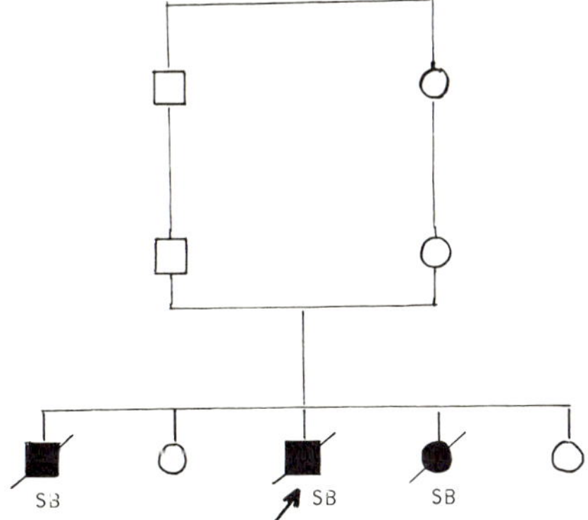

FIGURE 14.3 Pseudoachondroplastic spondyloepimetaphyseal dysplasia: recessive.

notch is normal and there is no narrowing of the lumbar spinal cord and no neurological complications. Cooper *et al.* (1973) have reported electron microscopic changes in cartilage from a patient suggestive of a storage disorder, perhaps of protein.

Diaphyseal disorders

The commonest diaphyseal disorder of bone is *osteogenesis imperfecta* which is dominant. Some hold the view that some cases of severe lethal osteogenesis imperfecta congenita are recessive, but most cases of this form of the disorder are undoubtedly sporadic. Only one well described family reported by Maloney in 1969 is suggestive of recessive inheritance.

Osteopetrosis congenita

This severe form of osteopetrosis, usually causing death in childhood from progressive pantacytopenia, is autosomal recessive. The first report by Sick in 1914 included affected sibs born to normal parents and numerous such families have been reported since. In addition several instances of parental consanguinity have been reported. Radiologically the main features are dense sclerotic bone without distinction of cortical and cancellous bone. Pathologically the essential anomaly appears to be a failure to reabsorb primary spongiosa and this spongiosa is dense and compact.

Pycnodysostosis

This condition was first defined by Maroteaux and Lamy in 1962, though previous cases had been reported under the label of cleidocranial dysostosis or osteopetrosis. In Maroteaux and Lamy's original report there were two affected sibs born to normal parents and many similar families have since been reported. Parental consanguinity has been reported on several occasions. About a quarter of the patients are mentally retarded. Lamy has made a good case that Toulouse Lautrec, a product of a cousin marriage, had this condition rather than osteogenesis imperfecta. There is short stature, widening of the cranial sutures with persistence of the anterior fontanelle, hypoplasia of the facial bones and a marked obtuseness of the angle of the jaw. Radiologically there is an increase in density of the whole skeleton, the distal phalanges are tapered. One family with nephew and uncle affected, suggestive of X-linked inheritance, was reported by Shuler (1963).

Craniotubular bone dysplasias and hyperostoses

I should also just mention the rare autosomal recessive forms of craniotubular bone dysplasias. These include *metaphyseal dysplasia* (*Pyle's disease*) and recessive *craniometaphyseal dysplasia* and *craniodiaphyseal dysplasia*. The recessive craniotubular hyperostoses include the severe form of *endosteal hyperostosis* which is also called juvenile Paget's disease and *hypophosophatasia congenita* but is now referred to as *osteoectasia* (on the analogy of bronchiectasis) and also a milder form, *van Bruchem's disease* or *hyperphosphatasia tarda*.

Conclusion

This brief survey has illustrated the wide range of inborn errors of the skeletal system yet to be precisely identified. It is likely that the identification will be a two-way process. As more is learnt about the normal mechanism of cartilage and bone formation, more of the specific metabolic errors in the osteochondrodystrophies will be found and at the same time their identification will throw more light on the normal mechanisms.

REFERENCES*

BANNERMAN, R. M. (1969). X-linked spondyloepiphyseal dysplasia tarda (S.D.T.). *Birth Defects*, **5**, **part 4**, 48

CARTER, C. and SUTCLIFFE, J. (1970). Genetic varieties of spondylo-epiphyseal dysplasia. In A. M. Jelliffe and B. Strickland (eds.), *Symposium Ossium*, p. 218 (Edinburgh : Livingstone)

CARTER, C. O. and FAIRBANK, T. J. (1974). *The Genetics of Locomotor Disorders.* (London : Oxford University Press)

COOPER, R. R., PONSETI, I. V. and MAYNARD, J. A. (1973). Pseudoanchondroplastic dwarfism: a rough surfaced endoplasmic reticular storage disorder. *J. Bone Joint Surg. (Am.)*, **55A**, 475

DENNIS, N. R. and RENTON, P. (1975). Severe recessive form of pseudo-achondroplasia. *Pediatr. Radiol*, **3**, 169.

LAXOVA, R., O'HARA, P. T., RIDLER, M. A. C. and TIMOTHY, J. A. D. (1973). Family with probable achondrogenesis and lipid inclusions in fibroblasts. *Arch. Dis. Child.*, **48**, 212

MALONEY, F. P. (1969). Osteogenesis imperfecta of early onset in three members of an inbred group. *Birth Defects*, **5**, **part 4**, 219

MCKUSICK, V. A. (1972). *Heritable Disorders of Connective Tissue*, 4th Ed. (St Louis : Mosby)

O'BRIEN, J. S. (1969). Generalised gangliosidis. *Birth Defects*, **5**, **part 4**, 219

SCOTT, C. I. (1972). *Prog. Med. Genet.*, **8**, 243

SHULER, S. E. (1963) Pycnodysostosis. *Arch. Dis. Child.*, **38**, 620

SPRANGER, J. W., LANGER, L. O. and WIEDEMANN, H. R. (1974). *Bone Dysplasias : An Atlas of Constant Disorders of Skeletal Development.* (Philadelphia : W. B. Saunders)

* References to other papers mentioned in the text, other than those listed above, will be found in Carter and Fairbank, 1974.

15

Idiopathic juvenile osteoporosis

D. P. Brenton and C. E. Dent

Introduction

When Dent and Friedman (1965) described six patients with osteoporosis of unknown aetiology beginning in the prepubertal years they commented on the paucity of previous descriptions of idiopathic osteoporosis in childhood, finding only two in the literature (Schippers, 1938; Berglund and Lindquist, 1960). The tendency has always been to regard children with unexplained osteoporosis as having some form of osteogenesis imperfecta (OI), i.e. as having a genetically determined disease. Our experience since 1965 still supports the concept that there is a very uncommon idiopathic form of childhood osteoporosis beginning acutely in previously healthy children which heals during their late pubertal development. This paper reviews the 17 patients with idiopathic juvenile osteoporosis (IJO) seen by us since 1957 including with follow-up the original six of Dent and Friedman (1965). None of the patients has had a family history of predisposition to fractures and on this basis there is nothing to suggest a genetic aetiology for their disease. Idiopathic juvenile osteoporosis might seem therefore to be an unsuitable topic for consideration by a Society dedicated to the study of inborn metabolic errors, but its distinction from inherited forms of osteoporosis is important.

Childhood osteoporosis

Table 15.1 lists the causes of childhood osteoporosis encountered by us and if other diseases do cause osteoporosis the severity must be usually mild. The classification of osteogenesis imperfecta is controversial. The classical dominant form with blue sclerae and deafness is well recognised and of very variable severity. The rarer patients with white sclerae in our experience may be severely affected with appreciable limb deformity. Ibsen (1969) found that in the majority of these patients with white

Table 15.1 *Childhood osteoporosis*

1. Osteogenesis imperfecta
   (a) Severe intrauterine with early postnatal death
   (b) Intrauterine with postnatal recovery
   (c) Classical dominant form with blue sclerae and deafness
   (d) Severe form with white sclerae
   (e) Cystic form
2. Idiopathic juvenile osteoporosis
3. Calcium deficiency osteoporosis
4. Other rare cases of unknown cause
5. Complicating other diseases
   (a) Endogenous or exogenous steroids
   (b) Homocystinuria
   (c) Anticonvulsants
   (d) Immobilisation
   (e) Malignant disease—leukaemia
   (f) Biliary atresia
   (g) Cyanotic heart disease

sclerae there was no family history making the differentiation from idiopathic juvenile osteoporosis more difficult. A cystic form of osteogenesis imperfecta was distinguished by Fairbank (1951), but its separate existence is not accepted by McKusick (1972). It is retained here because the three cases seen by us have been uniformly severe and quite different in other respects too from the others. Intrauterine fractures may occur in patients from families with typical dominant osteogenesis imperfecta with blue sclerae. However a lethal recessive form of osteogenesis imperfecta probably exists with severe intrauterine fractures and early postnatal death because of instances in the literature of affected siblings born to normal parents with a high incidence of parental consanguinity (Ibsen, 1969). There may exist an entirely separate and quite different intrauterine form of the disease since one case has been seen by us with intrauterine fractures and complete recovery after birth and we have two other similar ones incompletely documented. The other causes of osteoporosis listed are all well recognised except for calcium deficiency osteoporosis. This clinical entity has not yet been described but a 7-year-old boy with osteoporosis was seen at U.C.H. in 1958 who had been on a self-imposed diet containing less than 150 mg of calcium daily. He had not grown for one year and had suffered both vertebral and long bone fractures. His calcium balance was negative by 143–206 mg/day. On additional calcium and small doses of vitamin D the balance became positive, growth was restored and he returned to full activity. Subsequently he went through a normal pubertal development without any recurrence of his disease during this rapid growth phase (quoted in Dent, 1972).

A comparison of osteogenesis imperfecta and idiopathic juvenile osteoporosis is shown in Table 15.2. The limitations of family history in

Table 15.2

	Idiopathic juvenile osteoporosis	*Osteogenesis imperfecta*
Onset of symptoms	2–3 years before puberty	From birth
Duration	1–4 years depending on severity	Lifelong
Metaphyseal fractures	Common	Rare
Calcium balance	Marked negative in severe cases	Small positive
Connective tissue defects	None	Blue sclerae, hyperextensile joints, abnormal teeth
Family history	None	Maybe positive

the patients with white sclerae and osteogenesis imperfecta have been mentioned above. In this situation the history of a recent acute onset of the disease helps to differentiate the idiopathic juvenile osteoporosis. Apart from the differences listed in Table 15.2 there are some helpful radiological differences. Severe cases of osteogenesis imperfecta have abnormally narrow long bones and ribs which never attain a normal width. In severe idiopathic juvenile osteoporosis the overall width of the shafts of the long bones and ribs is normal although there may be extreme thinning of cortical bone. The fibula in osteogenesis imperfecta is often slender and variously curved as though too long for this tibia. This has not been seen in idiopathic juvenile osteoporosis except as a late stage of a severe case and the skull is always normal in this condition but may be deformed in osteogenesis imperfecta. These differences are readily explicable on the basis that osteogenesis imperfecta potentially disturbs bone formation and growth from conception onwards whereas idiopathic juvenile osteoporosis arises only in later childhood. In addition neo-osseous porosis (see later) only arises in the severe acute phase of IJO.

Idiopathic juvenile osteoporosis

The 17 patients studied by us are classified in Table 15.3 according to their clinical severity and the ages at which symptoms began are recorded in Figure 15.1. Two of the severely affected patients in Table 15.3 are unlike the other patients; one because his symptoms began at the age of 4 years and another because his osteoporosis coincided with biochemical, radiological and histological features of osteomalacia. Our experience has been that patients most commonly present 2–4 years before sexual development so that systems are developing in that period of time when normally the rapid phase of growth is beginning. It is possible that this experience of idiopathic osteoporosis in childhood is unrepresentative, disturbed perhaps by the diagnostic problem that the earlier its onset the more likely is the osteoporosis to be regarded as a form of osteogenesis imperfecta. If that confusion commonly happens then the onset of symptoms may be less dramatically concentrated in the immediate prepubertal years than indicated in Figure 15.1. The common presenting features are impaired growth and pain at one of three characteristic sites, the back, knees and ankles. Cessation of growth may not be noticed by either the patient or the patient's family. Direct questioning may reveal however that the patient's growth is not keeping up with contemporaries at school. Vertebral crush fractures may be suggested by pain and a discrepancy between the patient's arm span and his height (Figure 15.8, for example) or a discrepancy between the crown-pubis and pubis-heel lengths. The more mildly affected patients commonly have only back pain which radiologically is seen to be due to one or a small number of crush fractures of the vertebrae. Five of our patients fall into this group. Temporary limitation of activity restricting games is required, but the patients are well enough to remain mobile. The ultimate height loss is probably small judging from the discrepancy between the patient's span and height and all have either recovered well or look like doing so. Five other patients are classified as moderately severe. In this group vertebral fractures are more numerous (Figure 15.2), knee and ankle pains become more common with occasional long bone fractures due to mild trauma. Metaphyseal impaction fractures (Figure 15.3) cause the knee and ankle pains which are probably produced by the osteoporotic process when it severely affects the newly formed bone of the metaphyses (Figure 15.4). This process occurs all over the skeleton when new bone growth occurs, but is only symptomatic when weight bearing occurs. It illustrates well the sudden change in bone formation so characteristic of IJO as distinct from OI. We suggest the new name *neo-osseous*

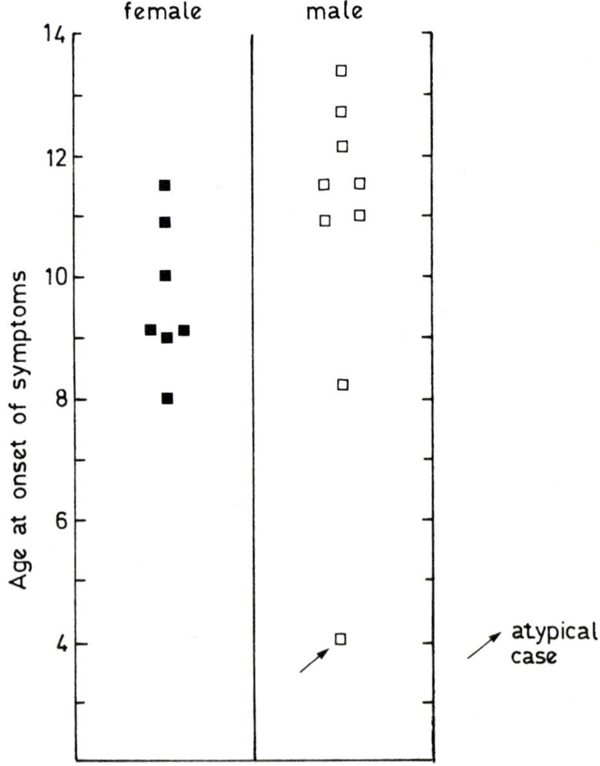

FIGURE 15.1 Idiopathic osteoporosis of childhood. Age of onset of symptoms in U.C.H. series. Note the strong suggestion of a puberty linkage with the girls about 2 years ahead of the boys.

Table 15.3

Clinical grading	*Number of patients*	*Pain*	*Fractures*	*Activity*	*Ultimate height loss**	*Recovery*
Mild	5	Back	1–3 crushed vertebrae	Temporary restriction; may need walking sticks	4 cm	Full activity
Moderate	5	Back, knees, ankles	Numerous vertebral, metaphyseal and occasional long bone	More prolonged restriction. Temporary use of wheelchair	4–12 cm	Full activity
Severe	7	Back, knees, ankles generalised	Numerous vertebral, metaphyseal and frequent long bone	Prolonged restriction. Temporary or permanent use of wheelchair	12–35 cm	Partial recovery. Cessation of spontaneous fractures

*Measured as the difference between standing height and arm span after puberty.

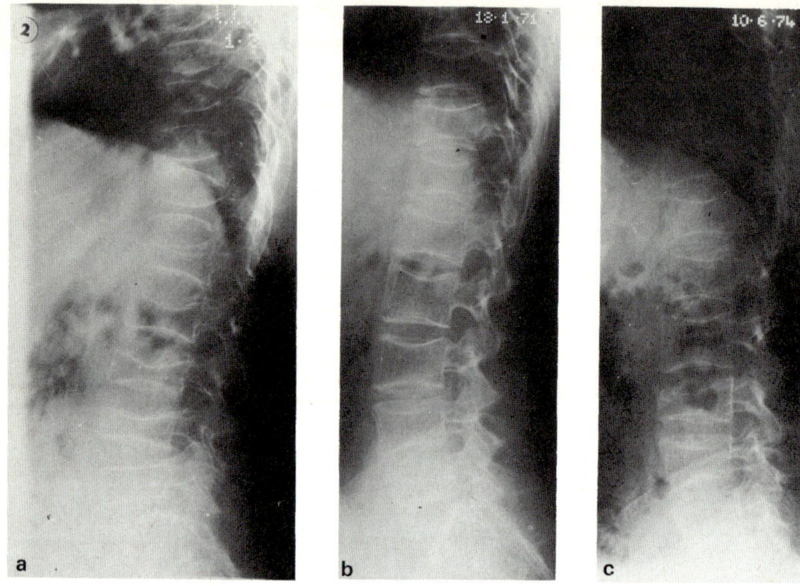

FIGURE 15.2 (a) March 1967. Vertebral crush fractures in Peter B.; (b) January 1971. Note the improvement since 1967. (c) June 1974. A much later fracture of L3 was produced by trying to lift a motorcycle.

porosis for this phenomenon. Such fractures severely limit activity so that sticks may be required for normal walking or even temporary existence in a wheel chair may be necessary when metaphyseal fractures are occurring during normal weight bearing. Because vertebral fractures are more widespread the ultimate height loss is some 4–12 cm. Nevertheless the recovery in this group is usually very good with the patients returning to full mobility and a normal occupation. Seven patients, including the two atypical ones are included in the severe group. A similar pattern of pains is present but more widespread because of the increasing incidence of fractures of the ribs and shafts of the long bones with minimal trauma. Nearly all the patients have spent long periods in wheel chairs and one of the original six patients of Dent and Friedman is permanently confined in this way due to deformity, wasting and pseudoarthroses caused by numerous fractures. The ultimate height losses are very great and the extensive vertebral collapse causes sternal protuberance and reduced vital capacity. During recovery spontaneous fractures cease but severe deformities remain and the patients' activities may be permanently restricted in this group.

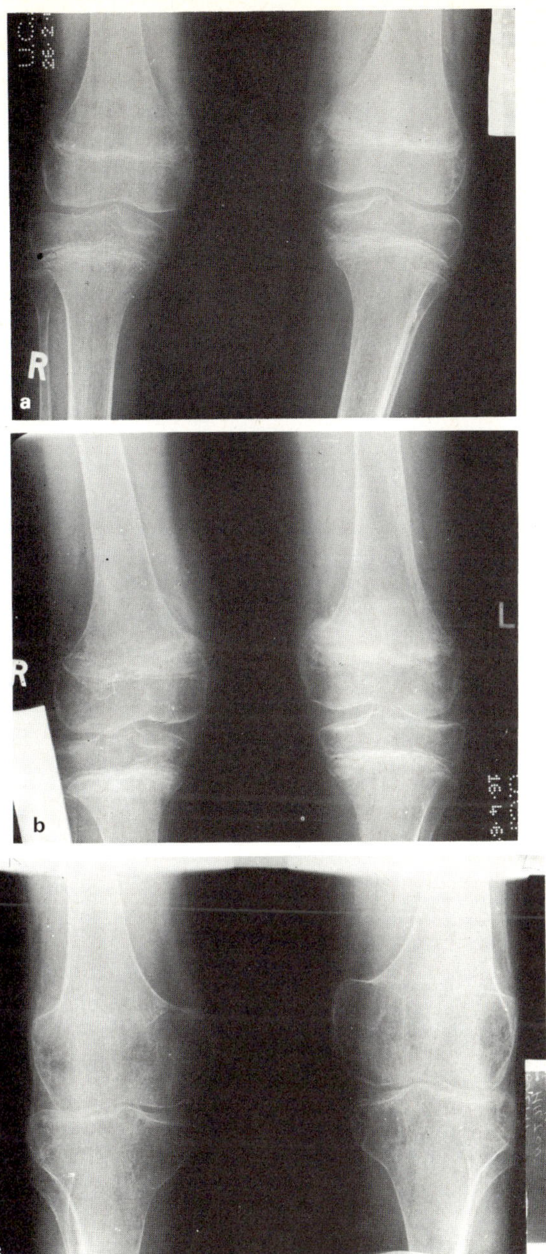

FIGURE 15.3 Metaphyseal fractures in Michael H.: (a) February 1969. Note the extremely thin cortex which is intact throughout the metaphysis except perhaps at the lower medial end of the left femur; (b) April 1969. Fractures have now occurred by impaction of the extremely thin metaphyses which now show as irregular dense areas with marked irregularities in the cortices; (c) April 1974. Healing of the fractures leaves the curious sharp angulation between diaphyseal and metaphyseal regions. The epiphyses are fused satisfactorily. The cortices are still thin.

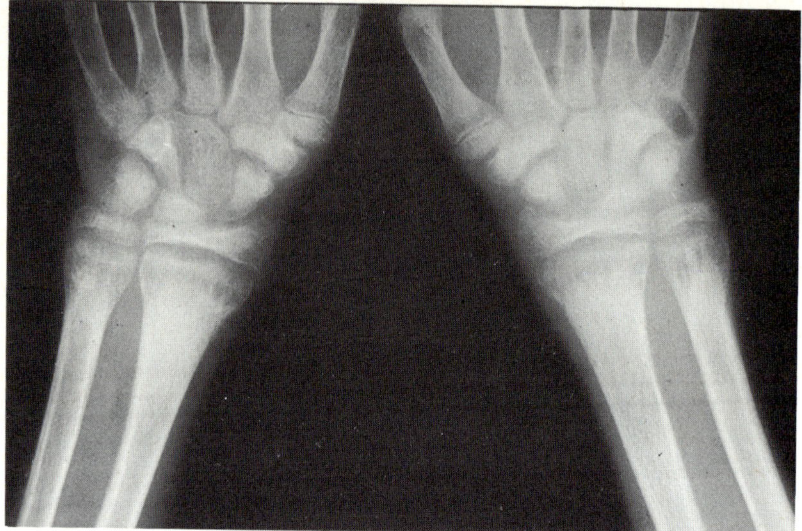

FIGURE 15.4 Wrist of Christopher G. Note the relative lucency of the newly formed metaphyseal bone—'neo-osseous porosis'. This patient was atypical in showing some radiological and histological features of rickets but the changes illustrated have been clearly seen in several of the other juvenile osteoporotic patients whose growth plates have not shown this mildly rachitic appearance.

Calcium balance studies have been carried out in 17 of the 18 patients referred to us. The only patient in whom a balance study was not performed was one of the mildly affected patients with two crushed vertebrae who rapidly recovered. The initial calcium balance results are summarised in Figure 15.5. The results of four mildly affected patients are shown all in positive balance although in some instances not as strongly positive as would be expected in normal children of this age (300–400 mg/day). The results on the severely affected patients are quite scattered. Three were in gross negative balance and one in rather less severe negative balance. A fifth patient, a girl, had been symptomatic for 2 years before the balance was carried out and began menstruation within six months of study so that her positive balance was probably a sign of recovery. The remaining two are the atypical patients mentioned above. Both were in positive balance, but it is emphasised that the extent was less than in a normal child. However, the boy with the onset of symptoms at 4 years was in small positive balance like patients with osteogenesis imperfecta. However, in the latter group of diseases he could only be classified in the severely affected group with white sclerae

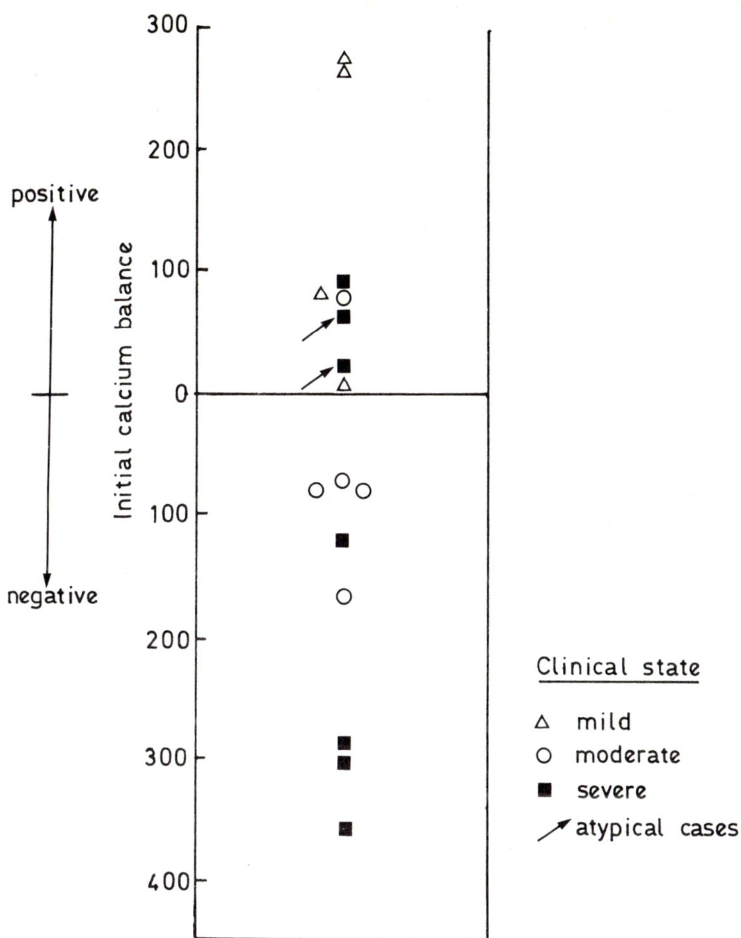

FIGURE 15.5 Initial calcium balance results before treatment.

and yet differs from other patients we have seen in this group because his dwarfism was extreme and affected long bones as well as trunk and because during 4 years of follow-up he has not grown at all nor gone into more positive calcium balance. Balance studies in the moderately affected group of patients tend to be intermediate between the other two groups. The usual finding is a negative balance of 50–150 mg/day. The results indicate that an initial severe negative balance is a bad prognostic sign and an initial positive balance a sign of mild or recovering disease.

Treatment and outcome

There is no treatment for any form of osteoporosis which has been convincingly shown to have increased the amount of normal bone. Views on the basic defect in osteoporosis most commonly see it primarily in terms of abnormalities in the rate of synthesis or breakdown of bone matrix. This contrasts with rickets and osteomalacia where the defect is seen as one of mineralisation. Unfortunately, this view of the defect in osteoporosis, even if it is correct, does not offer any exciting therapeutic possibilities except where excessive steroid secretion or administration is adversely affecting matrix physiology. The time of onset of idiopathic juvenile osteoporosis suggests that there may be temporary hormonal disturbances associated with puberty causing the bone disease but the earlier investigations did not reveal unequivocal evidence of it (Dent and Friedman, 1965); wider hormonal investigations are indicated. The forms of treatment used in the patients with idiopathic juvenile osteoporosis are listed in Table 15.4. Most have no

Table 15.4 *Treatment*

Clinical grading of patients	*None*	*I.V. calcium*	*Oral calcium*	*Oral calcium & vit. B*	*Calcitonin*	*Sex hormones*
Mild	4		1			
Moderate	1		2	2		
Severe	1	2		6	3	3

The figures indicate the number of patients undergoing each treatment. More than one treatment was often tried in the severely affected patients. Purified bone powder (Ossopan) was the most frequently used source of oral calcium and vitamin D includes in this context both D_2 and DHT.

good theoretical basis since there is no understanding of the aetiology of the disease, although it remains possible that a more specific defect of intestinal calcium absorption may be a factor in some patients. It can be said however that at the very least increasing the calcium absorption from the intestine with vitamin D and oral calcium supplements is probably valuable to meet the demand for mineral by the bone during the phase of spontaneous improvement. The risks of such treatments are well known, namely hypercalcaemia, hypercalcuria and renal stones.

Mildly affected patients have in general received no treatment, but they are advised to avoid potentially traumatic games. Other exercise, especially swimming, is encouraged. Growth is not severely affected and the patients return to full activity and normal occupations. Treatment has been attempted in the clinically severe group and the worst patients in the moderate group (Table 15.3). The results of sex hormone treatment were described by Dent and Friedman (1965) who used them on their first three severely affected patients. One of these (Lindy W.) was already recovering and treatment of the other two did not result in improvement of the calcium balance. More prolonged trials might have been attempted, but it was felt that the hormone treatment might be contributing to the severely dwarfed state of the earliest treated patients. Calcitonin was tried in three patients, but positive calcium balance was not achieved. Intravenous treatment with calcium salts is difficult in practice and the calcium although it is retained initially seems to be excreted in the urine after several days. With one exception oral supplements of calcium salts have not produced positive calcium balances. The exception is illustrated in Figures 15.6 and 15.7. He was a little different to the other cases in that his faecal calcium was always lower than his dietary calcium even during negative calcium balance, indicating significant net absorption of calcium. It is usual in active osteoporosis for the faecal calcium to equal or exceed the dietary intake. It may be that this relative preservation of intestinal absorption was important in his response to calcium salts. He grew well, returned to full activity and showed considerable radiological improvement (Figure 15.2). A combined treatment of DHT and purified bone powder has significantly altered the calcium balance results in all the five patients in whom it has been tried. Examples are shown in Figures 15.8 and 15.9. The patient Michael H. was very severely affected, his height being 6 cm less than his span when first seen (Figure 15.8) with a catastrophically severe negative calcium balance. He suffered crush fractures of all his vertebrae with recurrent metaphyseal and shaft fractures of the long bones. Treatment restored positive calcium balance from the age of 13 years onwards, but in general it was only positive 100–200 mg daily, less than for a normal boy of his age and much too little for the repair of

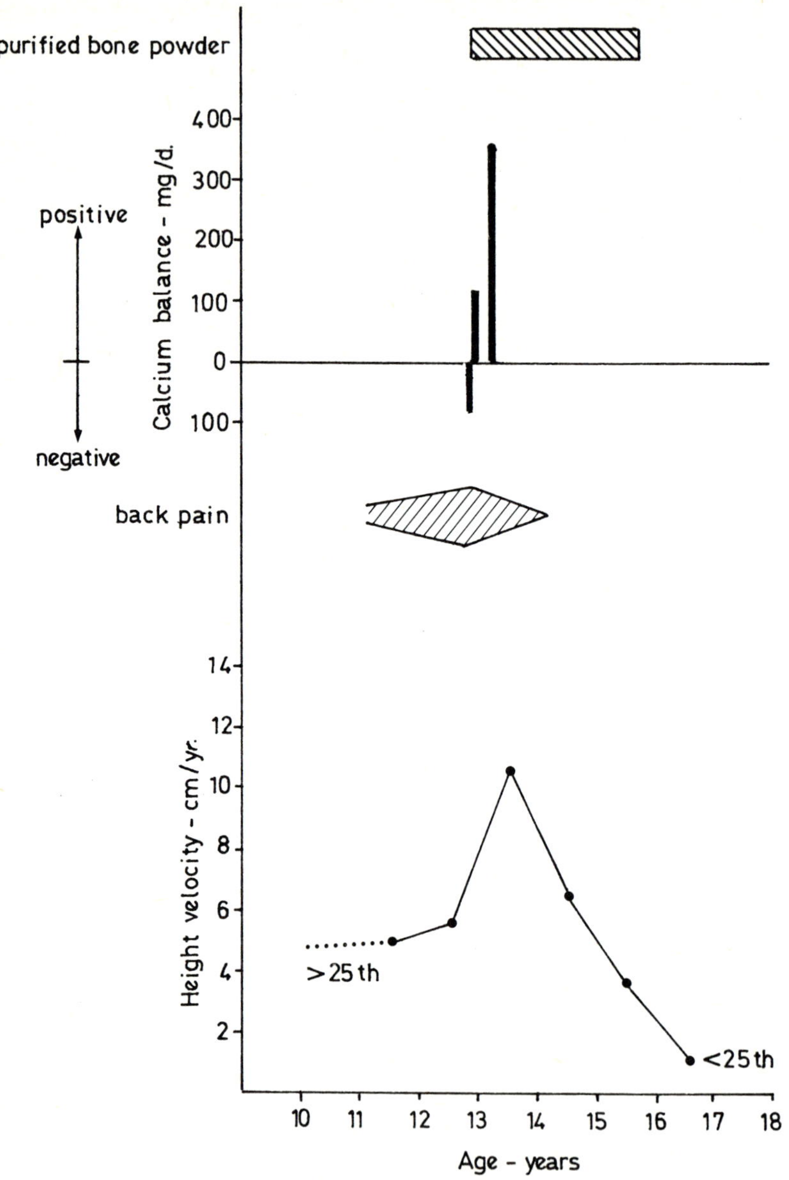

FIGURE 15.6 Patient Peter G. Overall calcium balance correlated with symptoms, growth and treatment. Note the good growth spurt, the initial height being just above the 25th percentile and the final height just below.

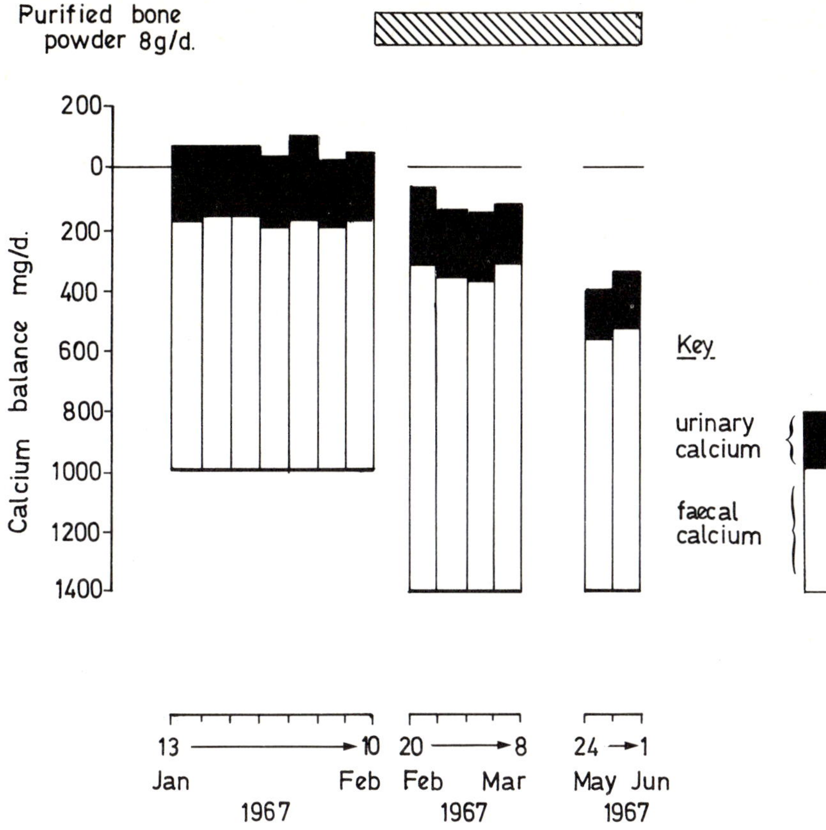

FIGURE 15.7 Patient Peter G. More detailed calcium balances. Intake is plotted downwards from the line of zero balance and excretion upwards from the level of the intake. When excretion exceeds intake the column rises above the zero line and the balance is negative.

his grossly demineralised bones. The dose of DHT ultimately chosen for long term treatment was small, 0·1 mg daily. Larger doses tried earlier when just over 13 years resulted in a positive daily balance of 400 mg, but induced hypercalcaemia. The dose of purified bone powder was 8 g/day. A few months before he was 16 years old bendrofluazide was briefly added to the regime which increased his positive balance to 370 mg/day, suggesting possible therapeutic advantage, but his sexual development was nearing completion and the bendrofluazide was discontinued. The bones remained radiologically very osteoporotic and he continued to lose height after his pubertal development was completed although he was much more mobile. Patient

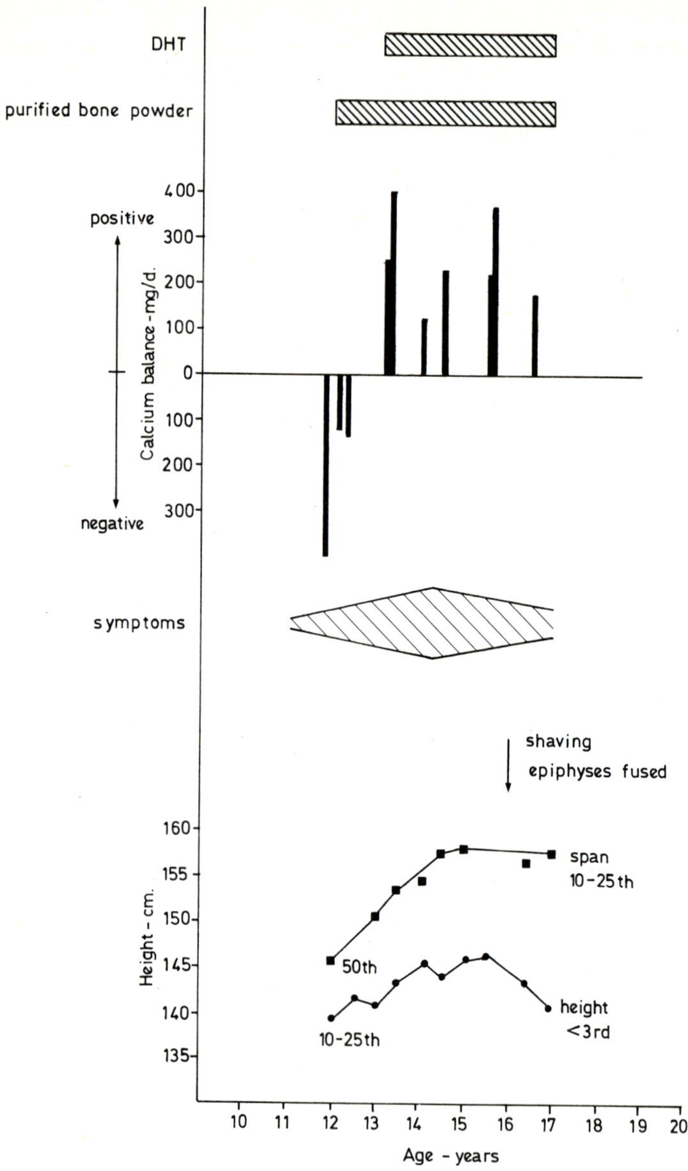

FIGURE 15.8 Patient Michael H. Net calcium balance correlated with symptoms, growth and treatment. Note that growth in height is more seriously impaired than growth in arm span. The percentile height figures shown at 12 and 17 years are those for his real standing height and for his span which presumably would have equalled his height if vertebral collapse had not occurred. For the dose of DHT see text. The dose of bone powder was 8 g/day.

Trevor W. is classified in Table 15.3 as a moderately severe case, but required temporary use of a wheelchair because of troublesome metaphyseal impaction fractures. He was in less severe negative calcium

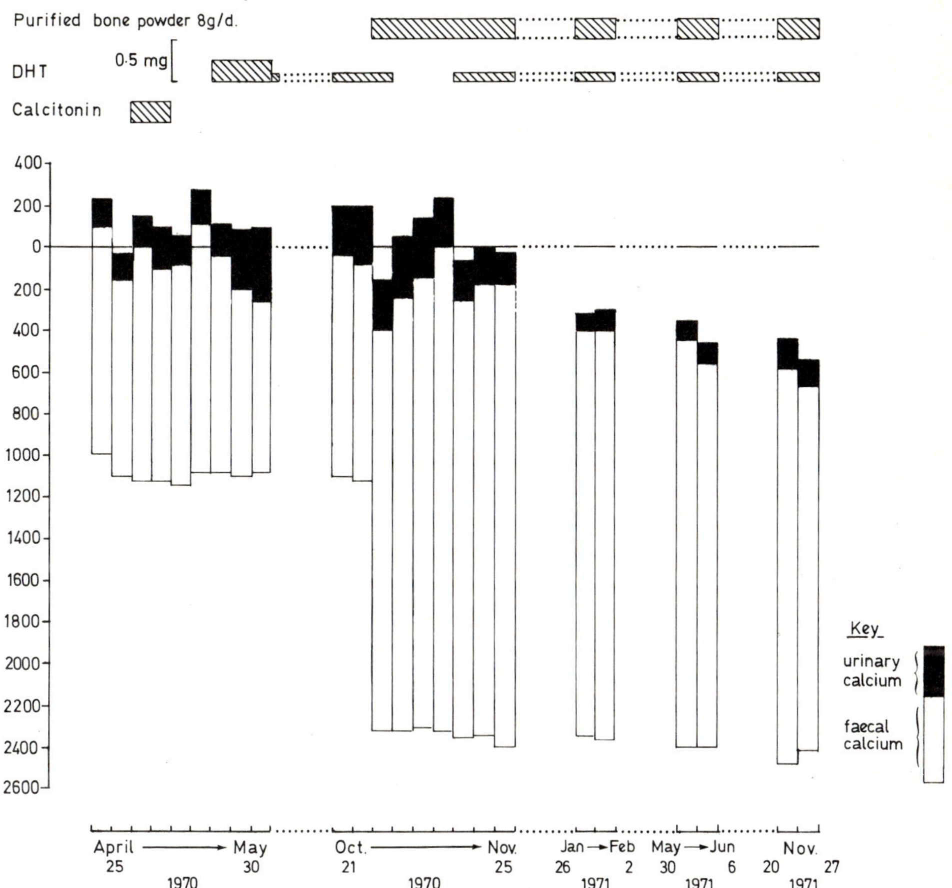

FIGURE 15.9 Patient Trevor W. Detailed calcium balances plotted as in Figure 15.7. Note that the early negative balance is not reversed by DHT or by purified bone powder given separately but becomes positive when both are given together.

balance than Michael H. when first seen and made a better growth response with evidence of radiological healing. A positive calcium balance of between 300 and 400 mg/day was achieved in his case (Figure 15.9) and he now works normally on a farm.

Summary

Seventeen children with idiopathic osteoporosis are described. Fifteen are regarded as having idiopathic juvenile osteoporosis including the original six patients described by Dent and Friedman (1965) when they defined the condition. Two patients are difficult to categorise because of an early age of onset in one and coincidental features of rickets and osteomalacia in another.

The concept of an acute attack of osteoporosis beginning just before puberty is upheld with improvement occurring as puberty develops. The variable severity is stressed. Recovery in the severely affected children occurs only slowly over 3-4 years and is incomplete with permanent deformities. Good recoveries occur in more mildly affected patients.

The new radiological sign 'neo-osseous porosis', i.e. severe porosis visible in all newly forming bone is present in severe cases. It leads to impaction fractures in weight bearing metaphyses with pain locally near the joint which must not be confused with arthritis.

No treatment has been successful in rapidly abating the active disease. Correct management is of great importance and consists in ensuring minimal immobilisation after fractures.

REFERENCES

BERGLUND, G. and LINDQUIST, B. (1960). Osteopenia in adolescence. *Clin. Orthop.*, **17**, 259

DENT, C. E. (1972). Keynote address. In B. Frame, A. M. Parfitt and H. Duncan (eds.), *Clinical Aspects of Metabolic Bone Disease*, p. 1. (Amsterdam : Excerpta Medica)

DENT, C. E. and FRIEDMAN, M. (1965). Idiopathic juvenile osteoporosis. *Quart. J. Med.*, **134**, 177

FAIRBANK, J. J. (1951). *An Atlas of Generalised Affections of the Skeleton*, p. 2. (Edinburgh : Livingstone)

IBSEN, K. H. (1969). Skeletal dysplasia. *Birth Defects*, **4**, 140

MCKUSICK, V. A. (1972). *Heritable Disorders of Connective Tissue*, 4th Ed., p. 392. (St Louis : C. V. Mosby)

SCHIPPERS, J. C. (1938). Spontaneous generalised osteoporosis in a girl 10 years old. *Maandschr. Kindergeneesk.*, **8**, 109

16

Metabolic effects of a diphosphonate in the treatment of ectopic calcification in children

N. R. Belton, W. S. Uttley. H. Sheppard and J. Syme

Inorganic pyrophosphate retards both the growth and dissolution of apatite crystals *in vitro* (Fleisch *et al.*, 1966). Diphosphonates are chemically related to pyrophosphate and their main structural similarity is the presence of a P—C—P bond and, like pyrophosphate they have been shown to inhibit calcium phosphate deposition and dissolution *in vitro* (Francis, 1969; Fleisch *et al.*, 1970; Russell *et al.*, 1970).

However unlike pyrophosphate, the diphosphonates are resistant to hydrolysis and enzymatic breakdown (Francis, 1969).

As a result of this basic experimental evidence, a diphosphonate, disodium ethane-1-hydroxy-1,1-diphosphonate (EHDP) or disodium etidronate (Figure 16.1) was demonstrated to have a beneficial effect in the treatment of two cases of myositis ossificans progressiva (Bassett *et al.*, 1969). Subsequently EHDP has been used in the treatment of diseases characterised by ectopic calcification associated with dermatomyositis (Cram *et al.*, 1971; Geho and Whiteside, 1973) and myositis ossificans progressiva (Weiss *et al.*, 1971; Russell *et al.*, 1972). However there is little information on the effect of EHDP on external mineral balance (Cram *et al.*, 1971; Weiss *et al.*, 1971; Smith *et al.*, 1973) and in total this represents only six patients, all of whom were adults except one, and these studies involved relatively short durations of therapy.

We have used EHDP as long-term therapy, in the treatment of three children with ectopic calcification and have performed serial calcium phosphate and magnesium balances in these children in order to provide more information on the effect and mechanism of action of EHDP.

Methods

Balance studies were carried out before and during EHDP therapy, and all extended over 5-day periods. Analysis for calcium, phosphate and magnesium was made on duplicate diets, stools and urine. Samples were

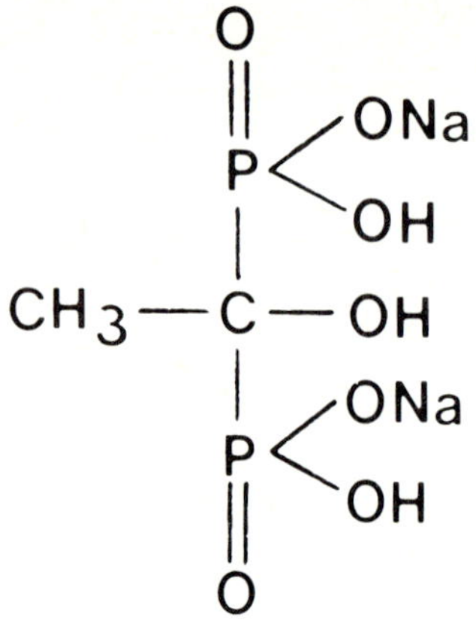

```
        O
        ‖   ONa
        P<
        |   OH
CH3 —   C — OH
        |   ONa
        P<
        ‖   OH
        O
```

FIGURE 16.1 The structure of disodium etidronate (EHDP).

homogenised and aliquots were digested with nitric acid, ashed in a furnace at 420 °C and finally dissolved in dilute nitric acid. Calcium and magnesium were estimated by atomic absorption spectrophotometry (Unicam Atomic Absorption Method Instruction Sheets Ca 1, Mg 1) and phosphate by a micro adaptation of the phosphomolybdate method of Fiske and Subbarow (1925).

Patients

Case 1

A male child of birthweight 4·2 kg began to develop lumps in the skin of the neck, anterior chest, abdominal walls and left arm and leg at 2 weeks of age. Although the lesions appeared to be tender and painful the baby was otherwise thriving. A biopsy from the anterior chest wall showed mature bone formation in the subcutaneous tissues. At 4 months of age the serum calcium was 9·6 mg/100 ml, phosphorus 6·9 mg/100 ml and serum alkaline phosphatase 48 King–Armstrong units.

A course of ACTH produced no obvious beneficial effect and the extent and severity of the ectopic calcification increased. Limitation of joint movements became more pronounced despite physiotherapy. Aluminium hydroxide (5 mls Aludrox gel q.i.d.) was then given for a 12-month period without effect. EHDP (10 mg/kg/day) was therefore commenced at age 1 year and 9 months. As there was no significant radiological evidence of reduced calcification nor of increase in joint mobility by 3 years of age, the dose of EHDP was increased to

20 mg/kg/day. Clinically it appeared that although there was no reduction in ectopic calcification, the rate of deterioration was reduced by therapy and skeletal bone continued to grow normally.

As shown in Figure 16.2, this child was in strongly positive calcium balance 5 months before and immediately before the start of EHDP treatment and remained so after 3 months of EHDP therapy. Thereafter faecal excretion of calcium was greatly increased and the overall balance became negative. These findings were roughly paralleled by changes in magnesium balance whereas phosphate balance, although being reduced after long-term EHDP therapy, remained positive.

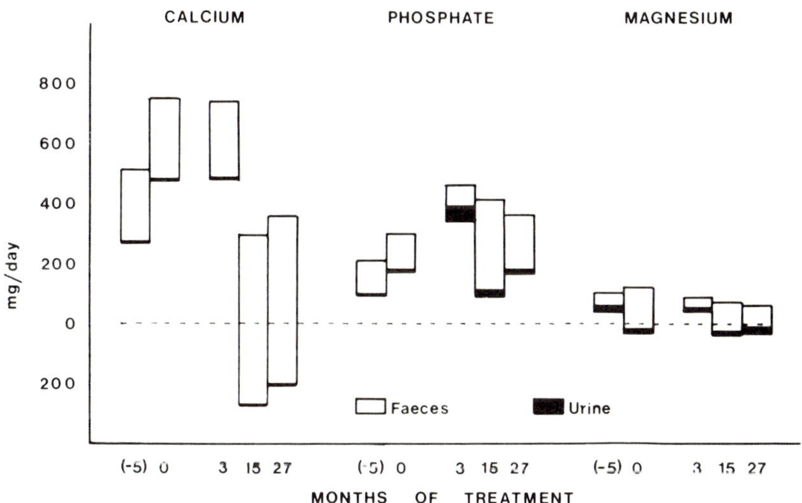

FIGURE 16.2 Case 1; 24-hour mineral balances before and during treatment with EHDP. All mineral balances are expressed as mg/24 hours and represent mean values for determinations over 5-day periods. *Intake* is shown by the upper limit of the enclosed block from the dotted base line. *Excretion* is represented by the distance between the upper and lower limits of the enclosed block. *Urinary Excretion* is represented by the dark section of the enclosed block and *Faecal Excretion* is shown by the remainder of the enclosed block (unshaded portion). *Mineral Balance* is thus the distance between the lower limit of the enclosed block and the dotted base line and is positive when the lower limit of the excretion block is above the line and negative when it is below.

Serum calcium in this child began to fall below the normal range about 6 months after the commencement of EHDP and fell to an all-time low of 3·4 mg/100 ml after withdrawal of EHDP at age 4 years. Serum phosphate always tended to be high and so did alkaline phosphatase. These biochemical changes led to the diagnosis of pseudo-hypoparathyroidism being considered and this was confirmed by a failure of the patient to increase the urinary excretion of cyclic adenosine monophosphate after stimulation by parathormone (Chase *et al.*, 1969).

Case 2

Dermatomyositis was diagnosed at 2½ years of age in a male child who presented with a rash over the upper eyelids and cheeks and who had joint and muscle pains.

Changes in the elctromyogram, a rise in serum aldolase and a muscle biopsy confirmed the diagnosis. Due to removal from the area, the child was not seen again until he was 11 years old. He then had extensive calcinosis of both lower limbs and bilateral equinus deformity. He had a number of subcutaneous calcium deposits and Figure 16.3 gives some

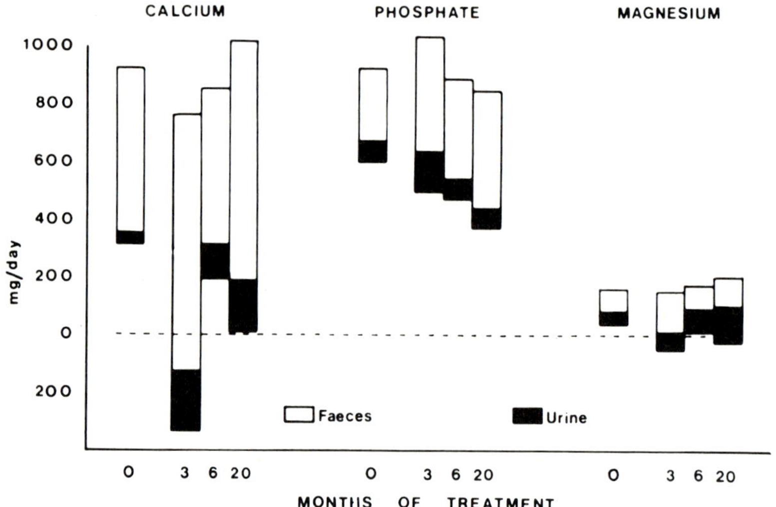

FIGURE 16.3 Case 2. 24-hour mineral balances before and during treatment with EHDP (details as Figure 16.2).

indication of their radiological appearance at this time. However his serum chemistry was now normal and estimation of erythrocyte sedimentation rate and serum creatine kinase showed that his primary disease was inactive. He had been receiving weekly injections of 1 mg synacthen gel for 3 years. This treatment was continued and EHDP (10 mg/kg per day) was commenced. Figure 16.4 shows the marked improvement in ectopic calcification after over 2 years of EHDP therapy and there was a concomitant improvement in the mobility of all the affected joints. As Figure 16.5 shows, he was in positive calcium

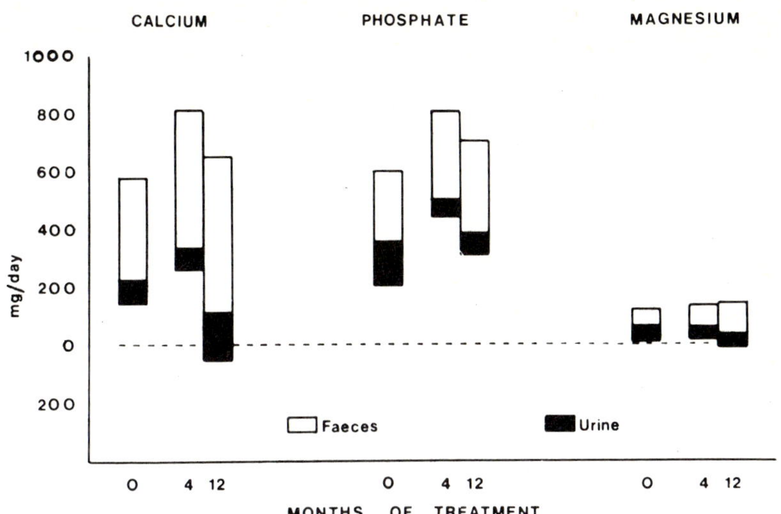

FIGURE 16.4 Case 3: 24-hour mineral balances before and during treatment with EHDP (details as Figure 16.2).

balance just before introduction of EHDP therapy. However he was in marked negative calcium balance, and also negative magnesium balance after 3 months therapy, and throughout the period of EHDP therapy the calcium and magnesium balances were reduced compared to the original balances before treatment. Some reduction also occurred in phosphate balance.

Case 3

This male child presented at 6 years of age with a facial rash with painful and tender muscles. Dermatomyositis was diagnosed after muscle biopsy, electromyography and estimation of creatine kinase. He was treated for 3 years with 10 mg of prednisolone daily. Ectopic calcification in the left thigh with marked limitation of joint movement in this limb was noted during the first year of this treatment. EHDP (10 mg/kg per day) therapy was therefore started at the age of 7 years. Despite therapy the extent of ectopic calcification has increased in the affected limb and other areas have shown calcification. In Figure 16.6 the balance studies show that this child went into negative calcium and magnesium balance after 12 months of EHDP therapy due to increased faecal excretion of both minerals. However the positive phosphate balance before treatment with EHDP was increased during this same period.

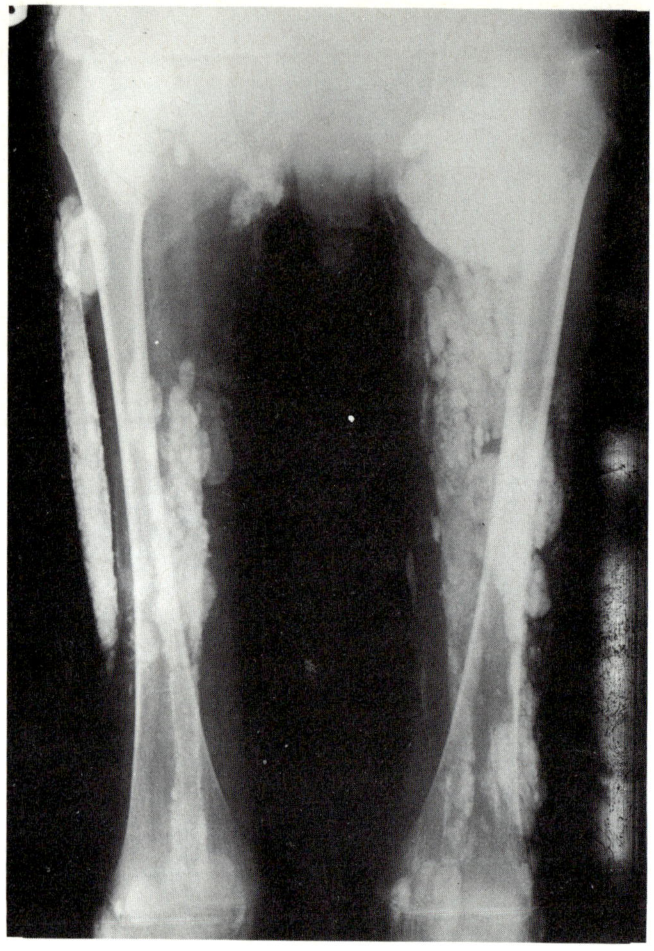

FIGURE 16.5 Soft tissue X-ray of both thighs of Case 2 before EHDP treatment.

Discussion

From these studies it appears that EHDP produces a reduction of calcium balance. This reduction was most marked after prolonged therapy, and a negative calcium balance occurred at some point in the treatment of all three patients. The cause appears to be an increase in the faecal excretion of calcium. The known influence of steroids in producing a reduction in calcium balance cannot be the factor involved even though cases two and three were receiving synacthen and pred-

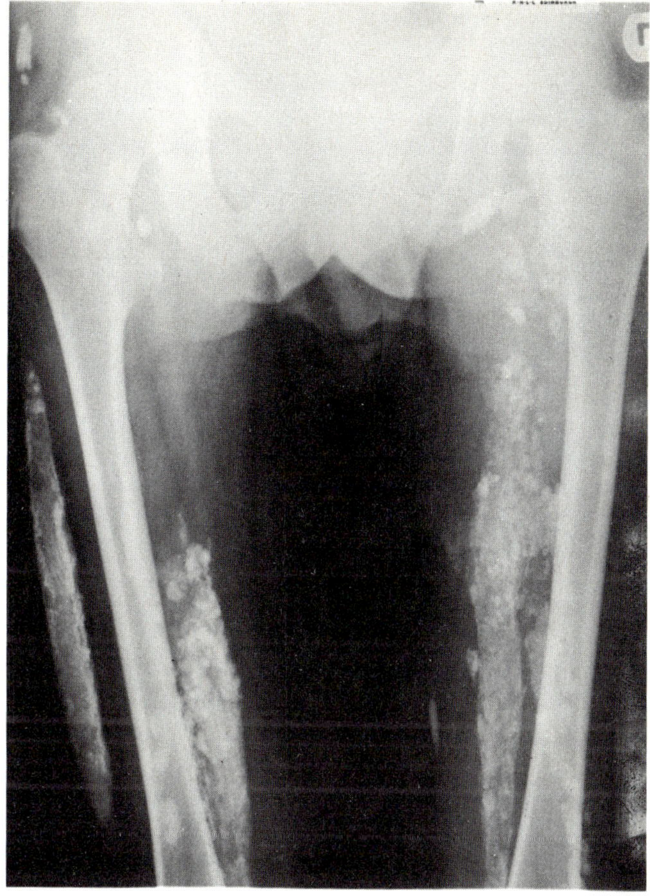

FIGURE 16.6 Soft tissue X-ray of both thighs of Case 2 after 2 years and 8 months of EDHP treatment.

nisolone respectively. This is because the patients had been receiving these drugs for over a year before EHDP therapy was commenced and their dosages were constant during the period of EHDP treatment. Similar changes in magnesium balance to those observed in calcium balance occurred. All three patients exhibited at least one period of negative magnesium balance during EHDP treatment and in general the magnesium changes paralleled those of calcium. Phosphate balance appeared to be much less influenced by EHDP and no constant pattern was evident.

Cram *et al.* (1971) investigated calcium and phosphorus excretion and balance before EHDP treatment and 22 weeks after the start of therapy in a 9-year-old girl with acute dermatomyositis and calcinosis universalis. They described that the net calcium balance changed from positive to neutral and that faecal calcium increased from 132 mg/day to 306 mg/day. Urinary calcium and phosphorus and faecal phosphorus were all increased although the phosphorus balance remained positive.

In a 21-year-old man with myositis ossificans progressiva, Weiss *et al.* (1971) found that the calcium balance was negative before therapy (−78 mg/day) and was essentially unchanged by EHDP therapy. Phosphorus balance showed a similar pattern being also negative before therapy (−48 mg/day) and was still negative during EHDP treatment. The patient showed progressive improvement during treatment and radiocalcium kinetic studies documented the reduction of bone mineral excretion and resorption rates. In the study by Smith *et al.* (1973), four adult males with Paget's disease were in negative calcium balance before treatment with EHDP and during treatment serial balances showed little change in three patients but in one patient the balance became positive. They suggested that more balance studies should be used to study the effect of EHDP particularly where the diphosphonate is given for more than 3 months.

The effect of EHDP on absorption still remains undecided. Morgan *et al.* (1971) stated that EHDP increased calcium absorption at smaller doses but reduced it strongly at higher doses producing rickets. Reversible rickets have been reported in some children treated with EHDP by Fleisch and Bonjour (1973) and an increase in unmineralised osteoid of excessive thickness has been shown in bone biopsy specimens after treatment with EHDP by Russell *et al.* (1974).

One possible explanation for the increased faecal excretion of calcium shown in our studies in patients treated with EHDP is the possibility that EHDP inhibits the formation of 1,25-dihydroxycholecalciferol. Animal experiments by Bonjour *et al.* (1973), by Hill *et al.* (1973) and by Bonjour *et al.* (1973) have all suggested such a possibility although the dose needed to produce such an effect may be greater than the doses used in man. Hill *et al.* (1973), for instance, administered 40 mg/kg per day subcutaneously to rats in order to produce an inhibition in the biosynthesis of 1,25-dihydroxycholecalciferol. However in our patients the fact that the most marked changes in calcium balance were produced after many months of EHDP therapy in two of the cases may mean that such an inhibitory effect may be produced in man by long-term oral therapy with lower doses, i.e. 10–20 mg/kg per day.

It has also been suggested that parathyroid hormone action in the kidney might be affected by EHDP. Plasma phosphate appears to be increased by the action of EHDP. However Recker *et al.* (1973) have concluded that EHDP causes hyperphosphataemia by increasing tubular reabsorption of phosphorus without causing inhibition of parathyroid hormone action on renal tubules.

Although similarities in the trends of the metabolic balance studies in the different patients have been observed in this study, these balance changes do not reflect the clinical success of EHDP therapy. In Case 1 new lesions continued to appear although perhaps at a slower rate than previously. A marked improvement was apparent in Case 2 whereas EHDP was not successful in Case 3.

It seems that although some users report no success in the use of EHDP in the management of ectopic calcification (Metzger, Singer, Bluestone and Pearson, 1974), this drug may still warrant a trial in the treatment of certain diseases which have proved refractory to other forms of treatment in the past. The manufacturers now suggest that the duration of a single course of treatment with EHDP should not exceed 12 months. It is therefore important that during future long-term therapy with EHDP, careful monitoring of serum chemistry, radiological assessment of bone development, the measurement of vitamin D metabolites such as 25-hydroxycholecalciferol and the use of metabolic balance studies are all carried out in order to further evaluate the effect of EHDP and help to provide information on the value and mode of action of this diphosphonate.

Acknowledgements

We thank the Procter and Gamble Company, Cincinnati, Ohio, for supplies of EHDP and Miss Barbara Atkinson for her help in the collection of specimens.

REFERENCES

BASSETT, C. A. L., DONATH, A., MACAGNO, F., PREISIG, R., FLEISCH, H. and FRANCIS, M. D. (1969). Diphosphonates in the treatment of myositis ossificans. *Lancet*, **ii**, 845

BONJOUR, J.-P., DELUCA, H. G., FLEISCH, H., TRECHSEL, U., MATEJOWEC, L. A. and OMDAHL, J. L. (1973). Reveral of the EHDP inhibition of calcium absorption by 1,25 dihydroxycholecalciferol. *Eur. J. Clin. Invest.*, **3**, 44

BONJOUR, J.-P., RUSSELL, R. G. G., MORGAN, D. B. and FLEISCH, H. (1972). Intestinal calcium absorption, Ca-binding protein and Ca-ATPase in diphosphonate treated rats. *Am. J. Physiol.*, **224**, 1011

CHASE, L. R., MELSON, G. L. and AURBACH, G. D. (1969). Pseudohypoparathyroidism: defective excretion of 3′,5′-AMP in response to parathyroid hormone. *J. Clin. Invest.*, **48**, 1832

CRAM, R. L., BARMADA, R., GEHO, W. B. and RAY, R. D. (1971). Diphosphonate treatment of calcinosis universalis. *N. Engl. J. Med.*, **285**, 1012

FISKE, C. H. and SUBBAROW, Y. (1925). The colorimetric estimation of phosphorus. *J. Biol. Chem.*, **66**, 375

FLEISCH, H. and BONJOUR, J.-P. (1973). Diphosphonate treatment in bone disease. *N. Engl. J. Med.*, **189**, 1419

FLEISCH, H., RUSSELL, R. G. G., BISAZ, S., MÜHLBAUER, R. C. and WILLIAMS, D. A. (1970). The inhibitory effect of polyphosphonates on the formation of calcium phosphate crystals *in vitro* and on aortic and kidney calcification *in vivo*. *Eur. J. Clin. Invest.*, **1**, 12

FLEISCH, H., RUSSELL, R. G. G. and STRAUMANN, F. (1966). Effect of pyrophosphate on hydroxyapatite and its implications in calcium homeostasis. *Nature*, **212**, 901

FRANCIS, M. D. (1969). The inhibition of calcium hydroxyapatite crystal growth by polyphosphonates and polyphosphates. *Calcif. Tissue Res.*, **3**, 151

GEHO, W. B. and WHITESIDE, J. A. (1973). Experience with disodium etidronate on diseases of ectopic calcification. In B. Frame, A. M. Parfitt and H. Duncan (eds.), *Clinical Aspects of Bone Disease*, p. 506. (Amsterdam : Excerpta Medica)

HILL, L. F., LUMB, G. A., MAWER, E. B. and STANBURY, S. W. (1973). Indirect inhibition of the biosynthesis of 1,25-dihydroxycholecalciferol in rats treated with a diphosphonate. *Clin. Sci.*, **44**, 335

METZGER, A. L., SINGER, F. R. BLUESTONE, R. and PEARSON, C. M. (1974). Failure of disodium etidronate in calcinosis due to dermatomyositis and scleroderma. *N. Engl. J. Med.*, **291**, 1294

MORGAN, D. B., BONJOUR, J.-P., GASSER, A. B., O'BRIEN, K. and FLEISCH, H. A. (1971). The influence of a diphosphonate on the intestinal absorption of calcium. *Isr. J. Med. Sci.*, **7**, 384

RECKER, R. R., HASSING, G. S., LAU, J. R. and SAVILLE, P. D. (1973). The hyperphosphatemic effect of disodium ethane-1-hydroxy-1, 1-diphosphonate (EHDP™): renal handling of phosphorus and the renal response to parathyroid hormone. *J. Lab. Clin. Med.*, **81**, 258

RUSSELL, R. G. G., MÜHLBAUER, R. C., BISAZ, S., WILLIAMS, D. A. and FLEISCH, H. (1970). The influence of pyrophosphate, condensed phosphates, phosphonates, and other phosphate compounds on the dissolution of hydroxyapatite *in vitro* and on bone resorption induced by parathyroid hormone in tissue culture and in thyroparathyroidectomised rats. *Calcif. Tissue Res.*, **6**, 183

RUSSELL, R. G. G., SMITH, R., BISHOP, M. C., PRICE, D. A. and SQUIRE, C. M. (1972). Treatment of myositis ossificans progressiva with a diphosphonate. *Lancet*, **i**, 10

RUSSELL, R. G. G., SMITH, R., PRESTON, C., WALTON, R. J. and WOODS, C. G. (1974). Diphosphonates in Paget's disease. *Lancet*, **i**, 894

SMITH, R., RUSSELL, R. G. G., BISHOP, M. C., WOODS, C. G. and BISHOP, M. (1973). Paget's disease of bone; experience with a diphosphonate (disodium etidronate) in treatment. *Quart. J. Med.*, **42**, 235

WEISS, I. W., FISHER, L. and PHANG, J. M. (1971). Diphosphonate therapy in a patient with myositis ossificans progressiva. *Ann. Intern. Med.*, **74**, 933

17

Cartilage chemistry in bone dysplasias with neonatal presentation

C. A. Pennock and A. C. Sewell

Diseases of bone may be divided into three main groups (Spranger, 1973).

(1) Secondary bone disease such as rickets.
(2) Regulatory bone disease such as hypoparathyroidism.
(3) Intrinsic diseases of bone or bone dysplasias.

The first two groups have been discussed in depth during this symposium and have complex biochemical mechanisms which are now more easy to understand. The bone dysplasias to which Dr Carter has already referred during this meeting are only at the first two stages of discovery of the inborn error.

Many of the bone dysplasias clearly originate in some abnormality of the basic structure and differentation of cartilage but the biochemical mechanisms have not been investigated. A considerable volume of literature has accumulated on the structure of cartilage and its principle protein, collagen, which is embedded in a proteoglycan matrix. Most of the work has been done on animal cartilage or on human articular cartilage with the objective of understanding the pathogenesis of osteoarthrosis in man. Several excellent reviews have been published in recent years (Barrett 1968; McDevitt, 1973; Muir, 1973) none of which discuss any work on cartilage in bone dysplasias or even normal cartilage in infants and children. Spranger (1973) has reviewed the biochemistry of bone dysplasias and was only able to discuss experimental work on osteogenesis imperfecta, hyposphosphatasia, osteoctasia, and the mucopolysaccharidoses as examples of biochemical abnormalities. He was forced to conclude that 'our knowledge about the biochemical basis of bone dysplasias is sparse'.

We have recently had the opportunity to study small pieces of epiphyseal cartilage taken from four infants who died with one of the bone dysplasias acting as a contributory cause. Those dysplasias which may cause death in the neonatal period or early infancy have recently been reviewed by Gordon (1974) and his classification is shown in Table 17.1.

Table 17.1 *Lethal bone dysplasias—Gordon (1974)*

TYPE I

Skeleton inadequate to withstand stress of delivery
Osteogenesis imperfecta congenita–Ekman (1788)
Hypophosphatasia–Rathbun (1948)
Achondrogenesis I–Parenti (1936)
Achondrogenesis II (Thanatophoric Dwarfism II)—Legrand (1956); Saldino (1971)

TYPE II

Development of ribs defective, resulting in a thoracic cage which is too small to permit adequate respiratory function
Infantile thoracic dystrophy—Jeune *et al.* (1955)
Thanatophoric dwarfism I—Maroteaux *et al.* (1967)
Camptomelic dwarfism—Maroteaux *et al.* (1971)
Chondroectodermal dysplasia—Ellis and Van Creveld (1940)
Spondylo-thoracic dysplasia—Jarcho and Levin (1938)
Dysplasia described by Saldino and Noonan (1972)

TYPE III

Hypoplasia of the odontoid process leading to atlanto-axial dislocation
Mucopolysaccharidosis Type IV—Morquio (1929)
Chondrodysplasia punctata—Conradi (1914)

At first sight it seemed that the amount of material available to us would be insufficient for a detailed and complex analysis which would include isolation of the collagen as well as light and heavy protein–polysaccharide complexes of the matrix. However, we were encouraged to find that Pedrini-Mille *et al.* (1967) had measured a few constituents of epiphyseal cartilage from children in a fairly simple manner. Furthermore, they had managed to demonstrate possible defective metabolism of chondroitin sulphate in two siblings with multiple epiphyseal dysplasia (Hunt *et al.*, 1967). We, therefore, felt that it should be possible to measure certain constituents of the macromolecules in cartilage and that these results might reflect alterations in the relative amounts of these macromolecules.

Cartilage consists of collagen fibres embedded in a matrix of glycosaminoglycans (chondroitin sulphate and keratan sulphate) as proteoglycan complexes with glycoproteins and a variety of minerals. We, therefore, decided to measure hydroxyproline which is unique to collagen, hexuronic acid which would reflect proteoglycan content and sialic acid which would reflect glycoprotein content. Analysis of hexosamines which are present in glycosaminoglycans and glycoproteins (glucosamine in keratan sulphate and glycoproteins and galactosamine in chondroitin sulphate) might reflect the relative levels of these constituents and estimation of neutral sugars would reflect glycoprotein content. In addition we estimated the important bone minerals calcium and magnesium. We wish to present these results and compare them with data obtained on cartilage from nine infants who died of conditions in which an abnormality of cartilage development was most unlikely.

Materials and methods

The lower epiphyseal cartilage was obtained at post mortem examination from the left femur of four infants with a bone dysplasia and nine infants who died of other causes. The samples were stored at −20 °C until they were processed. The cartilage was homogenised in 20 ml of absolute ethanol using a 'Polytron'* homogeniser at 15 000 rpm. The homogenate was kept at 4 °C overnight, then centrifuged and the supernatant discarded. 20 ml of diethyl ether was added to the pellet, mixed and allowed to stand for 4 hours. The samples were then centrifuged and the supernatant discarded and the cartilage sample was dried in a vacuum dessicator. Aliquots of 10 mg dry cartilage powder were carefully weighed and hydrolysed in duplicate in:

(1) 4 M hydrochloric acid at 100 °C for 18 hours and
(2) 0·05 M sulphuric acid at 80 °C for 1 hour.

The hydrochloric acid hydrolysates were analysed for hydroxyproline

* Kinematica GMBH Lucerne, Switzerland.

by an autoanalyser method (Pennock *et al.*, 1970) and for hexosamines by gas liquid chromatography of the hexosamines as alditol acetates (Murphy *et al.*, 1974). The sulphuric acid hydrolysates were used for the estimation of neutral sugars by the anthrone reaction using galactose as a standard (Humbel, 1974), sialic acid (Warren, 1959), hexuronic acid including a blank estimation on each sample without carbazole (Bitter and Muir, 1962) and calcium and magnesium by atomic absorption spectroscopy using a Perkin-Elmer Model 103 single beam instrument. The estimation of each constituent was done on all samples in a single batch.

Results

The results given in Table 17.2 are shown as the mean value for the duplicate estimations expressed as a percentage of the dry weight of the cartilage. They show a number of possibly abnormal results which are outside the observed range in the controls and which are shown in parentheses. There was no apparent change with age in any of the constituents measured in the control group.

Discussion

It has been shown that the collagen content of epiphyseal cartilage rises with age and the glycosaminoglycan content falls largely due to a decrease in chondroitin sulphate content (Simunek and Muir, 1971). Dramatic zonal differences in hexuronic acid content have been demonstrated in adult cartilage with greater concentrations in the deeper layers (Stockwell, 1970; Maroudas *et al.*, 1969). A recent paper by Stanescu *et al.* (1974) confirms these changes with age and zonal difference in the human foetus, neonate and children but they found that the zonal differences were not significant in the neonatal period. They measured hydroxyproline and hexosamine content on 13 samples of tibial cartilage from neonates. Our hydroxyproline results are slightly higher than theirs and our hexosamine results slightly lower. This may be due to methodological differences since our results are in close agreement with those obtained on three neonatal samples by Ponseti *et al.* (1968). Our hexuronic acid and neutral sugar results differ markedly from those given by Stockwell (1970). Our hexuronic acid results appear to be too low in relation to the total hexosamine and this could

Table 17.2 *Results from cartilage analysis expressed as percentage dry weight*

Normal controls	*Age*	*HP*	*HUA*	*NS*	*SA*	*HexN*	*GluN*	*GalN*	*Gal/Glu*	*Ca*	*Mg*
1	1 m	4·60	2·24	5·70	0·034	6·74	0·84	5·90	7·02	0·36	0·076
2	1 m	5·76	5·26	5·57	0·092	4·76	0·69	4·07	5·89	0·26	0·076
3	5 m	5·55	2·62	3·87	0·063	6·28	0·90	5·38	5·97	0·25	0·064
4	SB	5·36	3·71	3·77	0·070	5·15	0·70	4·45	6·35	0·31	0·071
5	SB	4·65	6·00	3·79	0·217	4·47	0·65	3·82	5·87	0·30	0·080
6	SB	4·80	3·70	4·07	0·129	6·39	0·93	5·46	5·87	0·39	0·080
7	2 d	4·85	4·37	4·87	0·166	5·43	0·68	4·75	6·98	0·47	0·094
8	2 m	5·50	2·39	2·74	0·716	4·64	0·59	4·05	6·86	0·30	0·067
9	7 d	5·30	4·52	8·32	0·467	4·48	0·59	3·89	6·59	0·23	0·068
Bone dysplasias											
1	1 y	(6.20)	2·72	2·75	0·313	6·60	(1·14)	5·46	(4·78)	0·38	(0·055)
2	3 m	(7·8)	(1·52)	1·78	0·034	4·72	(1·28)	(3·44)	(2·68)	0·23	(0·050)
3	12 hr	4·15	(1·75)	2·77	0·327	(4·05)	0·89	(3·16)	(3·55)	(2·99)	(0·063)
4	24 hr	(4·15)	3·10	(1·46)	0·151	(3·45)	(0·49)	(2·96)	6·04	0·43	(0·015)

Key: HP—hydroxyproline; HUA—hexuronic acid; NS—neutral sugar; HexN—hexosamine; GalN—galactosamine; GluN—glucosamine; Gal/Glu—galactosamine to glucosamine ratio; Ca—calcium; Mg—magnesium; SB—stillborn. Results outside the observed control values are shown in parentheses.

be due to destruction during hydrolysis. It is probably preferable to do a proteolytic digestion prior to the estimation of hexuronic acid. We are unable to comment on our other results as we were unable to find similar data in the literature.

The results on patients with bone dysplasias show a number of possible abnormalities. Since all analyses on controls and abnormals were done in a single batch these results are not due to between batch errors. It is difficult to place an interpretation on any of them since the number of controls is small. Furthermore, although the diagnosis in the two patients with chondrodysplasia punctata was unequivocal, the patient with 'thanatophoric dwarfism' is probably a case of anosteogenesis (Gordon 1974) and the other patient did not have hypophosphatasia (serum alkaline phosphatase was high) and there is considerable uncertainty about the actual diagnosis.

It is remarkable that the two samples from the patients with chondrodysplasia punctata show similar abnormal results but it must be appreciated that one infant was a year old and cartilage of that age was not available to us in our control group. We would be most appreciative of any comments on the interpretation of our data from members of the audience.

While it is clear that certain methodological problems must be investigated and a larger number of normal controls must be examined, we believe that the simple approach we have used has given sufficiently unusual results in patients with bone dysplasias to signify its potential. The methods used are all simple and the amount of material required is small such that analysis could be done on biopsy material from living patients and compared directly with histological findings.

REFERENCES

Barrett, A. J. (1968). Cartilage. In M. Florkin (ed.), *Comprehensive Biochemistry*, Vol. 26 B, p. 425. (Amsterdam : Elsener)

Bitter, T. and Muir, H. M. (1962). A modified uronic acid carbazole reaction. *Anal. Biochem.*, **4**, 330

Carter, C. O. (1975). Diseases of bone in search of an inborn error. This symposium, p. 214

Conradi, E. (1914). Vorzeitiges Auftreten von Knochen- und eigenartigen Verkalkungskernen bei Chondrodystrophia fötalis hypoplastica. Histologische und Röntgenuntersuchungen. *Jahrb. Kinderh.*, **80**, 86

Ellis, R. W. B. and Van Creveld, S. (1940). A syndrome characterised by ectodermal dysplasia, polydactyly, chondrodysplasia and congenital morbus cordis. Report of three cases. *Am. J. Dis. Child.*, **115**, 65

Ekman, O. J. (1788). Dissertatio medica descriptionem et casus aliquot osteomalaciae sistens. MD Thesis (Uppsala) quoted by V. A. McKusick (1972). *Heritable Disorders of Connective Tissue*, 4th Ed., p. 391. (St Louis : C. V. Mosby)

Gordon, I. R. S. (1974). Lethal bone dysplasias. Paper read at South Wales Bone Dysplasia register

Humbel, R. (1974). Identification and quantitation of keratan sulphate in urine. *Clin. Chim. Acta*, **52**, 173

Hunt, D. D., Ponseti, I. V., Pedrini-Mille, A. and Pedrini, V. (1967). Multiple epiphyseal dysplasia in two siblings. *J. Bone Joint Surg.* (*Am.*), **49A**, 1611

Jarcho, S. and Levin, P. M. (1938). Hereditary malformation of the vertebral bodies. *Bull. Johns Hopkins Hosp.*, **62**, 216

Jeune, M., Beraud, C. and Carron, R. (1955). Dystrophie thoracique asphyxiante de caractère familial. *Arch. Fr. Pediatr.*, **12**, 886

Legrand, J. (1956). Une cliché de foetus achondroplasique 'in utero'. *J. Radiol. Electrol. Med. Nucl.*, **37**, 82

Maroteaux, P., Lamy, M. and Robert, J. M. (1967). Le nanisme thanatophore. *Presse Med.*, **75**, 2519

Maroteaux, P., Spranger, J. Opitz, J. M., Kucera, J., Lowry, R. B., Schimke, R. N. and Kagan, S. M. (1971). Le Syndrome Campomélique. *Presse Med.*, **79**, 1157

Maroudas, A., Muir, H. and Wingham, J. (1969). The correlation of fixed negative charge with glycosaminoglycan content of human articular cartilage. *Biochim. Biophys. Acta*, **177**, 492

McDevitt, C. A. (1973). Biochemistry of articular cartilage. Nature of proteoglycans and collagen of articular cartilage and their role in ageing and in osteoarthrosis. *Ann. Rheum. Dis.*, **32**, 364

Morquio, L. (1929). Sur une forme de dystrophie osseuse familiale. *Bull. Soc. Pédiatr.* (Paris), **27**, 145

Muir, H. (1973). Biochemistry of cartilage. In M. A. R. Freeman (ed.), *Adult Articular Cartilage*, p. 100. (London : Pitman Medical Press)

Murphy, D., Pennock, C. A. and Longdon, K. J. (1974). Gas–liquid chromatographic measurement of glucosamine and galactosamine content of urinary glycosaminoglycans. *Clin. Chim. Acta*, **53**, 145

Parenti, G. C. (1936). La anosteogenesi (una verieta della osteogenesi imperfetta). *Pathologica*, **28**, 447

Pedrini-Mille, A. Pedrini, V., Hunt, D. D. and Ponseti, I. V. (1967). Chemical studies on the ground substance of human epiphyseal plate cartilage. *J. Bone Joint Surg.* (*Am.*), **49A**, 1628

Pennock, C. A., Moore, G. R. and Hoyle, M. D. (1970). Estimation of hydroxyproline in urine. *J. Med. Lab. Tech.*, **27**, 302

Ponseti, I. V., Pedrini-Mille, A. and Pedrini, V. (1968). Histological and chemical analysis of human iliac crest cartilage. *Calcif. Tissue Res.*, **2**, 197

Rathbun, J. C. (1948). 'Hypophosphatasia,' a new developmental anomaly. *Am. J. Dis. Child.*, **75**, 822

Saldino, R. M. (1971). Lethal short limbed dwarfism; achondrogenesis and thanatophoric dwarfism. *Am. J. Roentgenol.*, **112**, 185

Saldino, R. M. and Noonan, C. D. (1972). Severe thoracic dystrophy with striking micromelia, abnormal osseous development, including the spine, and multiple visceral anomalies. *Am. J. Rontgenol.*, **114** (2), 257

Simunek, Z. and Muir, H. (1971). Changes in the protein-polysaccharides of pig articular cartilage during prenatal life, development and old age. *Biochem. J.*, **126**, 515

Spranger, J. (1973). The biochemical basis of bone dysplasias. *Prog. Pediatr. Radiol.*, **4**, 29

Stanescu, V., Stanescu, R. and Maroteaux, P. (1973). Chemical studies on the human growth cartilage in fetuses and newborns. *Biol. Neonate*, **23**, 432

Stockwell, R. A. (1970). Changes in the acid glycosaminoglycan content of the matrix of ageing human cartilage. *Ann. Rheum. Dis.*, **29**, 509

Warren, L. (1959). The thiobarbituric acid assay of sialic acids. *J. Biol. Chem.*, **234**, 1971

18

Calcium and vitamin D metabolism during anticonvulsant therapy

T. C. B. Stamp

Heidelberg is an appropriate setting for this paper since anticonvulsant bone disease was first recognised in Germany by Schmid (1967), and in this hospital by Kruse (1968). Our own detailed description of anticonvulsant rickets and osteomalacia came in 1970 (Dent *et al.*, 1970), and since that time clinical reports from other centres have accumulated (Borgstedt *et al.*, 1972; Genuth *et al.*, 1972; Sotaniemi *et al.*, 1972).

When we first postulated that anticonvulsant rickets and osteomalacia were produced by hepatic enzyme induction, under the influence of anticonvulsant drugs, our suggestion was based on clinical observation coupled with knowledge of analogous changes in steroid metabolism (Kuntzmann, 1969). Most clinical and experimental data since that time, discussed below, have supported this original concept. Induced liver enzymes are mostly hydroxylases and conjugases, enzymes of the so-called detoxicating system; their activity diverts the metabolism of cholecalciferol from its normal major pathway (through 25-hydroxycholecalciferol), into abnormal amounts of other hydroxylated and inactive metabolites. A new form of ultimate vitamin deficiency is thus produced despite adequate diet and normal intestinal absorption. This chapter summarises the clinical features of anticonvulsant rickets and osteomalacia, documents the complication of tertiary hyperparathyroidism and presents studies of radioactive vitamin D metabolism in epileptic patients. In addition it reviews briefly other experimental data and highlights some of the outstanding questions which still remain to be answered.

During a survey of an epileptic colony Richens and Rowe (1970) recorded hypocalcaemia in 22% of their patients and raised alkaline phosphatase levels in 28%. Both bone and liver phosphatase isoenymes were significantly elevated. Of the 12 patients with clinical bone disease who have been in our care we have published clinical details of eight (Dent *et al.*, 1970; Stamp *et al.*, 1972; Stamp, 1974). Their ages have ranged from 20 months to over 60 years and the duration of their compound anticonvulsant therapy has ranged from 18 months to over 40 years.

A main feature of the disease is the relative resistance to treatment with vitamin D which these patients show. We have emphasised that this resistance may occur even when vitamin D is administered parenterally, showing that the disease is not due to malabsorption of vitamin D (Dent *et al.*, 1970). Figure 18.1 illustrates in a calcium balance study

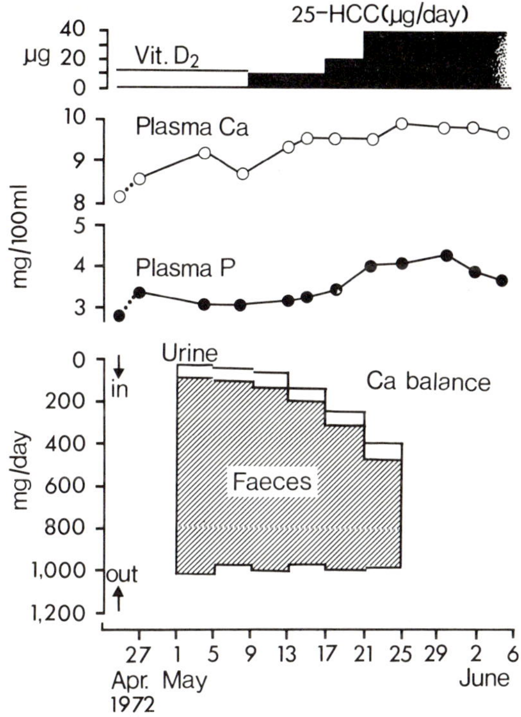

FIGURE 18.1 Metabolic balance data in a 57-year-old man with anticonvulsant osteomalacia. He had been on a vitamin D supplement providing 500 i.u. daily for one year. Note the steady improvement in calcium balance and plasma levels when 25-hydroxycholecalciferol at first in a dose of 10 µg daily, was substituted for calciferol 12·5 µg daily (from Stamp *et al.*, 1972).

how resistance to treatment is rapidly overcome using 25-hydroxycholecalciferol ($25(OH)D_3$) instead of vitamin D. Presumably oral $25(OH)D_3$ can bypass the liver and thus provide direct substrate for the kidney 1α-hydroxylase which elaborates the hormonal form of the vitamin. The most striking resistance in our series occurred in an 8-year-

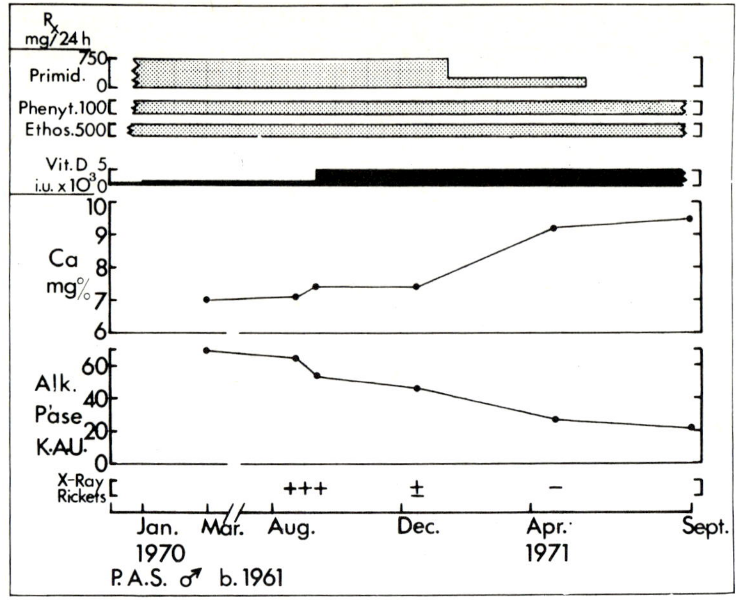

FIGURE 18.2 Progress in anticonvulsant rickets. See text for description (from Stamp, 1974).

old boy of Asian origin living in a residential school (Figure 18.2). Rickets had been diagnosed 2 years 9 months previously; for 2 years he had received vitamin D 1000 i.u. daily, he then received two injections of 15 000 i.u. daily and his supplement was increased to 1600 i.u. daily for a further 9 months; nevertheless, his rickets steadily worsened. In an attempt to titrate the dose of vitamin D required to heal his disease he was given 5000 i.u. daily and subsequently took 4–8 months to heal his rickets. This resistance to treatment is important when considering the advisability of prophylactic vitamin D treatment in epileptics; to be sure of prophylaxis in all patients may undoubtedly risk intoxication, which is even more dangerous, in some. It is important to be aware that anticonvulsant drugs may themslves tend to increase fit frequency because of the hypocalcaemia they may produce and the resultant excitatory effect of hypocalcaemia on the central nervous system. Anticonvulsant dosage in the patient illustrated in Figure 18.2 (which was controlled independently elsewhere) was materially reduced without worsening his epilepsy, after normocalcaemia had been restored. A significant reduction in fit frequency has also been reported in a clinical trial of vitamin D in epileptic patients (Christiansen *et al.*, 1974). The vicious circles that anticonvulsant therapy may produce are shown in Figure 18.3.

Tertiary hyperparathyrodism occurs when an autonomous parathyroid adenoma develops from long-standing secondary hyperparathyroidism due to osteomalacia (Davies *et al.*, 1968). This has not been previously described following long-term anticonvulsant therapy and documentation in the following case-report is thus warranted.

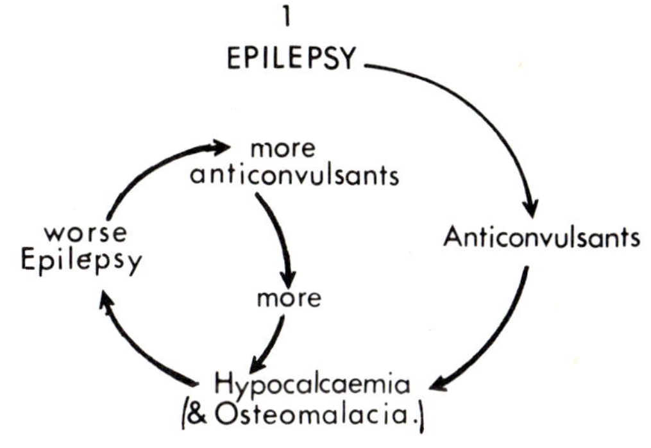

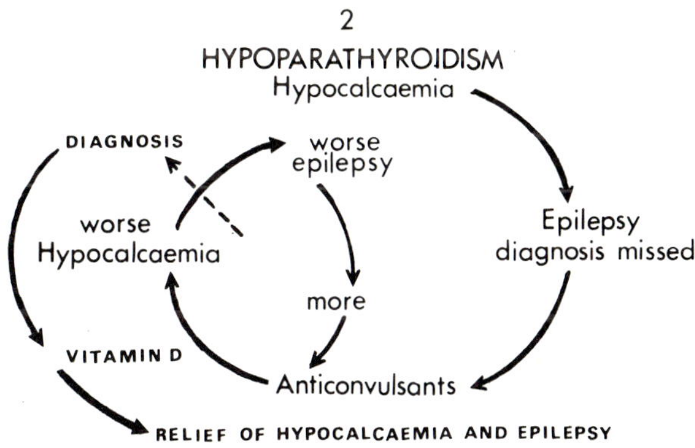

FIGURE 18.3 Diagrammatic representation of the vicious circles which may result from anticonvulsant therapy in epilepsy, and if the correct diagnosis is missed in hypoparathyroidism.

CASE REPORT

A 37-year-old female presented in September 1973 with a 3–4 month history of low back pain radiating to the groins. At the age of 21 she had suffered from miliary tuberculosis followed by tuberculous meningitis from which she recovered satisfactorily, but developed epilepsy at the age of 26. Since that time she had been receiving phenytoin 200 mg daily and diazepam 10 mg daily. There were no other abnormal symptoms. She travelled widely and ate a varied diet (estimated vitamin D content 102 i.u. daily). She had no bone tenderness or myopathy. Investigations showed: calcium 10·0 mg/100 ml (corrected for specific gravity), phosphorus 1·4 mg/100 ml, alkaline phosphatase 23 K.A. units; full blood count and routine plasma biochemistry were normal; plasma 25-hydroxyvitamin D was low at 4 ng/ml and immuno-reactive parathyroid hormone was raised at 2·4 ng/ml. Indices of hepatic enzyme induction were variably positive; serum γ-glutamyl transpeptidase mildly raised at 49 units, plasma antipyrine half-life very low at 6·6 hours (Dr A. McLean; normal range 13·2 $\pm$2·2 (S.D.) hours), quinine half-life 5·4 hours (within normal range of 6·6 $\pm$1·2 (S.D.) hours). Urinary total hydroxyproline was mildly raised at 78 mg/24 hours. Bone biopsy showed changes of gross osteomalacia accompanied by slight hyperparathyroidism. Test of gastro-intestinal function (faecal fat excretion, barium follow through, etc.) were well within the normal range. Treatment was begun with sodium phosphate 10 g daily and vitamin D_2 2 mg daily and her progress is shown in Figure 18.4. Hypercalcaemia developed in 9 days and persisted despite stopping vitamin D and continuing sodium phosphate which has a hypocalcaemic effect on its own. Plasma calcium did not fall during a standard hydrocortisone test, 40 mg 8-hourly (Dent and Watson, 1968). At operation, a parathyroid adenoma weighing 500 mg was removed. Post-operatively a striking 'hungry bones stage' developed which required a high dose of dihydrotachysterol and calcium supplements to restore her plasma calcium slowly to normal. Recovery was otherwise uneventful and her backache was relieved.

As would be expected, plasma levels of 25-hydroxyvitamin D (25 (OH)D) are abnormally low in drug treated epileptics (Stamp *et al.*, 1972; Hahn *et al.*, 1972b). When related to estimated vitamin D intake plasma 25(OH)D levels were strikingly lower among patients receiving chronic diphenylhydantoin therapy throughout the estimated range of vitamin D intake (Hahn *et al.*, 1976).

The effect of hepatic enzyme induction in vitamin D nutrition in epilepsy must be differentiated from a straightforward tendency for nutritional deficiency which is likely among epileptic patients. Solar ultraviolet irradiation is an important source of vitamin D in Britain, healthy populations showing marked seasonal variations in plasma levels of 25-hydroxyvitamin D (Stamp and Round, 1974). Any population whose outdoor activity is likely to be curtailed, such as epileptics, will therefore be at risk from developing nutritional deficiency. This problem may be more acute when patients are hopitalised or if they reside in a home. Richens and Rowe (1971) showed that epileptics who worked out of doors in one epileptic colony had higher plasma calcium levels than their fellow residents who remained inside. Surveys of bone

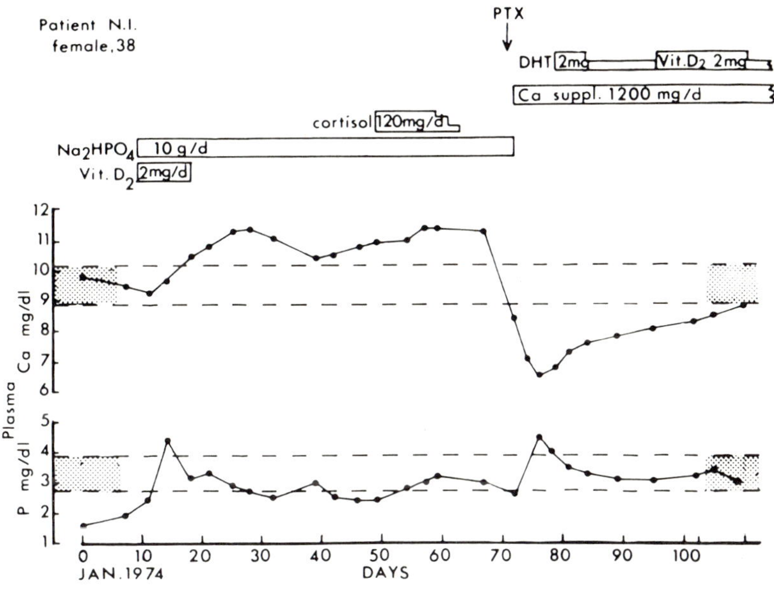

FIGURE 18.4 Tertiary hyperparathyroidism associated with anticonvulsant osteomalacia. Note the rapid development of hypercalcaemia after beginning vitamin D, its persistence despite treatment with full doses of sodium phosphate and hydrocortisone, and the marked 'hungry bones' stage following successful operation.

mineral mass using absorption densiometry have shown decreased bone mineral content among epileptics which improved steadily during treatment with vitamin D in a dose of 2000 i.u. daily (Christiansen *et al.*, 1972; Christiansen *et al.*, 1973).

A further clinical problem is the apparently raised incidence of pure osteoporosis alone in epilepsy (Dent and Watson, 1966). Seven of the latter workers' series of about 80 osteoporotic patients below the age of 50 had had grand mal seizures from idiopathic epilepsy. None of them had evidence of rickets or osteomalacia; it may well be that among epileptics osteoporosis is more common than osteomalacia and would also cause decreased bone mineral content.

The relative rarity of frank clinical rickets and osteomalacia among epileptic patients, 1% in the epileptic colony surveyed by Richens and Rowe (unpublished data), requires further consideration. The urinary excretion of D-glucaric acid has been used as a clinical index of enzyme induction (Hunter *et al.*, 1971) and among epileptic patients excretion was found to vary several hundred-fold; it may be therefore only those few patients who are susceptible to extreme degrees of enzyme induction who may be at risk from developing overt bone disease. An inborn error (potential) of metabolism may determine this susceptibility and the interesting possibility of its genetic transmissibility requires study.

Many experimental data concerning the effects of anticonvulsant therapy on vitamin D metabolism have also accumulated. Several studies have indicated that tritiated cholecalciferol disappears more rapidly from the plasma of anticonvulsant-treated patients than from normals (Hahn *et al.*, 1972; Schaefer, Flury *et al.*, 1972a; Mawer, 1974). Our data (adapted from Rowe, 1973) is shown in Figure 18.5 and gives changes in plasma [1–^{3}H, 4–^{14}C], cholecalciferol with time after injection in three epileptic patients and four patients with other disorders of calcium metabolism; their diagnoses are given in Table 18.1. Figure 18.6 shows the corresponding appearance of [1–^{3}H, 4–^{14}C], 25-hydroxycholecalciferol in these patients and it can be seen that the increase in this fraction was directly related to the speed of decrease in the vitamin D_3 fraction. The pattern of changes in plasma radioactivity after administration of labelled cholecalciferol has previously been showed to depend primarily on the patient's state of vitamin D nutrition (Mawer *et al.*, 1971), rather than necessarily reflecting any alteration in cholecalciferol metabolism. This relationship between ^{3}[H]-vitamin D_3 half-life and nutritional status is also shown in the table. Further work is therefore required to prove whether cholecalciferol turnover is more rapid in states of enzyme induction *than would be expected* for the patients nutritional status. Liver microsomes from phenobarbitone-induced rats convert cholecalciferol not to 25-hydroxycholecalciferol but to more polar and inactive metabolites (Hahn *et al.*, 1972a); intestinal absorption of radioactive cholecalciferol is not impaired in humans or in phenobarbitone-treated rats (Schaefer *et al.*, 1972b) although intestinal calcium transport is inhibited by phenytoin as would be expected (Koch *et al.*, 1972). Enhanced biliary excretion of conjugated cholecalci-

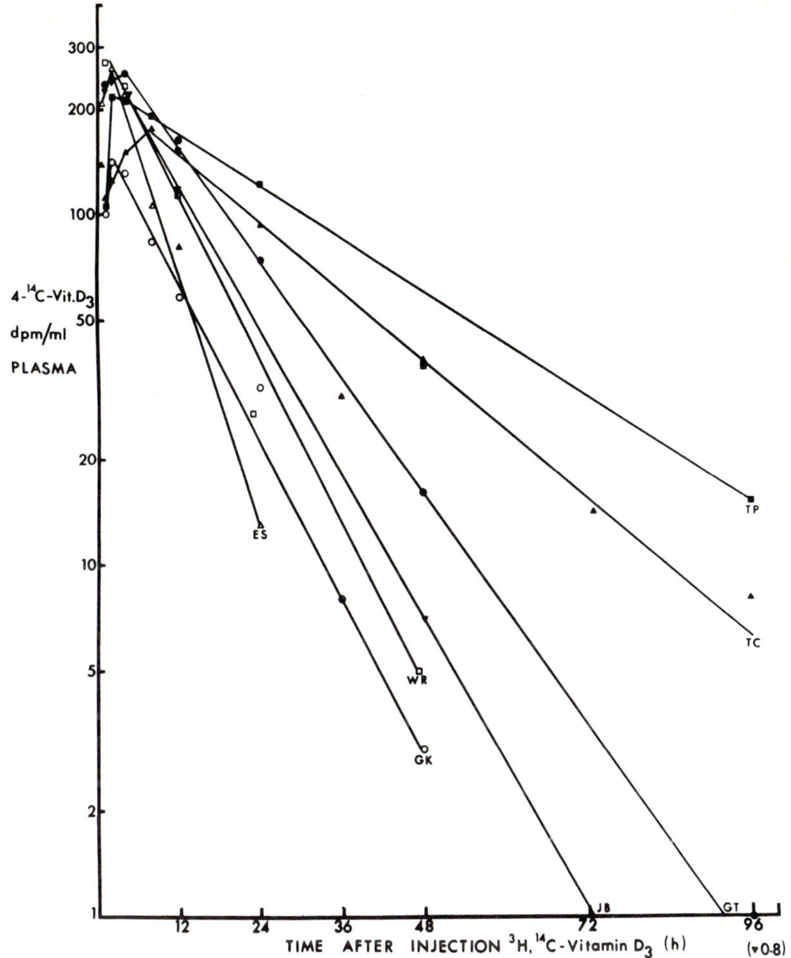

FIGURE 18.5 Disappearance of plasma 1–^{3}H, 4–^{14}C, cholecalciferol following intravenous injection in seven patients with disordered calcium metabolism. Open symbols represent patients with anticonvulsant osteomalacia; closed symbols represent patients with other disorders of calcium metabolism (see Table 18.1).

ferol and its metabolites has also been demonstrated in phenobarbitone-treated mammals, and following administration of radioactive vitamin D tissue radioactivity is more rapidly depleted in rats which have received prolonged treatment with phenobarbitone (Silver *et al.*, 1974). Finally, there is evidence that hepatic microsomal 25-hydroxylation itself is *not* induced by anticonvulsant drugs (De Luca, 1974). Resistance to parathyroid hormone-induced bone resorption has been found during in-

Table 18.1 *Clinical details and diagnoses of patients shown in Figures 18.4 and 18.5. All measured plasma 25(OH)D_3 levels (courtesy Dr J. G. Haddad) were grossly deficient irrespective of season (cf. Stamp and Round, 1974). Pre-treatment levels of plasma 25(OH)D_3 were not measured in the other patients but there was no reason to suspect they were abnormal except in patient T.P.*†

Subject	*Age*	*Sex*	*Diagnosis*	^{14}*C-Vit.*D_3 *t/2 (h)*	*Plasma 25(OH)*D_3 (ng/ml)
E.S. (△)	47	F	Anticonvulsant osteomalacia	5	1·4
W.R. (□)	56	M	Anticonvulsant osteomalacia	7	2·1
G.K. (○)	78	M	Anticonvulsant osteomalacia	8	‘< 2·6’
J.B. (▼)	19	F	Idiopathic hypoparathyroidism	9	(0·08 i.u./ml)*
G.T. (●)	46	M	Milk-alkali syndrome	11	—
T.C. (▲)	31	M	Hypercalcaemic sarcoidosis	18	—
T.P.† (■)	11	M	Vitamin D-dependent rickets	24	—

* Bioassayed antiricketic activity at very low level (courtesy Dr E. M. Cruickshank); the patient was midly epileptic and receiving treatment with phenobarbitone.

† Long-term pharmacological dosage with vitamin D, stopped 6–9 months previously.

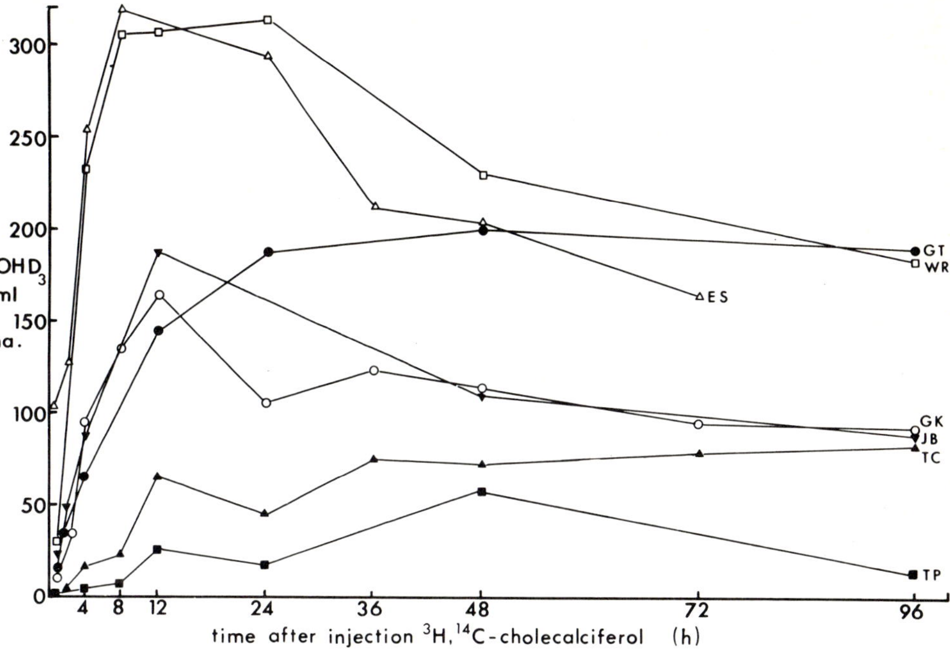

FIGURE 18.6 Appearance of radioactively-labelled 25(OH)D_3 following intravenous injection of 1^{3}H, 4–^{14}C cholecalciferol (see Figure 18.4 and Table 18.1).

cubation with phenytoin (Jenkins *et al.*, 1973) and a form of functional hypoparathyroidism associated with end organ resistance may be a further factor in the production of hypocalcaemia during anticonvulsant therapy.

Acknowledgements

The author is grateful to Professor C. E. Dent for permission to report these patients and to his other collaborators including Dr D. J. F. Rowe, Miss J. M. Round, Dr J. G. Haddad and Dr D. E. M. Lawson. Support from the Wellcome Trust is also gratefully acknowledged.

REFERENCES

BORGSTEDT, A. D., DRYSON, M. F., YOUNG, L. W. and FORBES, G. B. (1972). Long term administration of antiepileptic drugs and the development of rickets. *J. Pediatr.*, **81**, 9

CHRISTIANSEN, C., KRISTENSEN, M. and RØDBRO, P. (1972). Latent osteomalacia in epileptic patients on anticonvulsants. *Br. Med. J.*, **3**, 738

CHRISTIANSEN, C., RØDBRO, P. and LUND, M. (1973). Effect of vitamin D on bone mineral mass in normal subjects and in epileptic patients on anticonvulsants: a controlled therapeutic trial. *Br. Med. J.*, **2**, 208

CHRISTIANSEN, C., RØDBRO, P. and SJO, O. (1974). Anticonvulsant action of vitamin D in epileptic patients. A controlled pilot study. *Br. Med. J.* **2**, 258

DAVIES, D. R., DENT, C. E. and WATSON, L. (1968). Tertiary hyperparathyroidism. *Br. Med. J.*, **3**, 395

DeLuca, H. F. (1974). Vitamin D—1973. *Am. J. Med.*, **57**, 1

Dent, C. E. and Watson, L. (1966). Osteoporosis. *Postgrad. Med. J.*, Oct. Suppl.

Dent, C. E. and Watson, L. (1968). The hydrocortisone test in primary and tertiary hyperparathyroidism. *Lancet*, **ii**, 662

Dent, C. E., Richens, A., Rowe, D. J. F. and Stamp, T. C. B. (1970). Osteomalacia with long-term anticonvulsant therapy in epilepsy. *Br. Med. J.*, **4**, 69

Genuth, S. M., Klein, L., Rabinovitch, S. and King, K. C. (1972). Osteomalacia accompanying chronic anticonvulsant therapy. *J. Endocrinol. Metab.*, **35**, 378

Hahn, T. J., Birge, S. J., Scharp, C. R. and Avioli, L. V. (1972a). Phenobarbital-induced alterations in vitamin D metabolism. *J. Clin. Invest.*, **51**, 741

Hahn, T. J., Hendin, B. A., Scharp, C. R. and Haddad, J. G. (1972b). Effect of chronic anticonvulsant therapy on serum 25-hydroxycalciferol levels in adults. *N. Engl. J. Med.*, **287**, 900

Hunter, J., Maxwell, J. D., Stewart, D. A., Parsons, V., Williams, R. (1971). Altered calcium metabolism in epileptic children on anticonvulsants. *Br. Med. J.*, **4**, 202

Jenkins, M. V., Harris, M. and Wills, M. R. (1973). The effect of anticonvulsant drugs *in vitro* on bone calcium mobilization by parathyroid hormone. *Clin. Sci. Mol. Med.*, **45**, 1 P

Koch, H.-U., Kraft, D., von Herrath, D. and Schaefer, K. (1972). Influence of diphenylhydantoin and phenobarbitone on intestinal calcium transport in the rat. *Epilepsia*, **13**, 829

Kruse, R. (1968). Osteopathien bei antiepileptischer Langzeittherapie. *Monatschr. Kinderheilkd.*, **116**, 378

Kuntzmann, R. (1969). Drugs and enzyme induction. *Annu. Rev. Pharmacol.*, **9**, 21

Mawer, E. B., Lumb., G. A., Schaefer, K. and Stanbury, S. W. (1971). The metabolism of isotopically labelled vitamin D3 in man: the influence of the state of vitamin D nutrition. *Clin. Sci.*, **40**, 39

Mawer, E. B. (1974). The metabolism of vitamin D in man. *Biochem. Soc. Spec. Publ.*, **3**, 27

Richens, A. and Rowe, D. J. F. (1970). Disturbance of calcium metabolism by anticonvulsant drugs. *Br. Med. J.*, **4**, 73

Richens, A. and Rowe, D. J. F. (1971). Anticonvulsant osteomalacia. *Br. Med. J.*, **4**, 684

Rowe, D. J. F. (1973). A study of disordered calcium and vitamin D metabolism in members of an epileptic colony and of the causal effects of their anticonvulsant drug therapy. Ph.D. Thesis, University of London

Schaefer, K., Flury, W. H., von Herrath, D., Kraft, D., Schweingruber, R. (1972a). Vitamin-D-Stoffwechsel und Antiepileptika. *Schweiz. Med. Wochenschr.*, **102**, 785

Schaefer, K., Kraft, D., von Herrath, D., Opitz, A. (1972b). Intestinal absorption of vitamin D_3 in epileptic patients and phenobarbital-treated rats. *Epilepsia*, **13**, 509

Schmid, F. (1967). Osteopathien bei antiepileptischer Dauerbehandlung. *Fortschr. Med.*, **85**, 381

Silver, J., Neale, G., Thompson, G. R. (1974). Effect of phenobarbitone treatment on vitamin D metabolism in mammals. *Clin. Sci. Mol. Med.*, **46**, 433

Sotaniemi, E. A., Hakkarainen, H. K., Puranen, J. A. and Lahti, R. O. (1972). Radiologic bone changes and hypocalcaemia with anticonvulsant therapy in epilepsy. *Ann. Intern. Med.*, **77**, 389

Stamp, T. C. B., Round, J. M., Rowe, D. J. F. and Haddad, J. G. (1972). Plasma levels and therapeutic effect of 25-hydroxycholecalciferol in epileptic patients taking anticonvulsant drugs. *Br. Med. J.*, **4**, 9

Stamp, T. C. B. (1974). Effects of long-term anticonvulsant therapy on calcium and vitamin D metabolism. *Proc. R. Soc. Med.*, **64**, 69

Stamp, T. C. B. and Round, J. M. (1974). Seasonal changes in human plasma levels of 25-hydroxyvitamin D. *Nature*, **247**, 563

19

α-Aminoadipic aciduria, a new inborn error of lysine metabolism

T. Gerritsen and M. H. Fischer

During routine screening of urine and blood samples of mentally deficient patients seen at the outpatient clinic of a state institution for the retarded, a 10-year-old boy was found to excrete a ninhydrin-positive compound, which on further analysis was demonstrated to be α-aminoadipic acid. The boy, KDM, was referred to the clinic for a special learning disability. According to the attending physicians, he was physically healthy and well grown, without obvious anomalies; he had an essentially normal EEG, and a full scale IQ of 86. (Full details about this patient have been reported by Fischer *et al.*, 1974.)

KDM had a 9-year-old brother, LSM, who was healthy and of normal intelligence. On analysis of urine samples of the brothers, the parents and other siblings of the propositus, KDM and LSM were found to excrete α-aminoadipic acid. The amino acid was undetectable in the urine of the other three siblings or the parents.

Amino acid studies

1. *Analyses of urine and blood*

On the one-dimensional paper chromatogram of urinary amino acids in BuAc (n-butanol, acetic acid and water, 150:10:50, v/v) the unknown compound had an Rf value of 29; in Ph (phenol in water, 4:1, w/v) the Rf value was 41. On quantitative analysis by column chromatography, using a Beckman Amino Analyser Model 119, a large peak was visible on the chromatogram where α-aminoadipic acid is normally eluted. Co-chromatography with synthetic α-aminoadipic acid at different pH levels resulted in a single symmetrical peak while hydrolysis of the urine (20 hours at 100 °C in 6N HCl) did not change the size of this peak.

Quantitative amino acid analysis was performed on several 24 hour urine collections from the two brothers and on one blood sample. Table

19.1 shows the urinary excretion levels and blood level of α-aminoadipic acid. Normally this compound is undetectable in blood.

Table 19.1 *α-Aminoadipic acid excretion and serum levels in patients with α-aminoadipic aciduria and controls*

Subject	*Urine* (mg/24 h)	*Plasma* (mg/100 ml)
III-3	158; 399	0·8
III-4	96; 117	N.D.
Controls (all ages)	0–10	Traces

2. *Lysine loading experiments*

α-Aminoadipic acid is an intermediate in the metabolic breakdown pathway of the essential amino lysine in mammals (Figure 19.1). The pathway via pipecolic acid is longer known but probably less important,

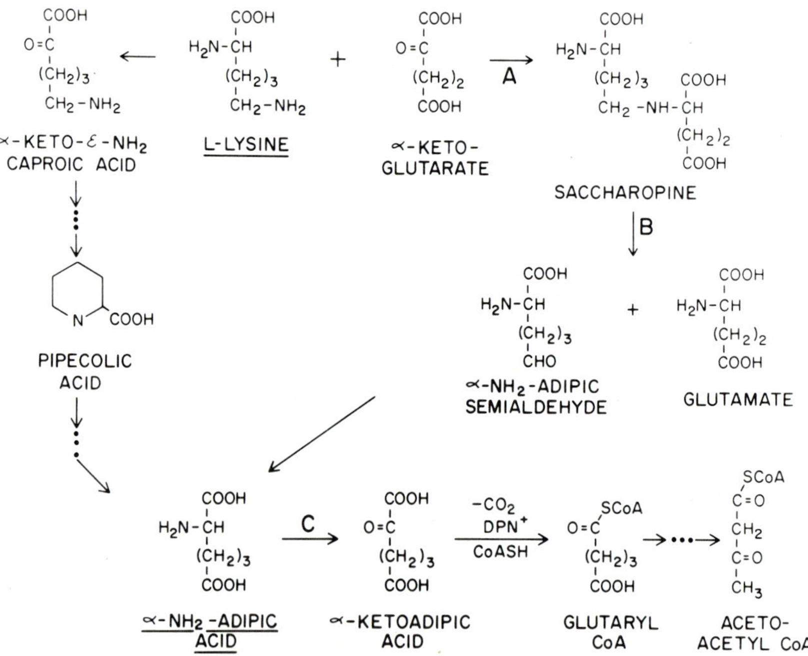

FIGURE 19.1 Metabolism of L-lysine in mammals. Indicated enzyme defects: A—Hyperlysinaemia; B—Saccharopinuria; C—Proposed site of α-aminoadipic aciduria.

while in the pathway through saccharopine (Fellows & Lewis, 1973) two enzyme defects are known, hyperlysinaemia and saccharopinuria. Based upon this information, loading experiments with L-lysine were performed, and quantitative amino acid analysis of urine collected during the 12 hours after 100 mg L-lysine/kg body weight was administered, demonstrated a significant increase in α-aminoadipic acid. This fact can be considered additional support for the identification of the latter amino acid.

The possible enzyme defect

The enzyme defect in this new aminoaciduria is as yet unknown. α-Aminoadipic acid is supposed to be metabolised via α-ketoadipic acid to glutaryl CoA and finally to acetoacetyl CoA. If the mutation were to be analogous to the defect in branched chain ketoaciduria, where accumulation of leucine, isoleucine and valine in the cell is a consequence of a block at the site of oxidative decarboxylation of the analogous branched-chain ketoacids, one could expect to find large amounts of α-ketoadipic acid in the urine of the two boys. Careful organic chemical and gas chromatographic analysis, however, could not detect this ketoacid in the urine.

The suggestion that a block exists in the formation of α-ketoadipic acid from α-aminoadipic acid, would mean that this transemination is activated by a specific aminotransferase, and such an enzyme has not been described as yet. A mutation affecting the synthesis of the α-aminoadipic acid active site of an otherwise nonspecific aminotransferase is another rather improbable possibility.

It seems more logical to presume that there are other pathways in the metabolism of lysine and α-aminoadipic acid, which have not yet been elucidated (Alton Meister, personal information), and that further investigation of the metabolic defect reported here may throw more light on this problem.

Summary and conclusion

According to our information, urinary excretion of α-aminoadipic acid in the amounts reported here, has not been described before. Shih *et al.* (1974) in a recent letter to the Lancet, reported the presence of α-aminoadipic acid in the urine of patients with Reye's syndrome, but no quantitative data were available.

The enzymic cause of the new inborn defect of amino acid metabolism in two brothers of 9 and 10 years old reported here, α-aminoadipic aciduria, has not yet been identified. The defect causes excretion of α-aminoadipic acid in the urine, but there seems to be no reason to attribute the slight mental retardation of one of the two boys to this genetic abnormality.

Table 19.2 *Urinary amino acid excretion (mg/12 h) before and after* L-*lysine load in individuals with α-aminoadipic aciduria*

	Basal		*After lysine load**	
Subject	*AAA*	*Lys*	*AAA*	*Lys*
III-3	124	28·3	302	51
III-4	72	10·1	105	4·4

* 100 mg/kg body weight.

REFERENCES

Fellows, F. C. and Lewis, M. H. R. (1973). Lysine metabolism in mammals. *Biochem. J.*, **136**, 329

Fischer, M. H., Gerritsen, T. and Opitz, J. M. (1974). Alpha-aminoadipic aciduria, a non-deleterious inborn metabolic defect. *Humangenetik*, **24**, 265

Shih, V. E., Glick, T. H. and Bercu, B. B. (1974). Lysine metabolism in Reye's syndrome. *Lancet*, **ii**, 163

20

α-Ketoadipic aciduria — a new inborn defect of lysine degradation

H.J. Bremer, S. K. Wadman, Hildegard Przyrembel, U. Wendel and Ingrid Lombeck

Several hereditary defects of lysine degradation have been detected. These are hereditary hyperlysinaemia, saccharopinuria, lysine intolerance with periodic ammonia intoxication, and hyperpipecolataemia. This is a report of an additional defect of lysine metabolism with an increased urinary excretion of α-ketoadipic acid, α-hydroxyadipic acid, α-aminoadipic acid and a reduced degradation of α-ketoadipic acid in fibroblasts.

Case report

The patient, a girl, now 20 months old, is the first child of a 21-year-old mentally retarded mother and an unknown father who, we have reason to suspect, is a near relative of the mother. The mother herself is of subnormal intelligence. As a young child the mother had been seen three times at our hospital because of respiratory tract and skin infections. At the age of 15 months she was noted to have psychomotor retardation and showed muscular hypotonia. A pneumoencephalogram performed at that age showed dilatation of the cerebral ventricles. The mother has attended four classes of a school for the mentally retarded, she lives with her parents but is able to earn her own living. Her sister is reported to have normal intelligence, her brother to be retarded. As the family is not co-operative no additional investigations besides those on one urine sample from the mother and one urine sample from the maternal grandmother were possible.

Our patient was born spontaneously at term after a pregnancy complicated by some vomiting and slightly elevated blood pressure during the last months. The Apgar score was 9, the birth weight 2950 g, the length 50 cm. The child was a typical 'collodium baby' (Figure 20.1). On the first day of life she had a generalised convulsion. This, together

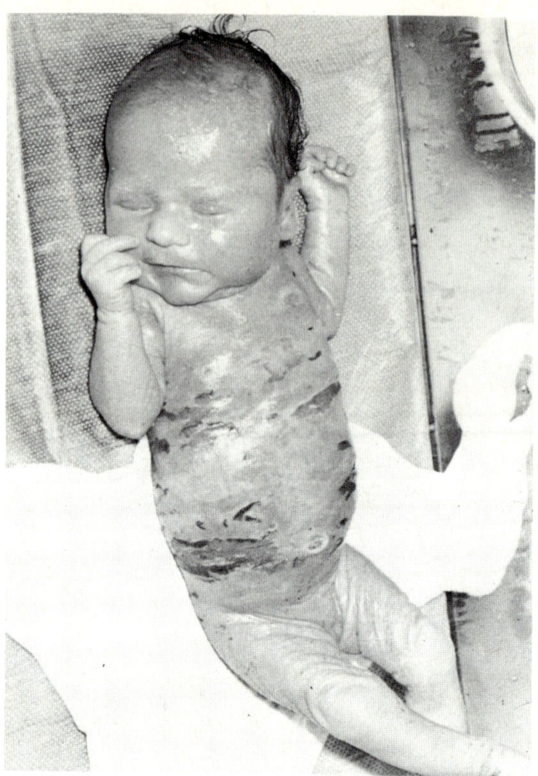

FIGURE 20.1 The patient at age 4 days. Note the typical apperance of a 'collodium baby'.

with the dermatological abnormalities, was the cause for transfer to our hospital. The aetiology of this convulsion remains obscure, further convulsions have not occurred.

The girl thrived well on normal feeding and the skin changes responded to symptomatic treatment with application of salicylic acid-vaseline. Echoencephalography, electroencephalography and the eye fundi were normal at the new-born age. A metabolic abnormality was first suspected because of a positive dinitrophenylhydrazine test and the appearance of an unknown ninhydrin-positive spot in the position of α-aminoadipic acid on the thin-layer chromatogram of amino acids in the child's urine. The sample was submitted to our screening programme because of the family history and the convulsion in the neonatal period. Further investigations were impossible at that time as the family insisted on taking the child out of our hospital.

On readmittance at the age of $5\frac{1}{2}$ months retarded development was obvious. We saw a floppy baby with oedema of the dorsum of hands and feet. Deep tendon reflexes were hyperactive, the Babinksi sign was negative. Parachute and Landau reflexes were negative. Motor nerve conduction velocity was normal and no definite abnormality was found in the electromyography. The head circumference was normal.

At the age of 13 months muscular hypotonia was still present (Figure 20.2). The child showed slow reactions to her surroundings and reached for objects, but she did not lift her head when in a prone position and did not sit up. Echoencephalography at that time indicated dilatation of all ventricles. After institution of physical therapy there was some improvement in the motor development. At the age of 18 months the girl now sits without help and shows good head control. She turns from the supine to the prone position but does not attempt to crawl or to stand.

According to the grandmother the similarity in behaviour of the child

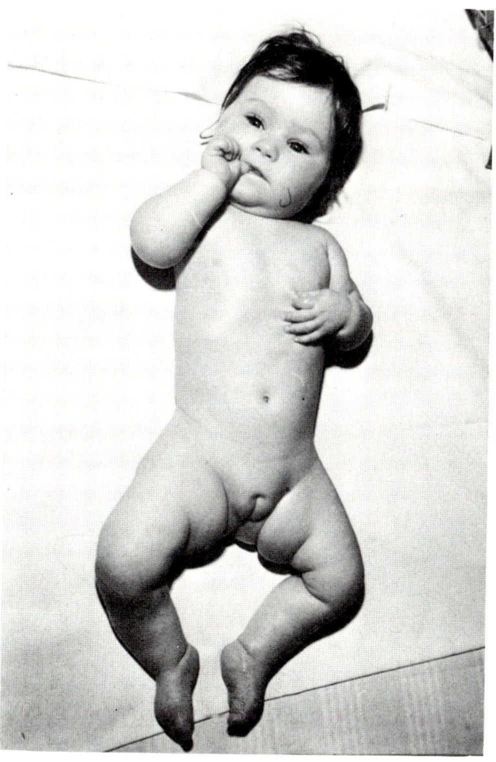

FIGURE 20.2 The patient at age 13 months, showing muscular hypotonia.

and her mother at the same age is quite obvious. Routine laboratory investigations in the child were normal with the exception of moderately varying disturbances of blood coagulation and thrombocyte function and a persistent compensated metabolic acidosis (base excess up to −9 mEq/l) which was aggravated by a lysine load.

Biochemical investigations

Special biochemical investigations showed an inconsistently positive dinitrophenylhydrazine test in urine and an unusual spot on thin-layer chromatograms (Figure 20.3). By separating the urinary amino acids by an amino-acid analyser (Unichrom, Beckman) using the two column method of Spackman *et al.* (1958) the unknown compound appeared in the position of α-amino-n-butyric acid. Separation from α-amino-n-butyric acid and quantitation was achieved by changing the initial column temperature from 30 °C to 34 °C or 37 °C (Figure 20.4). Depending on column temperature the unknown compound showed retention time changes typical of authentic α-aminoadipic acid. To isolate the unknown substance the acidic and neutral amino acids were separated from the basic ones by the method of Kakimoto and Akazawa (1970). The unknown ninhydrin-positive substance was isolated from

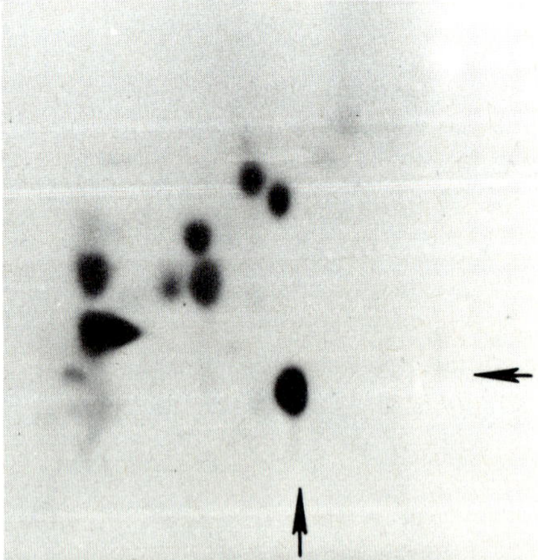

FIGURE 20.3 Thin-layer chromatogram of the patient's urinary amino acids. → indicates α-aminoadipic acid. (10 × 10 cm microcristalline cellulose plates (Merck, Darmstadt), solvent I: pyridine/dioxane/ammonia/water (35/35/15/15; v/v) solvent II: n-butanol/acetone/glacial acetic acid/water (35/35/10/20; v/v). Stain 0·2% ninhydrin in acetone/glacial acetic acid (80/20; v/v).)

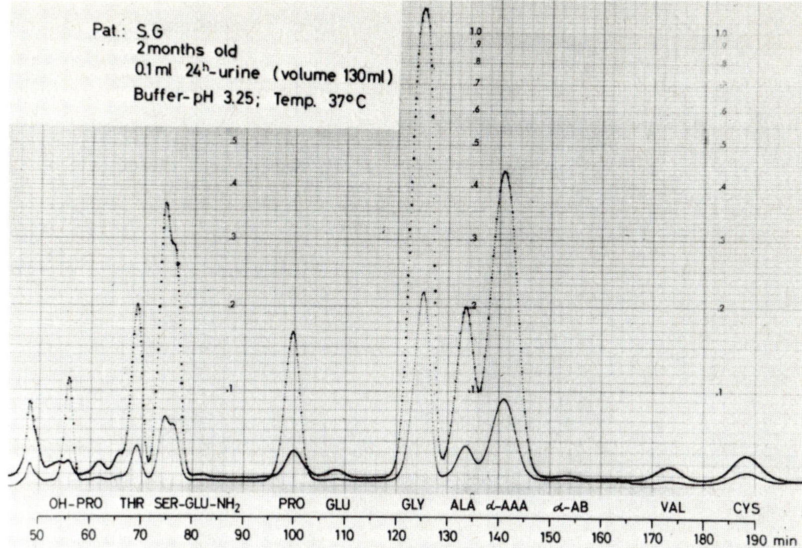

FIGURE 20.4 Separation of the patient's urinary amino acids on the autoanalyser Multichrom (Beckman Instruments, Munich) at 37 °C. Gly = glycine; Ala = alanine; α-AAA = α-aminoadipic acid; α-AB = α-amino-n-butyric acid.

the fraction of the acidic and neutral amino acids by a combination of preparative column chromatography (using 0·2 normal sodium acetate buffer, pH 3·25) and preparative thin-layer chromatography. The identity of the isolated substance was tested by one- and two-dimensional TLC against reference substances and by chromatography on the amino acid autoanalyser at different column temperatures. The isolated and

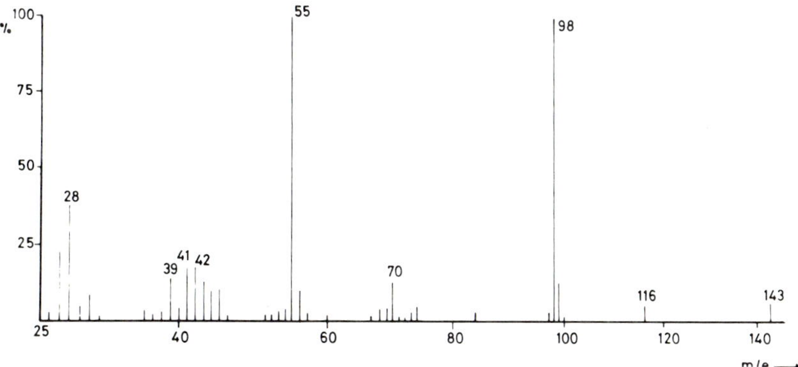

FIGURE 20.5 Mass spectrum of α-aminoadipic acid, isolated from the urine of patient S.G. Parent peak M = 161 not visible; M–H_2O = 143; M–COOH = 116; M–H_2O–COOH = 98; $(CO_2–CH{=}C{=}O)^+$ = 55.

purified compound was also subjected to direct inlet mass spectrometry (Jeol Mass Spectometer D 100, 75 eV, ion chamber temperature 140–150 °C). The mass spectrum was identical with that of synthetic α-aminoadipic acid (Figure 20.5). The search for urinary keto acids was started by thin-layer chromatography of the corresponding urinary 2,4-dinitrophenylhydrazones, prepared according to Cotte *et al.* (1967), on precoated cellulose plates (Merck, Darmstadt). The patient's urine showed a spot with the same Rf value as authentic α-ketoadipic acid (Figure 20.6). Extraction and trimethylsilylation of organic acids were performed according to Wadman *et al.* (1972). Gas chromatography was done on a F & M 810 apparatus with dual column, double FID, using a Hewlett-Packard 3370 A integrator. Columns were of stainless steel, 8 ft × $\frac{1}{8}$ inch containing 5% GESE-52 on Chromosorb W AW DMCS, 100–120 mesh. Temperatures: oven, 75 °C isothermal for 10 minutes, then 2 °C/min to 220 °C, finally isothermal for 10 minutes at 220 °C; injection port 190 °C; detector 220 °C. Gasflow: N_2, 27 ml/min; H_2, 28

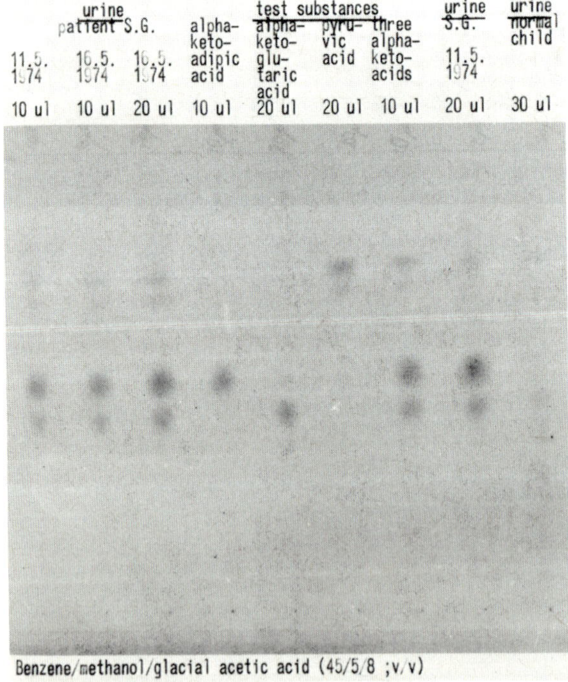

FIGURE 20.6 TLC of acidic dinitrophenylhydrazones from the patient's urine and from test substances (20 × 20 cm precoated silica gel plates). Solvent: benzene/methanol/glacial/acetic acid (45/5/8; v/v).

ml/min; air g450 ml/min. Range 10^2; attentuation 8; chart speed $\frac{1}{2}$ inch/min. Sample size 1 μl of final solution. Internal standard phenylbutyric acid. Figure 20.7 shows the gas chromatographic separation of the nonvolatile organic acids of the child's urine. The concentration of α-ketoadipic acid is at least 232 mg/ml or 215 mg/g of creatinine (no recovery experiments performed). Identity with α-ketoadipic acid was established by mass spectrometry (Figure 20.8).

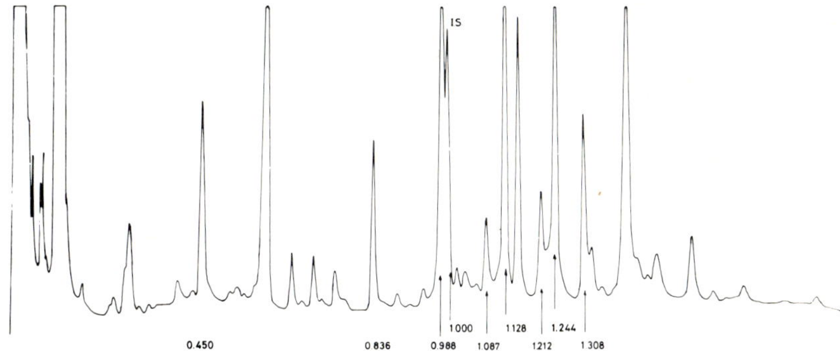

FIGURE 20.7 Gas chromatogram of TMS-derivatives of urinary acids in patient S.G.: peak demonstrated 1·244 = α-ketoadipic acid; peak demonstrated 1·212 = α-hydroxyadipic acid; peak demonstrated 0·988 = 1,2-butane dicarboxylic acid; peak demonstrated 0·450 = β-hydroxybutyric acid; peak demonstrated 0·836 = glutaric acid; peak demonstrated 1·087 = alpha-hydroxyglutaric acid; peak demonstrated 1·128 = alpha-ketoglutaric acid; peak demonstrated 1·308 = aconitic acid.

Figure 20.7 shows two additional unusual peaks occurring with relative retention times of 1·212 and 0·988. These substances were identified by mass spectrometry as α-hydroxyadipic acid and probably as 2-hexenedioic acid, respectively. The concentration of α-hydroxyadipic acid was one-third of that of α-ketoadipic acid. The peak of 2-hexenedioic acid contained another as yet unidentified substance. All the substances listed in the legend of Figure 20.7 were present in increased amounts in this urine sample. In each case their identity has been proved by mass spectrometry.

Degradation studies in skin fibroblasts

The pattern of urinary metabolites suggested a defect in the main lysine degradative pathway (for comparison see Figure 20.9). Cultured skin fibroblasts of the patient and of normal individuals were incubated with D,L-[1-^{14}C]-α-aminoadipate, [1-^{14}C]-α-ketoadipate, or [1,5-^{14}C]glutarate

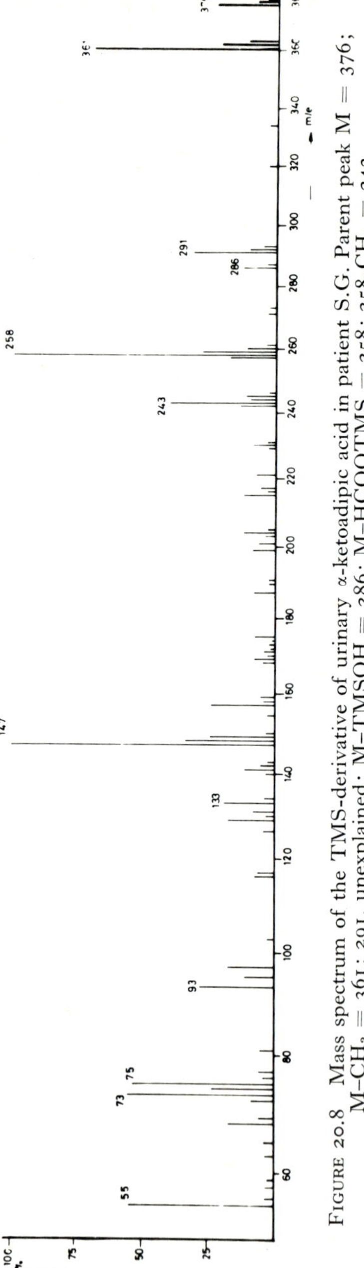

FIGURE 20.8 Mass spectrum of the TMS-derivative of urinary α-ketoadipic acid in patient S.G. Parent peak M = 376; M–CH_3 = 361; 291, unexplained; M–TMSOH = 286; M–HCOOTMS = 258; 258-CH_3 = 243.

and evolved $^{14}CO_2$ was measured. $^{14}CO_2$ production was linear within the first 6 hours from each substrate, and correlated well with the amount of cell protein. The results are depicted in Figure 20.10. The degrading activity of the patient's cells compared to normal cells was 14% for D,L-[1-^{14}C)α-aminoadipic acid, 7% for [1-^{14}C]-α-keto-adipic acid, and normal for [1,5-^{14}C]glutaric acid.

Two lines of cultured amniotic cells from the 15th and 16th week of gestation showed a comparable degrading activity for α-ketoadipic acid as normal adult skin fibroblasts do.

Dietary studies

As yet we can only present our results on the influence of lysine intake on α-aminoadipic acid plasma levels and urinary excretion. As shown in Table 20.1 there is no influence of lysine intake on the α-aminoadipic acid levels in plasma demonstrable in our patient. In the plasma of four

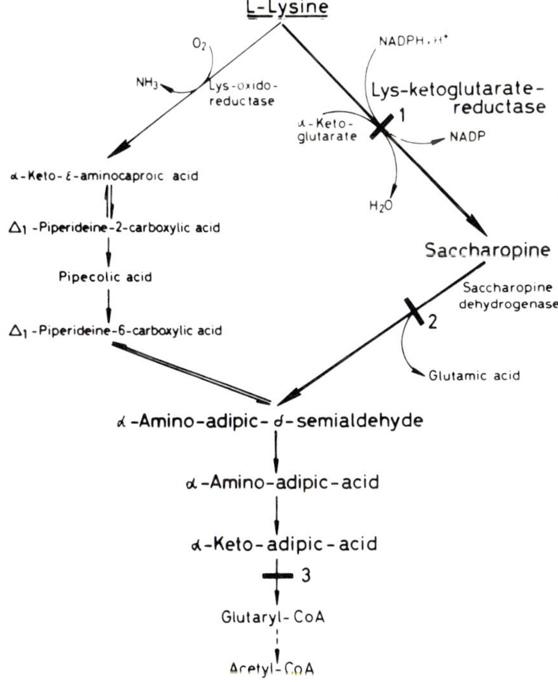

FIGURE 20.9 Pathways of lysine degradation; 1 = enzyme defect in hyperlysinaemia; 2 = enzyme defect in saccharopinuria; 3 = enzyme defect in patient S.G., 4 = enzyme defect in lysine intolerance with periodic ammonia intoxication.

healthy adults and four healthy infants we could not detect α-aminoadipic acid. But urinary excretion of this compound is clearly dependent on lysine administration as seen in Table 20.2.

An oral L-lysine load (0·1 g/kg body weight) led to acute diarrhoea, to very high and prolonged lysine increases in plasma and urine and to marked elevation of α-aminoadipic acid in plasma and urine. The same load in a normal age matched control produced only a very small rise in urinary lysine and α-aminoadipic acid excretion (Figures 20.11 and 20.12).

The patient's mother excretes 77 μmoles of α-aminoadipic acid per day; no α-aminoadipic acid was detectable in the plasma of the grandmother. The urine of the mother did not contain α-ketoadipic acid.

Discussion

Observation of one patient does not allow a comment on the clinical significance of a demonstrated metabolic abnormality. The fact that the

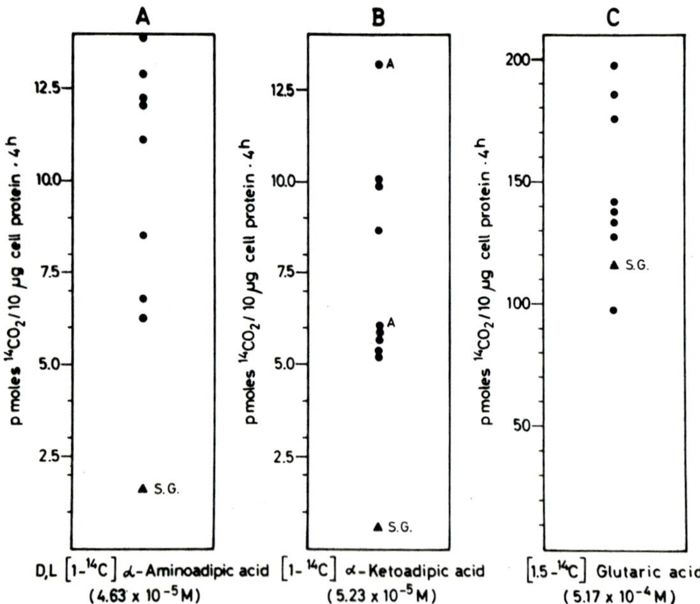

FIGURE 20.10 Degradation of α-aminoadipic acid (3A), α-ketoadipic acid (3B), and glutaric acid (3C) (expressed as amounts of $^{14}CO_2$ liberated by 10/μg cell protein in 4 hours) by fibroblasts of normal subjects (●) and the patient S.G. (▲). Degradation of α-ketoadipic acid was also measured in two amniotic cell lines (circles with letter A).

Table 20.1 *α-aminoadipic acid and lysine plasma levels in relation to protein intake*

	α-aminoadipic acid (μmol/ml plasma)	*lysine* (μmol/ml plasma)
Patient S.G.		
Age 1½ months		
Protein intake 4·1 g/kg b.w./day		
Lysine intake 390 mg/kg b.w./day	0·063	0·177
Age 10 months		
Protein intake 1·9 g/kg b.w./day		
Lysine intake *ca.* 140 mg/kg b.w./day	0·079	0·194
Age 13 months		
Protein intake 1·3 g/kg b.w./day		
Lysine intake *ca.* 80 mg/kg b.w./day	0·050	0·062
Normal children*		
Age 4–30 months old	—	0·227 ± 0·091

* Ghadimi and Pecora, 1964.

clinical picture of the patient resembles that of her mother might be due to other genetic factors.

α-Ketoadipic aciduria is the 5th instance of a disturbance at a defined step of lysine degradation. The others are after persistent hyperlysinaemia (Woody, 1964; Woody *et al.*, 1966; Ghadimi *et al.*, 1965; Armstrong and Robinow, 1967; van Gelderen and Teijema, 1973), defective lysine-ketoglutarate reductase, lysine intolerance with periodic ammonia intoxication (Colombo *et al.*, 1967) with a decreased activity of L-lysine dehydrogenase (Bürgi *et al.*, 1966) and saccharopinuria (Carson *et al.*, 1968; Simell *et al.*, 1973; Fellows and Carson, 1974). An additional metabolic defect, presumably in the pipecolic acid pathway of lysine degradation, may be suspected to underly the clinical picture of a patient with hyperpipecolataemia (Gatfield *et al.*, 1968).

Although the mode of lysine degradation in man is incompletely known, there is no real doubt that α-ketoadipic acid is a metabolite of the main degradation pathway and probably also occurs in those for

Table 20.2 *Urinary α-aminoadipic acid and lysine excretion in relation to lysine administration*

	α-aminoadipic acid (μmol/min/1·73 m²)	(μmol/24 h)	*lysine* (μmol/min/1·73 m²)	(μmol/24 h)
Patient S.G.				
Age 1½ months				
Protein 4·5 g/kg b.w.				
Lysine 390 mg/kg b.w.	3·153	519·7	0·736	121·3
Age 5½ months				
Protein 2·3 g/kg b.w.				
Lysine 170 mg/kg b.w.	0·601	155·1	0·205	52·9
Age 6 months				
Protein 2·3 g/kg b.w.				
Lysine ø 8	0·189	48·8	0·056	14·5
Controls				
Male, age 5½ months	0·082	20·9	0·133	33·9
Male, age 16 months	0·058	20·9	0·144	51·6
Male, age 24 months	0·140	58·3	0·210	87·4
Values from the literature				
Stein (1953), adults		*ca.* 6·2		
Scriver (1965), 3–10 years			0·113	51·6
Brodehl (1968), ½–4 months			0·171	
Brodehl (1968), 2–13 years			0·151	

tryptophan and hydroxylysine (Nishizuka *et al.*, 1965; Hiles *et al.*, 1970). That lysine is the main precursor of the excreted substances is shown by feeding experiments, e.g. the increased urinary excretion of α-amino-adipic acid after a lysine load and the decreased urinary excretion after omitting lysine from the food for some days. The lysine concentration in blood after an oral lysine load increased much more in this patient than had been expected from load tests in normal individuals. Because α-ketoadipic acid is not in direct equilibrium with lysine no simple

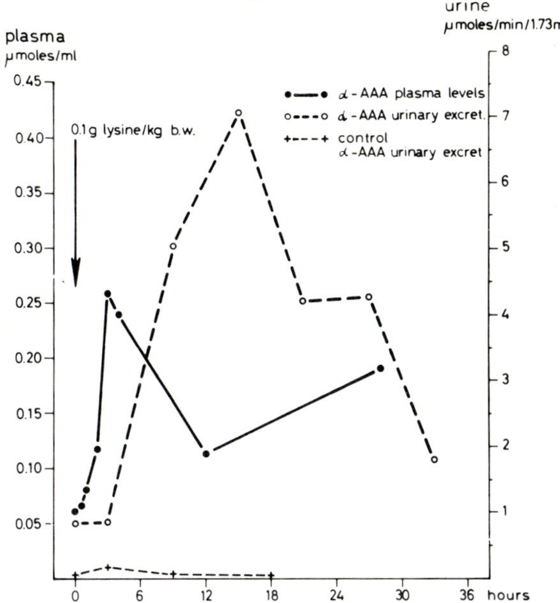

FIGURE 20.11 Oral lysine load test showing α-aminoadipic acid levels in plasma and urine of the patient and in the urine of a normal control.

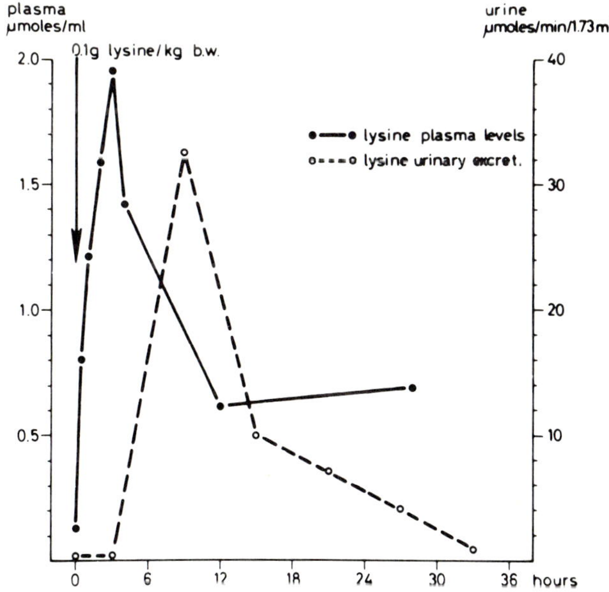

FIGURE 20.12 Oral lysine load test showing lysine levels in plasma and urine of the patient. The lysine excretion of the control child was too low for the scale used in this figure.

explanation can be suggested for this finding. Load tests with tryptophan and hydroxylysine have not yet been done.

The metabolic pattern in this defect deserves some comments: Because α-aminoadipic acid occurs in the patient's blood in unequivocally increased amounts and is markedly increased in the urine, there seems to be a similar relation between the keto- and the amino acid as occurs in MSUD and in PKU. The relation between α-hydroxyadipic acid and α-ketoadipic acid is unknown. There could be a simple equilibrium between both substances catalysed by one enzyme or a more complex relation, as has been found between phenylpyruvate and phenyllactate which is determined by two enzymes. The 2-hexenedioic acid may be a product of the oxidative deamination of α-aminoadipic acid. At the moment it is uncertain whether it is synthesised by an oxidative deaminase for α-aminoadipic acid occurring in human tissues or by a bacterial enzyme which acts on the α-aminoadipic acid in the intestinal lumen of the body.

No information on lysine degradation in fibroblast cultures beyond α-aminoadipate semialdehyde was available. As could be shown in this investigation degradation occurs at least beyond the glutaryl-CoA step. This is also true for amniotic cell lines from the 14th and 15th week of pregnancy.

As in α-ketoadipic aciduria the keto-and hydroxy- acids constitute the essential part of the metabolic pattern this defect is to be regarded as an organic acidopathy.

Acknowledgements

Appreciation is expressed to Miss Dorothea Bachmann for her expert technical assistance during these investigations and to the 'Landesamt für Forschung des Ministeriums für Wissenschaft und Forschung des Landes Nordrhein-Westfalen' for a research grant.

REFERENCES

ARMSTRONG, M. D. and ROBINOW, M. (1967). A case of hyperlysinemia: Biochemical and clinical observations. *Pediatrics*, **39**, 546

BRODEHL, J. and GELLISSEN, K. (1968). Endogenous renal transport of free amino acids in infancy and childhood. *Pediatrics*, **42**, 395

BÜRGI, W., RICHTERICH, R. and COLOMBO, J. P. (1966). L-lysine dehydrogenase deficiency in a patient with congenital lysine intolerance. *Nature*, **211**, 854

CARSON, N. A. J., SCHALLY, B. G., NEILL, D. W. and CARRE, I. J. (1968). Saccharopinuria: A new inborn error of lysine metabolism. *Nature*, **218**, 679

COLOMBO, J. P., BÜRGI, W., RICHTERICH, R. and ROSSI, E. (1967). Congenital lysine intolerance with periodic ammonia intoxication: A defect in L-lysine degradation. *Metabolism*, **16**, 910

COTTE, J., COLLOMBEL, C., CUIVRE, M. and PADIS, L. (1967). Séparation chromatographique sur couche mince des acides alphacétoniques urinaires. *Rev. Fr. Etudes Clin. Biol.*, **12**, 496

Fellows, F. C. I. and Carson, N. A. J. (1974). Enzyme studies in a patient with saccharopinuria: A defect of lysine metabolism. *Pediatr. Res.*, **8**, 42

Gatfield, P. D., Taller, E., Hinton, G. G., Wallace, A. C., Abdelnour, G. M. and Haust, M. D. (1968). Hyperpipecolatemia: A new metabolic disorder associated with neuropathy and hepatomegaly: A case study. *Can. Med. Assoc. J.*, **99**, 215

Ghadimi, H., Binnington, V. I. and Pecora, P. (1965) Hyperlysinemia associated with retardation. *N. Engl. J. Med.*, **273**, 723

Ghadimi, H. and Pecora, P. (1964). Plasma amino acids after birth. *Pediatrics*, **34**, 182

Hiles, R. A., Triebwasser, K. C. and Henderson, L. M. (1970). The degradation of hydroxyl-L-lysine in liver via its phosphate ester. *Biochem. Biophys. Res. Commun.*, **41**, 662

Kakimoto, Y. and Akazawa, S. (1970). Isolation and identification of N^G,N^G- and N^G,N'^G-dimethylarginine, N-mono-, di-, and trimethyllysine, and glucosylgalactosyl- and galactosyl-5-hydroxylysine from human urine. *J. Biol. Chem.*, **235**, 5751.

Nishizuka, Y., Ichiyama, A., Gholson, R. K. and Hayaishi, O. (1965). Studies on the metabolism of the benzene ring of tryptophan in mammalian tissues. *J. Biol. Chem.*, **240**, 733

Scriver, C. R. and Davies, E. (1965). Endogenous renal clearance dates of free amino acids in pre-pubertal children. *Pediatrics*, **36**, 1592

Simell, O., Johannsson, T. and Aula, P. (1973). Enzyme defect in saccharopinuria. *J. Pediatr.*, **82**, 54

Simell, O., Visakorpi, J. K. and Donner, M. (1972). Saccharopinuria. *Arch. Dis. Child.*, **47**, 52

Spackman, D. H., Stein, W. H. and Moore, S. (1958). Automatic recording apparatus for use in the chromatography of amino acids. *Anal. Chem.*, **30**, 1190

Stein, W. H. (1953). A chromatographic investigation of the amino acid constituents of normal urine. *J. Biol. Chem.*, **201**, 45

van Gelderen, H. H. and Teijema, H. L. (1973). Hyperlysinaeamia. A harmless inborn error of metabolism? *Arch. Dis. Child.*, **48**, 892

Wadman, S. K., van der Heiden, C., Ketting, D. and van Sprang, F. J. (1971). Abnormal tyrosine and phenylalanine metabolism in patients with tyrosyluria and phenylketonuria; gas-liquid chromatographic analysis of urinary metabolites. *Clin. Chim. Acta*, **34**, 277

Woody, N. C. (1964). Hyperlysinemia. *Am. J. Dis. Child.*, **180**, 543

Woody, N. C., Hutzler, J. and Dancis, J. (1966). Further studies of hyperlysinemia. *Am. J. Dis. Child.*, **112**, 577

21

Phenylketonuria variants

C. Toothill, J. M. H. Buckler and B. Winokur

The development of screening procedures in which blood is examined (Guthrie and Sussi, 1963; Scriver *et al.*, 1964; Ireland and Read, 1972; Holton, 1972) has resulted in the early detection of hyperphenylalaninaemia, including phenylketonuria (PKU). Investigations of patients with all types of hyperphenylalaninaemia have resulted in increased awareness of the variants of phenylketonuria (Hsia, 1970).

Hyperphenylalaninaemia may be associated with tyrosinaemia, whilst a transient form results from the slow development of the enzyme phenylalanine hydroxylase; but the largest group contains the persistent forms of the disorder. This last category includes the 'classical' and 'atypical' (Yu *et al.*, 1970) forms of phenylketonuria and the variant hyperphenylalaninaemia without PKU. Classical and atypical PKU patients both excrete abnormal quantities of phenylpyruvic acid (PPA) when blood phenylalanine concentrations in excess of 0·8–1·0 mmol/l are achieved; however, these two groups are different in that the blood phenylalanine levels on an unrestricted diet in the atypical cases is usually less than this critical range.

There appear to be two distinct zones of blood concentration of phenylalanine at which excretion of phenylpyruvic acid in abnormal amounts occurs. The lower, 0·8–1·0 mmol/l, applies to classical and atypical phenylketonuria whilst a blood concentration in excess of 2 mmol/l has to be achieved in order to produce phenylpyruvic aciduria in normal subjects (Jervis, 1960; and personal observations) and probably those with hyperphenylalaninaemia without PKU.

In addition to the excretion patterns of PPA there is a wide degree of tolerance to phenylalanine intake in cases of persistent hyperphenylalaninaemia. Table 21.1 shows the results of the recent management of seven of our patients. Three, K.P., H.T. and N.W. need low dietary phenylalanine in order that acceptable blood levels be maintained, this has proved difficult in the case of patient K.P. Patient N.A., although

Table 21.1 *Results of the recent management of seven patients with hyperphenylalaninaemia showing current phenylalanine intake and the range of plasma phenylalanine levels recorded over the last 6–8 months.*

Patient	*Age* (y)	*Phe intake* (mg/kg)	*Plasma Phe* (mmol/l)
H.B.	2	70	0·12–0·61
M.H.	2	60	0·18–0·61
*N.A.	$1\frac{1}{4}$	50	0·37–0·49
A.McC.	5	normal diet	0·55–0·79
*K.P.	$2\frac{1}{2}$	20	0·73–1·11
*H.T.	5	28	0·18–0·67
*N.W.	5	18	0·24–0·91

* 'classical' PKU.

tolerating higher dietary phenylalanine, has recently been confirmed to be a classical phenylketonuric by means of a loading test.

A.McC., now aged 6 years, was diagnosed at birth as a case of PKU and managed for $3\frac{1}{2}$ years as such. Two years ago she was challenged with a load of phenylalanine (100 mg/kg) and found not to excrete PPA in excess even at a blood level in excess of 1 mmol/l; her phenylalanine intake was gradually increased, currently she is receiving an unrestricted diet and has satisfactory blood levels of phenylalanine.

Table 21.2 *Case history of one patient (M.H.) with hyperphenylalaninaemia without phenylketonuria*

M.H.	(d.o.b. 14.9.72)
Sept. 1972	+ve Guthrie test (×2)
	NO PPA detected in urine
Nov. 1972	Phe loading test, highest value (5 h) 1·58 mmol/l
	TYR normal, no PPA in urine
	on PKU diet Plasma Phe < 0·06 mmol/l
Present treatment:	60 mg/kg Phe – plasma Phe 0·18–0·61 mmol/l

The remaining two patients (M.H. and H.B.) are similar and well illustrated by the brief history (Table 21.2) of one of them. These we regard as patients with hyperphenylalaninaemia without phenylketonuria along with A.McC.

Normal urinary excretion of phenylpyruvic acid in patients with blood concentrations of phenylalanine in excess of 1 mmol/l stimulated us to investigate two groups of patients with phenylketonuria who are not being treated; hospitalised patients, who have never been treated, and two patients taken off diet 2 years ago. The results of this investigation are presented in Table 21.3. Both groups of patients have blood phenylalanine levels in the range 0·85–1·52 mmol/l on unrestricted diet, these values are considerably lower than those found in young cases of classical phenylketonuria.

Figure 21.1 shows blood phenylalanine concentrations in the various types of persistent hyperphenylalaninaemia cases on a normal diet. It is noteworthy that the blood concentration range of phenylalanine- is similar in the case of the two groups of untreated PKU patients, and our patients with hyperphenylalaninaemia without PKU (non-PKU—HPhe). The principal biochemical difference between these two

Table 21.3 *Phenylketonuria patients not on treatment: 1—untreated and hospitalised (18); 2—treated but now off diet (2)*

	Age (y)	*Blood Phe* (mmol/l)	*Urine PPA*
1. Never treated—hospitalised			
Hospital a (10)	20–58	0·83–1·11	5 −ve
			2 ±
6F : 4M			3 +ve
Hospital b (9)	17–30	1·20–1·52	8 +ve
5F : 3M			
2. Treated—now off diet			
M.W.	11	1·18	+ve
		1·22	+ve
I.W.	11	1·27	+ve
		0·97	+ve

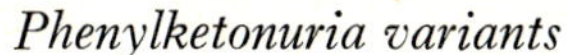

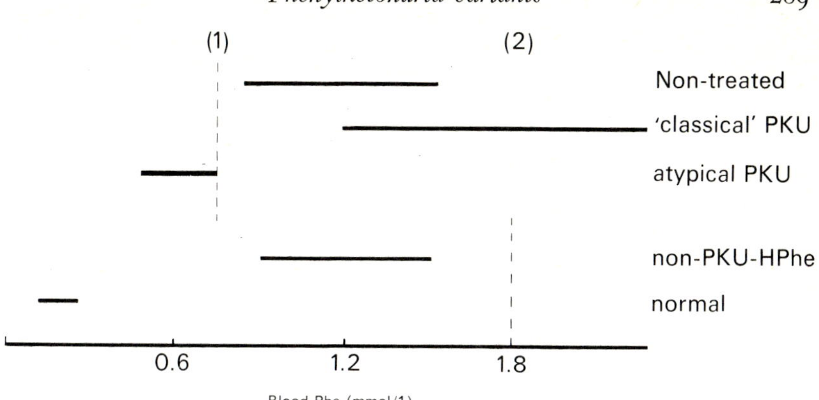

FIGURE 21.1 Ranges of plasma phenylalanine concentration in patients and normal subjects receiving normal diet. The vertical lines indicate plasma concentrations corresponding to phenylpyruvic aciduria in PKU (1) and normals and non-PKU-HPhe (2).

groups is that the latter do not produce excess urinary PPA at these blood phenylalanine levels.

These observations pose an interesting question regarding phenylalanine aminotransferase activity in PKU. It is suggested that this enzyme may have enhanced activity in this disorder (Figure 21.2); this may explain the clinical difference between classical PKU and

Reduced activity common to all variants

PHE —1→ TYR

Enhanced activity in PKU when blood PHE > 12–15 mg/100 ml

2

Enzymes:
1 PHE hydroxylase
2 PHE aminotransferase

PPA

FIGURE 21.2 Hyperphenylalaninaemia—a hypothesis.

other forms of persistent hyperphenylalaninaemia. To speculate further, PKU may be a variant of hyperphenylalaninaemia, all cases of the latter result from a deficiency of phenylalanine hydroxylase activity. The concept of a multiple specific enzyme defect in PKU has been suggested by Boscott and Bickel (1953).

An alternative explanation to account for the three patients (A.McC., M.H. and H.B.) would be a deficiency of phenylalanine aminotransferase as discussed by Auerbach and DiGeorge (1971), this deficiency accounting for the failure of PPA excretion. It is hoped that current studies on leukocyte enzymes will be of help in resolving our speculation and hypothesis.

Acknowledgements

The Authors wish to express their gratitude to Dr D. A. Spencer and Dr J. Blake for allowing them to investigate their patients and to the Leeds R.H.A. for financial assistance.

REFERENCES

Auerbach, V. H. and Di George, A. M. (1971). Defective phenylalanine transaminase as a cause of phenylalaninaemia. In H. Bickel, F. P. Hudson and L. I. Woolf (eds.), *Phenylketonuria*, p. 87. (Stuttgart : Thieme)

Boscott, R. J. and Bickel, H. (1953). Detection of some new abnormal metabolites in the urine of phenylketonurics. *Scand. J. Lab. Clin. Invest.*, **5**, 380

Guthrie, R. and Susi, A. (1963). A simple phenylalanine method for detecting phenylketonuria in large populations of newborn infants. *Pediatrics*, **32**, 338

Holton, J. B. (1972). A large scale composition of the bacteriological inhibition assay and the automated fluorometric method for phenylketonuria screening. *Ann. Clin. Biochem.*, **9**, 118

Hsia, D. Y-Y. (1970). Phenylketonuria and its variants. *Prog. Med. Genet.*, **7**, 29

Ireland, J. T. and Read, R. A. (1972). A thin layer chromatographic method for use in neonatal screening to detect excess aminoacidaemia. *Ann. Clin. Biochem.*, **9**, 129

Jervis, G. A. (1960). Detection of heterozygotes for phenylketonuria. *Clin. Chim. Acta*, **5**, 471

Scriver, C. R., Davis, E. and Cullen, E. (1964). Application of a simple micromethod to the screening of plasma for a variety of aminoacidopathies. *Lancet*, **ii**, 230

Yu, J. S., Stuckey, S. J. and O'Halloran, M. T. (1970). Atypical phenylketonuria: An approach to diagnosis and management. *Arch. Dis. Child.*, **45**, 561

Phenylalanine hydroxylase determinations in patients with phenylketonuria and hyperphenylalaninaemia

K. Bartholomé

Phenylalanine hydroxylase was first shown to be deficient in subjects with phenylketonuria (PKU) by Udenfriend and Cooper (1952) and this was confirmed by Jervis (1953). The complex mechanism of the phenylalanine hydroxylation system has been elucidated from 1956 onwards, mainly by Kaufman and Max (1971) and by La Du and Zannoni (1971).

True PKU requires early dietary treatment to prevent mental retardation. Hyperphenylalaninaemia, a condition which simulates PKU biochemically, is considered by most authors not to cause retardation. The differential diagnosis and decision regarding treatment is based upon biochemical parameters some of which are still ambiguous. Of additional value might be the determination of phenylalanine hydroxylase activity as a diagnostic parameter. There have been only a few reports in which enzyme activity has been measured in PKU and so-called variant patients.

Phenylalanine hydroxylase converts phenylalanine to tyrosine. For this reaction oxygen and two hydrogen atoms are needed, which are transferred from tetrahydrobiopterin. Tetrahydrobiopterin is regenerated by dihydrobiopterin reductase and NADPH. Our assay is based on the procedure of Kaufman (1969). His assay uses labelled phenylalanine, the naturally occurring cofactor biopterin and approximately optimised reaction conditions. We modified his assay by using dithioerythritol instead of an enzymatic dihydrobiopterin regenerating system. Our procedure is as follows: about 30 mg liver tissue is obtained by percutaneous needle biopsy and frozen immediately in liquid nitrogen. The samples are stored at −70 °C for 1–4 weeks before being assayed. Control specimens were either obtained during laparotomies for cholecystectomy or from needle biopsies performed in children with non-metabolic diseases. The extraction is done in 150 mM KCl using a

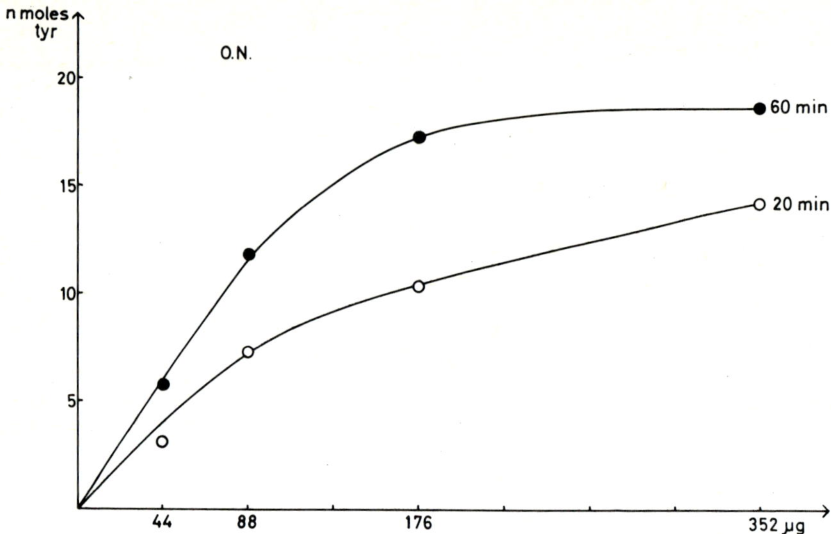

FIGURE 22.1 Dependence of the amount of tyrosine formed on the enzyme concentration (subject O.N.). 20 nmoles of tyrosine would represent a 100% conversion of the substrate.

Branson sonifier. The supernatant is assayed after centrifugation at 40 000 g.

The following reaction mixture is used for the enzyme assay: phosphate buffer 150 mM, lysolecithine 1 mM, phenylalanine 0·1 mM, ^{14}C-labelled phenylalanine 0·2 μCi, dithioerythritol 2 mM and biopterin 0·025 mM.

The test volume is 200 μl, the incubation time 60 minutes, the temperature 25 °C, and the reaction mixture is agitated. The reaction is stopped by boiling or by adding concentrated perchloric acid. Aliquots of the deprotenised supernatants are spotted on cellulose TLC plates and run in a mixture of chloroform–methanol–concentrated ammonia–water (58:32:8:2, v/v) for 20 minutes. Radio activity is scanned directly then the phenylalanine and tyrosine areas are scraped off and measured in a liquid scintillation counter.

Firstly, we looked at the amount of tyrosine formed at different concentrations of enzyme in the assay (Figure 22.1). Up to 20 μl of supernatant, corresponding to approximately 180 μg of protein, there is a fairly good correlation. The flattening of the curve may be due to substrate utilisation during the progress of the reaction.

Secondly, tyrosine formation as a function of the reaction time was

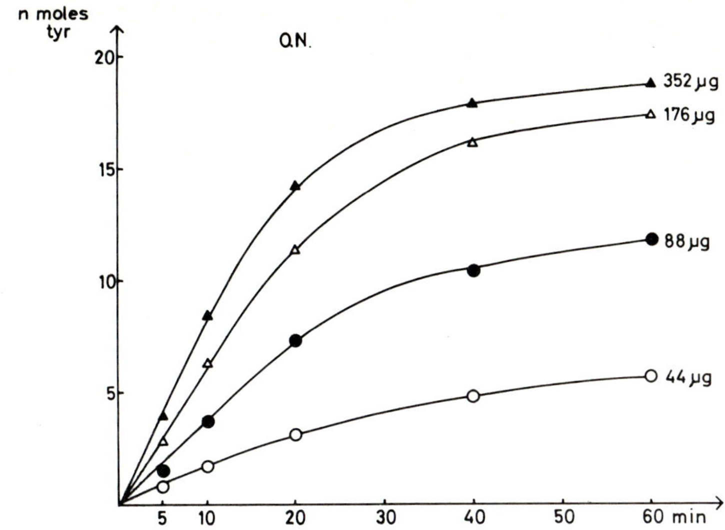

FIGURE 22.2 Dependence of the amount of tyrosine formed on the reaction time (subject O.N.).

measured (Figure 22.2). Linearity is found for up to 20–40 minutes, depending on the enzyme concentration. This, too, indicates substrate exhaustion.

Thirdly, the natural cofactor biopterin was used instead of dimethylpteridine (Figure 22.3). Biopterin optimises the assay for low residual activities. The use of biopterin necessitates the addition of lysolecithin.

From our results, patients can be divided into three major groups (Figure 22.4); (1) activity not detectable, (2) reduced activity and (3) normal activity. Correlating the enzyme activity with the clinical picture, the patients with no detectable activity (first group) suffered from true PKU both clinically and biochemically. Up to now, we have had only one exception. This patient is a 3-month-old boy. A standard phenylalanine loading test did not raise his phenylalanine blood level beyond 13 mg/100 ml (0·8 mmol/l), suggesting the diagnosis of a hyperphenylalaninaemia. This diagnosis was strengthened when identical results were obtained by loading his 6-year-old brother, who is apparently healthy though he never received treatment. He has not yet been studied for enzyme activity. However, the possibility of faulty handling of the specimen should be kept in mind.

The second group with reduced enzyme activity covers the broad range 0·8–31 μmol/g protein per 60 minutes. This group is apparently

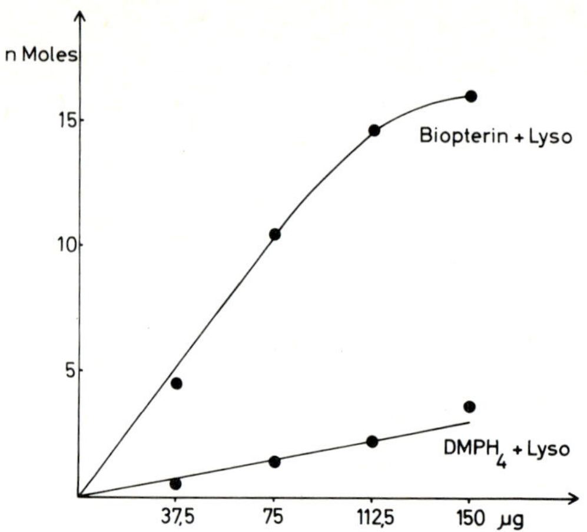

FIGURE 22.3 Influence of the naturally occurring cofactor biopterin compared to that of the synthetic cofactor 6,7-dimethylpteridine on the amount of tyrosine formed at varying enzyme concentrations.

heterogeneous. Three examples may serve to illustrate this statement: we found three seriously retarded patients with enzyme activities below 5 μmol/g protein per 60 minutes, two of them having siblings with comparably low values who were diagnosed early and developed normally under treatment. Another family whose enzyme activity has been studied was picked up by Dr Wolf in Kassel. One boy in this family has been treated for PKU. His 17-year-old sister showed phenylalanine blood levels up to 13 mg/100 ml on a normal diet, and has a normal IQ. Both the untreated sister and the treated boy exhibited an enzyme activity in the low residual group. In both cases a phenylalanine loading test over 3 days showed identical curves characteristic of hyperphenylalaninaemia. A third sibling exhibited normal enzyme activity and a normal phenylalanine loading curve. The mother, on the other hand, was found to have a normal loading curve but only 49% residual enzyme activity. The father has so far not been tested. This family resembles a family described by Kang *et al.* (1970) in which the presence of two mutant alleles for phenylalanine for phenylalanine hydroxylase was postulated, one coding for a hydroxylase devoid of enzyme activity and one for a variant of the enzyme. There are two further cases in the lower residual activity group which fit the clinical diagnosis of hyperphenylalaninaemia.

The second group also includes a subgroup consisting of four patients with higher residual enzyme activity ranging from 8·9–31 μmol/g

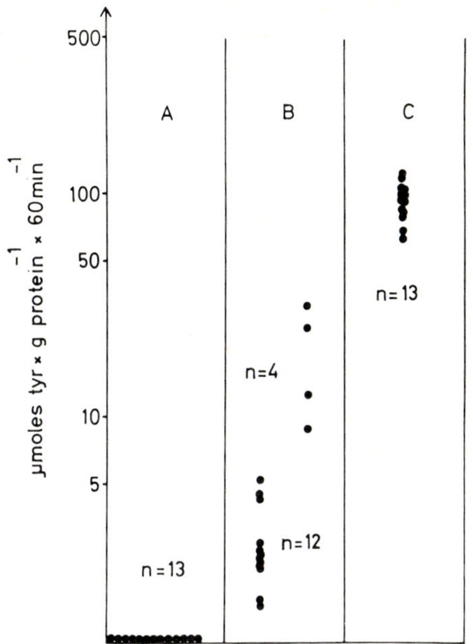

FIGURE 22.4 Enzyme activities found in 42 liver biopsies, listed in three ranges: A—no detectable activity; B—residual activity; C—normal activity (controls).

protein per 60 minutes. In all of them the diagnosis of hyperphenylalaninaemia had already been made by the usual criteria. They correspond to the two cases investigated by Justice *et al.* (1967).

During our study we made an observation which is quite exceptional and deserves further investigation. A boy now 8 months old exhibits all the biochemical signs of classical PKU. When, at the age of 6 weeks and 4 months, a needle biopsy was taken, hydroxylase determinations showed values of 75 and 55 µmol/g protein per 60 minutes respectively, which are in the low normal range. We believe that he has probably a different molecular defect (Bartholomé, 1974). Phenylalanine hydroxylase is part of a multienzyme system and therefore other defects in this complex system may be anticipated. Although this child received dietary treatment from the age of 2 weeks and his phenylalanine blood levels were well controlled, he now appears mentally retarded and suffers from severe tetraplegia.

In conclusion, patients with no detectable enzyme activity practically always have classical PKU. Patients with very low residual activity cannot yet be classified by the enzyme levels alone. Patients with residual activity greater than 10% of normal correspond to the diagnosis of hyperphenylalaninaemia. Normal phenylalanine hydroxylase values in the *in vitro* assay do not necessarily imply a normal function of the whole hydroxylation system in the liver, because the assay is specific for hydroxylase activity only.

REFERENCES

BARTHOLOMÉ, K. (1974). A new molecular defect in phenylketonuria. *Lancet*, **ii**, 1580

JERVIS, G. A. (1953). Phenylpyruvic oligophrenia: deficiency of phenylalanine-oxidising system. *Proc. Soc. Exp. Biol. Med.*, **82**, 574

JUSTICE, P., O'FLYNN, M. E. and HSIA, D. Y-Y. (1967). Phenylalanine hydroxylase activity in hyperphenylalaninaemia. *Lancet*, **i**, 928

KANG, E. S., KAUFMAN, S. and GERALD, P. S. (1970). Clinical and biochemical observations of patients with atypical phenylketonuria. *Paediatrics*, **45**, 83

KAUFMAN, S. (1969). Phenylalanine hydroxylase of human liver: assay and some properties. *Arch. Biochem. Biophys.*, **134**, 249

KAUFMAN, S. and MAX, E. E. (1971). Studies on the phenylalanine hydroxylating system in human liver and their relationship to pathogenesis of PKU and hyperphenylalaninaemia. In H. Bickel, F. P. Hudson and L. I. Woolf (eds.), *Phenylketonuria*, p. 13. (Stuttgart : Thieme)

LA DU, B. N. and ZANNONI, V. G. (1971). Basic biochemical disturbance in aromatic amino acid metabolism in phenylketonuria. In H. Bickel, F. P. Hudson and L. I. Woolf (eds.), *Phenylketonuria*, p. 6. (Stuttgart : Thieme)

UDENFRIEND, S. and COOPER, J. R. (1952). The enzymatic conversion of phenylalanine to tyrosine. *J. Biol. Chem.*, **194**, 503

23

A patient with a permanent chemical phenylketonuria and a normal phenylalanine tolerance

S. K. Wadman and M. Th. Grimberg

Introduction

In untreated classical phenylketonuria (PKU) patients have highly increased plasma phenylalanine concentrations (up to 50 mg/100 ml and even higher) and excrete large amounts of phenylalanine (Phe), phenylpyruvic acid (PPyA), phenyllactic acid (PLA), *o*-hydroxyphenylacetic acid (*o*-OHPAA) and phenylacetic acid (PAA), completely or mainly as a glutamine conjugate. Mandelic acid (MA) is also increased. Milder variants of this disorder are known, showing the same chemical picture but at a lower level. The mildest form is hyperphenylalaninaemia, without phenylketonuria, an asymptomatic trait. The chemical features are: increased plasma and urinary Phe only; the first less than 1 mM. In the urine the excretions of PPyA, PLA, *o*-OHPAA, PAA and MA are normal. For a survey of the hyperphenyl alaninaemic traits in man see reference Scriver and Rosenberg (1973).

In the present paper we describe a new, probably inherited variant of phenylalanine metabolism, characterised by a permanently increased excretion of PPyA, PLA, *o*-OHPAA and MA, but normal blood and urinary phenylalanine and urinary PAA concentrations. This abnormality was discovered in a nearly 14-year-old mentally normal girl with transient and probably non-specific neurological complaints. Her 12-year-old healthy sister showed the same chemical abnormality. A more detailed account of this work will be published elsewhere (Wadman *et al.*, 1975).

Case report

The patient W.Z. was a girl admitted at the age of 13 years 10 months for mainly meningitis-like symptoms such as headache (which had already lasted for 2 months), fever, drowsiness, apathy, neck stiffness and pains in neck and limbs. The symptoms of Kernig and Brudzinski were positive. She recovered after treatment with antibiotics.

According to the electroencephalographer the EEG showed diffuse post-traumatic changes, without definite focal abnormalities. At the age of 7 years she had twice had a commotio cerebri and, post-traumatically, a damaged cervical vertebra. Psychomotor development was without problems. Intelligence is average. Physical development is somewhat below normal: she was at the 30th percentile of her age group. Routine laboratory investigations were normal, except for urinary phenylpyruvic acid. The urine appeared to have a somewhat peculiar smell—therefore the ferric chloride reaction was done, and was repeatedly positive. Plasma phenylalanine however was normal, which excluded classical phenylketonuria or a milder variant. At this stage detailed gas chromatographic and related quantitative methods were applied, which

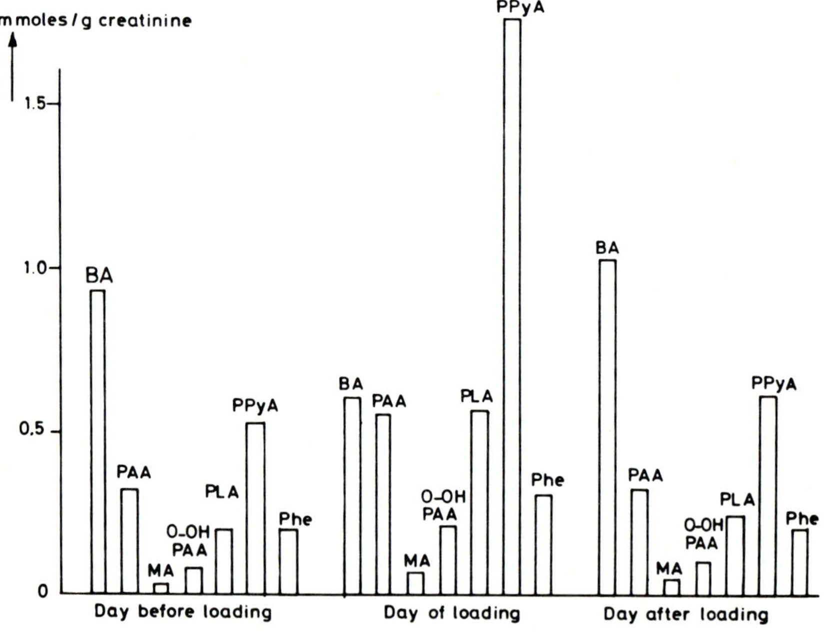

FIGURE 23.1 Excretory pattern of phenylalanine metabolites in patient W.Z. before, during and after loading with L-phenylalanine, 100 mg/kg. Gas chromatography of PPyA, PLA, *o*-OHPAA and PAA (trimethylsilyl derivatives) was done as described previously (Wadman *et al.*, 1971). PAA represents free plus conjugated PAA (obtained by alkaline hydrolysis).

Table 23.1 *Serum phenylalanine and tyrosine in W.Z. (mg/100 ml) as determined by rapid column chromatography using a Technicon TSM1 apparatus*

	Phenylalanine	*Tyrosine*
Fasting sample on 12.9.1973	1·3	0·7
Fasting sample before loading on 28.11.1973	0·8	1·0
30 min after loading	6·5	1·8
60 min after loading	7·1	2·3
120 min after loading	4·8	2·7
360 min after loading	1·6	1·6
24 h after loading	1·2	1·9

yielded the results given below. In the patient's parents and in two older brothers of 17 and 18 years no abnormal excretory pattern was present.

Results and discussion

In Figure 23.1 the urinary profiles of patient W.Z. before, during and after loading with 100 mg phenylalanine/kg are given. PPyA, PLA *o*-OHPAA and MA were all increased and responded to phenylalanine loading. PAA was normal and increased only weakly after loading. Urinary phenylalanine was practically normal, as was benzoic acid (BA), a metabolite produced from non-absorbed phenylalanine by the intestinal flora (Heiden *et al.*, 1971). Fasting serum phenylalanine was not increased. The response of serum phenylalanine to oral loading (see Table 23.1) was completely normal and different from that of PKU heterozygotes (Justice *et al.*, 1967). Blood phenylalanine did not exceed the renal threshold and on the day of loading the urinary concentration raised only slightly. Blood tyrosine responded well, indicating that *p*-hydroxylation was intact for the greater part. Figure 23.2 shows a thin layer chromatogram of the urinary phenolic acids of W.Z. on the day of loading with L-phenylalanine. Apart from the orange spot of *o*-OHPAA and the pink spot of PPyA, a large greyish-brown spot of an unknown compound was seen. This compound was probably also

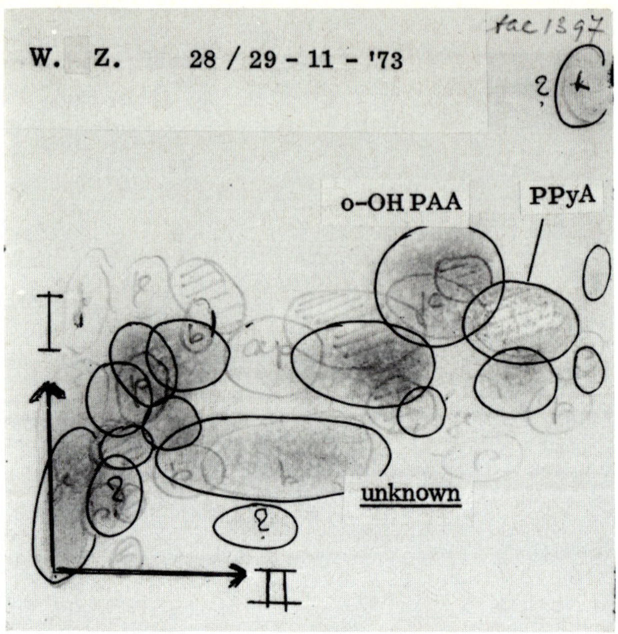

FIGURE 23.2 Thin layer chromatogram of urinary phenolic acids in W.Z. on the day of loading with phenylalanine, 100 mg/kg. *Phenolic acids* were analysed by two-dimensional chromatography according to Armstrong *et al.* (1956), but instead of filter paper 10 × 10 cm thin layer plates (D. C. Alufolien Cellulose 0·1 mm, E. Merck, A.G., Darmstadt No. 5552) were used. First solvent: isopropanol/ammonia 5% (8:2). Second solvent: benzene/glacial acetic acid/water (125:72:3). Spray: diazotised sulphanilic acid 0·5 g in 100 ml sodium carbonate 10%.

present on the days before and after loading, but at a much lower level. So far this compound has not been identified.

The patient's 12-year-old sister, E.Z., showed the same urinary abnormality. She also had a normal fasting phenylalanine level. In this healthy girl no phenylalanine loading has been done so far.

The patient's excretory pattern resembles that of patients with phenylketonuria in a number of respects: PPyA, PLA, *o*-OHPAA and MA clearly increased, to a lesser extent however. But differences also exist: urinary and blood phenylalanine are practically normal and urinary PAA is not increased. The excretory pattern of patient W.Gi., described by Chalmers and Watts (1974) was comparable to some extent with that of W.Z., but fasting phenylalanine was increased (3·8 mg/100 ml) whilst PAA was not analysed. In Figures 23.3 and 23.4 the urinary profiles of a phenylketonuric child and of a child with hyperphenylalaninaemia only are given for comparison.

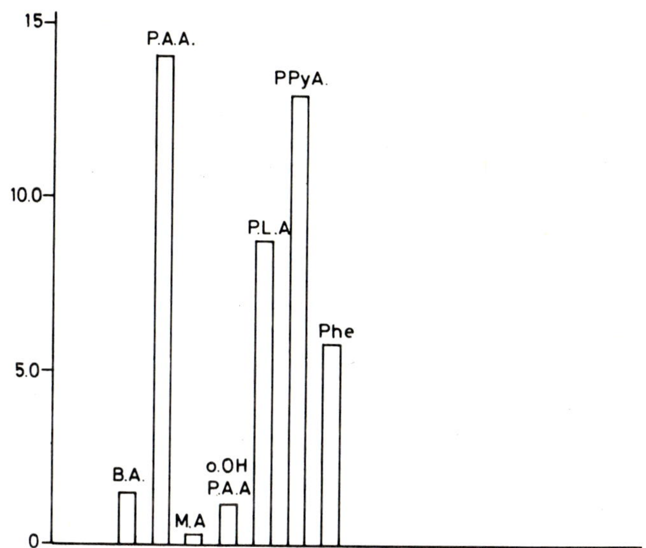

FIGURE 23.3 Excretory pattern of phenylalanine and metabolites in H.S., a patient with untreated phenylketonuria. Serum phenylalanine 38·5 mg/100 ml; urinary creatinine 490 mg/l. Compare with Figure 23.1.

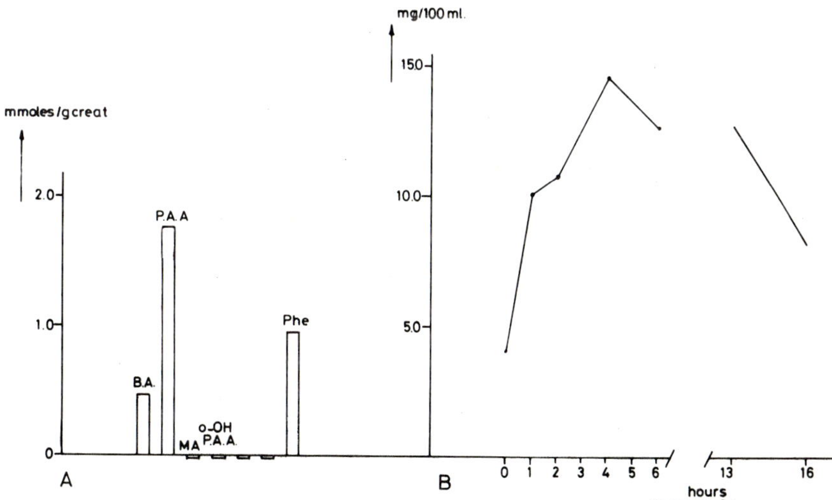

FIGURE 23.4A Urinary metabolites of patient M.H. Excretory pattern of phenylalanine and metabolites in hyperphenylalaninaemia. Dietary phenylalanine 92 mg/kg. Urinary creatinine 90 mg/l.

FIGURE 23.4B Serum phenylalanine after loading in the same patient. Phenylalanine load 100 mg/kg.

From Figure 23.5 the interrelationship of the above mentioned metabolites can be seen. The most simple hypothesis would be a decreased oxidative decarboxylation of phenylpyruvic acid, assuming that normally urinary PAA is partly formed from phenylpyruvic acid and partly by oxidative deamination of phenylethylamine. With this hypothesis in mind we tested whether the daily administration of 100 mg thiamine for one month would correct the anomaly in W.Z. However, no thiamine response could be demonstrated. On the whole very little quantitative information is available about the endogenous formation of phenylacetic acid from phenylpyruvic acid in normal and phenylketonuric individuals. It is believed to occur in the liver (Moldave and Meister, 1957).

The hypothesis of a decreased phenylalanine transaminase activity in liver only (and not in peripheral tissues) cannot explain the abnormality in W.Z. In her case plasma phenylalanine would be expected to be increased and this was not so.

It is difficult to say, whether the anomaly of our patient W.Z. is harmful. She did not exhibit symptoms likely to be connected with the

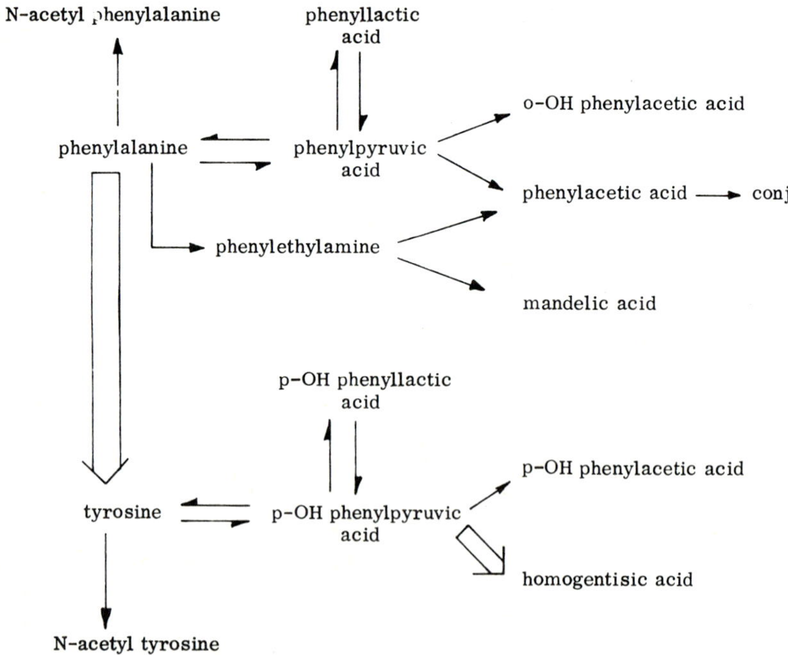

FIGURE 23.5 Endogenous phenylalanine and tyrosine metabolism.

chemical abnormality and her sister seems to be healthy. On the other hand, intracellular accumulation of phenylpyruvic acid may be dangerous to the developing central nervous system, as it is well known that this compound can inhibit several metabolic enzymes. Furthermore we must ask what would be expected from a combination of the underlying gene and a gene of the phenylketonuria-type or its variants.

In order to answer these questions, more cases will have to be detected. This can be done by systematic screening by the ferric chloride test or with more elaborate techniques for phenolic acid chromatography. If plasma phenylalanine alone is screened for, abnormalities such as those described here will remain undiscovered.

REFERENCES

ARMSTRONG, M. D., SHAW, K. N. F. and WALL, P. E. (1956). The phenolic acids of human urine. Paper chromatography of phenolic acids. *J. Biol. Chem.*, **218**, 293

CHALMERS, R. A. and WATTS, R. W. E. (1974). Quantitative studies on the urinary excretion of unconjugated aromatic acids in phenylketonuria. *Clin. Chim. Acta*, **55**, 281

HEIDEN, C. VAN DER, WAUTERS, E. A. K., KETTING, D., DURAN, M. and WADMAN, S. K. (1971). Gas chromatographic analysis of urinary tyrosine and phenylalanine metabolities in patients with gastro-intestinal disorders. *Clin. Chim. Acta*, **34**, 289

JUSTICE, P., O'FLYNN, M. E. and HSIA, D. Y-Y. (1967). Phenylalanine-hydroxylase activity in hyperphenylalaninaemia. *Lancet*, **i**, 928

MOLDAVE, K. and MEISTER, A. (1957). Synthesis of phenylacetylglutamine by human tissue. *J. Biol. Chem.*, **229**, 463

SCRIVER, C. R. and ROSENBERG, L. E. (1973). *Amino Acid Metabolism and its Disorders*, p. 290. (Philadelphia : W. B. Saunders)

WADMAN, S. K., HEIDEN, C. VAN DER, KETTING, D. and SPRANG, F. J. VAN (1971). Abnormal tyrosine and phenylalanine metabolism in patients with tyrrosyluria and phenylketonuria; gas-liquid chromatographic analysis of urinary metabolites. *Clin. Chim. Acta*, **34**, 277

WADMAN, S. K., KETTING, D., BREE, P. K. DE, HEIDEN, C. VAN DER, GRIMBERG, M. TH. and KRUYSWIJK, H. (1975). Permanent chemical phenylketonuria and a normal phenylalanine tolerance in two sisters with a normal mental development. *Clin. Chim. Acta.*, **65**, 197

24

Use of a semi-synthetic amino acid, 3-methoxyphenyl-L-alanine to measure amino acid absorption

J. W. T. Seakins and R. S. Ersser

Introduction

All existing methods for the measurement of the absorption of protein or of amino acids have both practical and theoretical disadvantages. Some, for example involving perfusion of a section of the small intestine may be used in adults, but are quite unsuitable for use with sick children, others employing ^{15}N-labelled amino acids and proteins require very expensive apparatus and are time consuming; radioactively labelled amino acids are ethically unacceptable and would introduce the further complication of recycling. Protein or amino acid loads require unphysiological amounts to give satisfactory plasma response.

It was hoped that the measurement of the metabolites of anisylalanine —a semi-synthetic amino acid which is absorbed in the small intestine and in the renal tubule by the same transport system as the other aromatic amino acids (Huang, 1961; 1962)—would reflect any defects in intestinal transport in the same way as the urinary excretion of 3-*O*-methyl-glucose parallels the absorption of glucose and galactose in the small intestine (Anderson *et al.*, 1965). In the event, this was not found to be so, but the determination of the plasma decay curves could give useful information.

The Ethical Committee of the Hospital for Sick Children and the Institute of Child Health gave permission for anisylalanine to be used to investigate amino acid absorption in children with cystic fibrosis. The nature and purpose of the investigation were explained to the parents before their consent was sought and obtained.

Materials and methods

Anisylalanine (3-methoxyphenyl-L-alanine; *O*-methyl-L-tyrosine) was either synthesised by the method of Seidel *et al.* (1963) or purchased (Koch-Light, Colnbrook, England).

Urinary aromatic acid excretion was investigated by the gas-liquid chromatography of ether or ethylacetate extracts of acidified urine. Trimethylsilyl ether/ester derivatives were run on silicone phases (OV1 and OV17) and identification was made by comparison with authentic samples. Plasma amino acids were quantitated on a Technicon TSM amino acid analyser using a short programme in which only phenylalanine, tyrosine and anisylalanine were measured.

The safety of the amino acid was tested in growing rats over a three-week period at increasing levels (100 mg/kg per day to 800 mg/kg per day) and compared with two control groups one receiving equivalent amounts of phenylalanine plus tyrosine, the other a completely normal diet. Ten normal adults each took one gram doses, and one of the authors (J.S.) took the amino acid on five occasions.

Procedure

After an overnight fast, the loading dose of anisylalanine (25 mg/kg) was taken with sucrose in place of breakfast. In adult subjects blood samples were taken at half-hourly intervals for 3 hours and subsequently at hourly intervals during the next 4 hours. In children fewer samples were taken. The midday meal was taken at the usual time.

Results and discussion

No differences were observed in the rates of growth of the three groups of rats. No adverse effects were observed by the adult volunteers who took anisylalanine.

Analysis by gas–liquid chromatography of urine specimens passed after ingestion of anisylalanine in a normal adult showed that the amino acid was excreted as three main metabolites namely *p*-methoxyphenylpyruvic acid, *p*-methoxyphenyllactic acid and acetylanisylalanine. Only trace amounts of the parent amino acid were detected in urine by thin-layer chromatography. The time course of the excretion of these metabolites was sufficiently erratic in the normal subject to make this parameter unsuitable as a measure of amino acid absorption.

In the six normal subjects a maximum rise of about 5 mg/100 ml plasma was observed, which occurred between 30 and 45 minutes after ingestion. Thereafter, the plasma concentration followed a strict exponential decline. There was little difference between the normal subjects.

In the eight subjects with cystic fibrosis who were studied (aged 3–10 years) two groups were discernible. In the larger (six subjects) the maximum plasma concentration achieved was significantly lower than in normal subjects and its occurrence was delayed somewhat. Subsequently the plasma concentration decayed exponentially. In the smaller group (two subjects) the time at which the maximum occurred was very delayed ($3\frac{1}{2}$ hours). These results indicate that the intestinal absorption of amino acids in cystic fibrosis may be impaired to varying extents, and offers an explanation of disappointing results often observed in patients who are given free amino acids or protein hydrolysates either as supplements to (or as replacements for) dietary proteins in order to obviate the deficiency of digestive enzymes in cystic fibrosis. As yet no satisfactory explanation of the absorption of anisylalanine (and presumably of other amino acids) can be offered.

A very poor absorption of anisylalanine was observed in the one patient with Hartnup disease.

Summary

This paper describes investigations on the absorption of 3-methoxyphenyl-L-alanine (anisylalanine) in normal subjects, children with cystic fibrosis and in one child with Hartnup disease.

Anisylalanine was slowly metabolised mainly to acetyl anisylalanine, and *p*-methoxyphenyl-pyruvic and lactic acids which were excreted. In normal adult subjects anisylalanine (25 mg/kg body weight) was rapidly absorbed, maximum plasma concentrations being obtained 0·5–1·0 hour after ingestion. Thereafter the plasma concentration declined exponentially. In the group of eight children with cystic fibrosis, the maximum plasma concentration was lower than observed in the control group, and was delayed. A very poor response was observed in an infant with Hartnup disorder.

REFERENCES

Anderson, C. M., Kerry, K. R. and Townley, R. R. W. (1965). An inborn defect of intestinal absorption of certain monosaccharides. *Arch. Dis. Child.*, **40**, 1

Huang, K. C. (1961). Renal excretion of L-tyrosine and its derivatives. *J. Pharmacol. Exp. Ther.*, **134**, 257

Huang, K. C. (1962). Intestinal transport of L-tyrosine and its derivatives. *J. Pharmacol. Exp. Ther.*, **136**, 361

Seidel, W., Sturm, K. and Geiger, R. (1963). Synthese eines vassopressorisch wirkenden Peptids. *Chem. Ber.*, **96**, 1436

25

Animal models for histidinaemia

L. A. Tyfield and J. B. Holton

Histidinaeamia is caused in man (Auerbach *et al.*, 1967) and the mouse (Kacser *et al.*, 1973) by a deficiency of the liver enzyme L-histidine ammonia–lyase (EC 4.3.1.3), or histidase. This enzyme catalyses the conversion of histidine to urocanic acid on the main pathway of histidine metabolism, which proceeds beyond urocanic acid to formiminoglutamic acid and glutamic acid (Figure 25.1). Because of a block at the level of histidase, histidine accumulates and there is an abnormal production of the metabolites imidazole pyruvic acid, imidazole lactic acid and imidazole acetic acid, which appear in the urine.

In respect of these main biochemical features histidinaemia has been compared to phenylketonuria. However, it is now apparent that the clinical manifestations of the two conditions are quite different. It seems certain that untreated phenylketonuria almost invariably causes mental retardation, usually severe. On the other hand, the natural history of histidinaemia has yet to be established, but it is clearly not as harmful as phenylketonuria.

Neville *et al.* (1972) reviewed the published cases of histidinaemia and concluded that a clear association between the biochemical disorder and any clinical abnormality could not be demonstrated. This led them to undertake a prospective study of the condition in infants detected by newborn screening but given no form of treatment. Their experiences so far support their original view (Clayton, 1974).

The finding of mental retardation and speech defect in about half the reported cases of histidinaemia might be the result of a bias in screening because, on the whole, the condition has only been looked for in children with this sort of history. To eliminate this bias, a recent paper examined only the sibs of children most of whom were screened and detected initially because of their retardation (Popkin *et al.*, 1974). This showed that, in these families, a histidinaemic sib had a 40% probability of being retarded, which was ten times greater than the probability of a non-histidinaemic sib being abnormal. Thus, this analysis appears to suggest

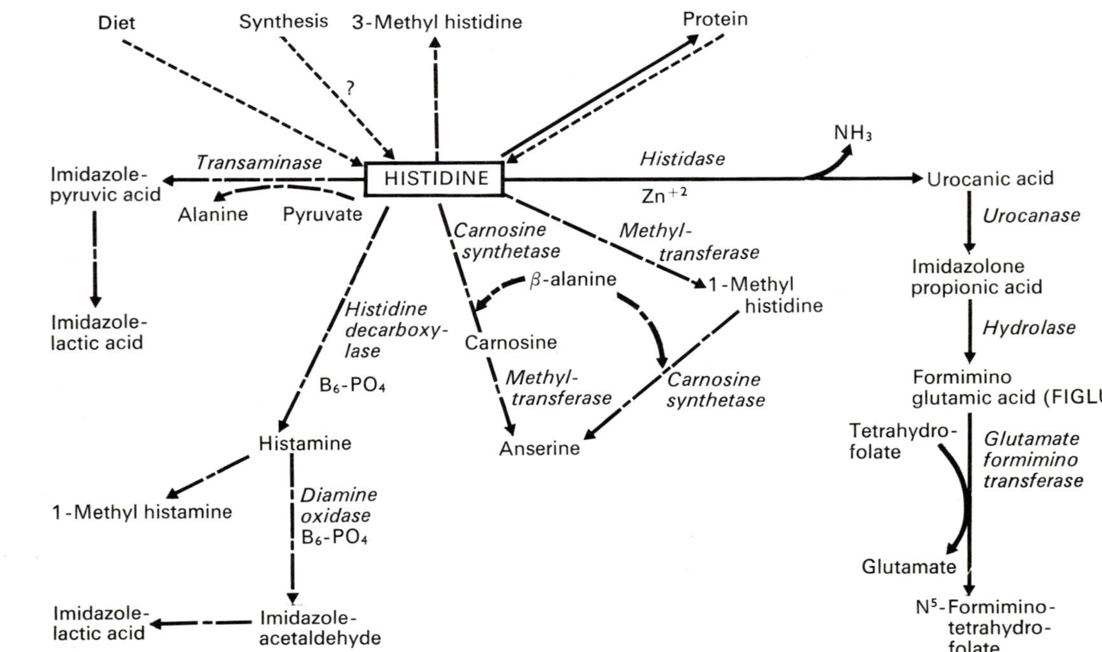

FIGURE 25.1 Metabclic pathways of histidine (from Stifel and Herman, 1971).

an association between histidinaemia and some intellectual impairment.

Another interesting aspect of the problem of the significance of histidinaemia was introduced by the work of Kacser *et al.* (1973) in a strain of mice exhibiting a similar genetically determined defect of the histidase enzyme, in association with a balance defect manifesting itself with head tilting and rolling. On closer study, it was found that the balance defect occurred in the offspring of mothers homozygous for the enzyme defect, although it was more severe in infant mice who were also homozygous for the biochemical abnormality. This damage to the foetus by the histidinaemic mother is analogous to the situation in maternal phenylketonuria.

The possibility that maternal histidinaemia is harmful in humans was supported by a recent family study by Lyon *et al.* (1974). However, a case of a normal child being born to a histidinaemic mother has been recorded previously (Neville *et al.*, 1971).

It is apparent that the clinical significance of histidinaemia is very uncertain but this should be largely resolved in time by the prospective studies currently being undertaken. In the meantime it has been our aim to explore the metabolic consequences of histidinaemia with animal models, in order to try to define what variations in the biochemical expression exist, which might be important in producing differences in the clinical manifestation. Similar experiments have often been done to simulate phenylketonuria and other amino acid disorders and so these comparative studies may be useful also in elucidating the pathogenesis of these other conditions.

The principal effect which has been examined is that of experimentally produced hyperhistidinaemia on the cerebral concentration of other amino acids. Other workers have demonstrated that a high level of one amino acid in the circulation can lead to a significant reduction in the concentration of other amino acids in the brain and this may have considerable pathological implications. In the first series of experiments, adult rats were injected intraperitoneally with histidine (0·5 mg/g body weight). Control rats were injected with similar volumes of physiological saline. The animals were sacrificed 1 hour after the injection for examination of the brain and plasma amino acids. In preliminary experiments, it was found that the plasma histidine concentration rose to 10 times the level found in the control animals, an increase which was comparable to that in histidinaemic patients. The brain concentration was about seven times that in the control animals.

Figure 25.2 shows the results for the amino acids whose brain concentration was significantly altered. The aromatic and branched-chain amino acids, and methionine, were all reduced by amounts ranging from 16–34%. In a second series of experiments the dose of histidine was increased to 1 mg/g body weight. It was interesting to note that, although there was a dose dependant increase in the plasma and brain

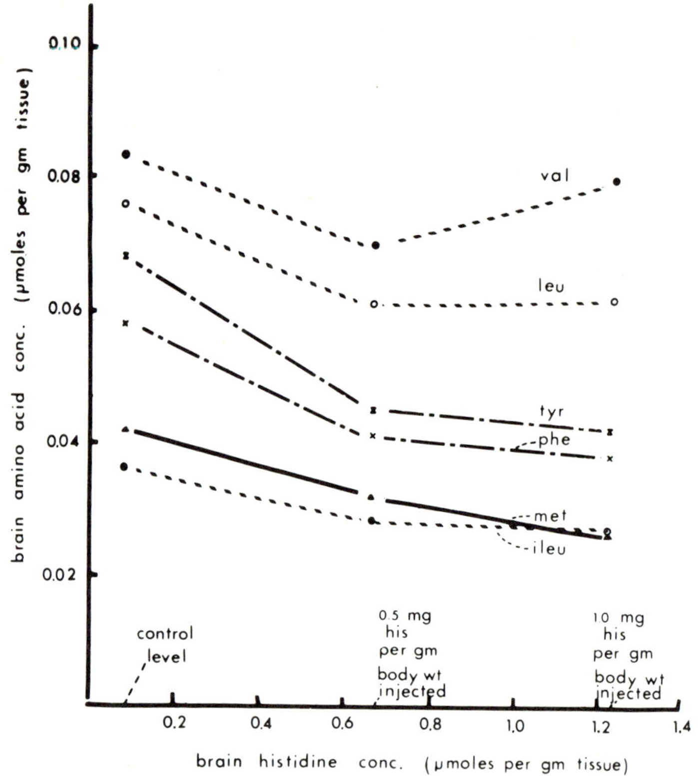

FIGURE 25.2 Changes in amino acid levels in rat brain one hour after intraperitoneal injections of histidine at two dose levels.

concentration of histidine, there was no further consistent change in the levels of the other amino acids (Figure 25.2). The existence of at least two transport mechanisms for histidine, one specific and the other shared with other amino acids, would explain this phenomenon. These would need to have different kinetic properties, the specific transport enzyme having the higher K_m for histidine. The concept of separate and shared mechanisms has been described by Scriver and colleagues (Mohyuddin and Scriver, 1970) for the transport of the amino acid and glycine in renal tissue.

The plasma levels of the other amino acids did not alter significantly in the injection experiments so, when the ratio of brain: plasma concentration of these compounds was plotted (Figure 25.3) it was to be expected that this would fall in response to histidine. This has demonstrated *in vivo*, what others have shown *in vitro* (Neame, 1964), namely an effect of histidine on the transport of other amino acids into brain tissue.

In the preceding experiments, mature animals were used. Since in this type of disorder we are more likely to be concerned with the vulnerability of the immature brain, the response of young animals to the same sort of biochemical insult was examined. When 8-day-old rats

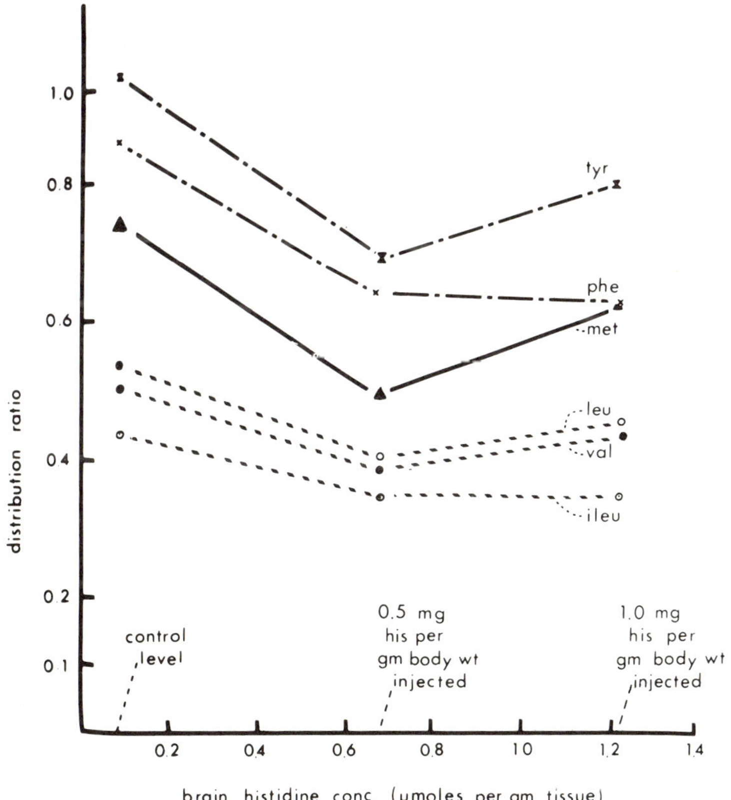

FIGURE 25.3 Ratios of brain/plasma concentration of some amino acids 1 hour after intraperitoneal injections of histidine at two dose levels.

were injected with histidine (0·5 mg/g body weight) and decapitated 1 hour after the injection, very similar results were obtained to those using adult rats (Figure 25.4). The brain concentration of the aromaic, branched-chain amino acids, and methionine, were all significantly reduced.

These observations are interesting in relation to the concept of the blood brain barrier in the immature brain. Early ideas about this were that it was poorly developed, allowing substances to pass through which were normally excluded from adult brain and accounting for the greater susceptibility of the immature brain to biochemical insult. This view

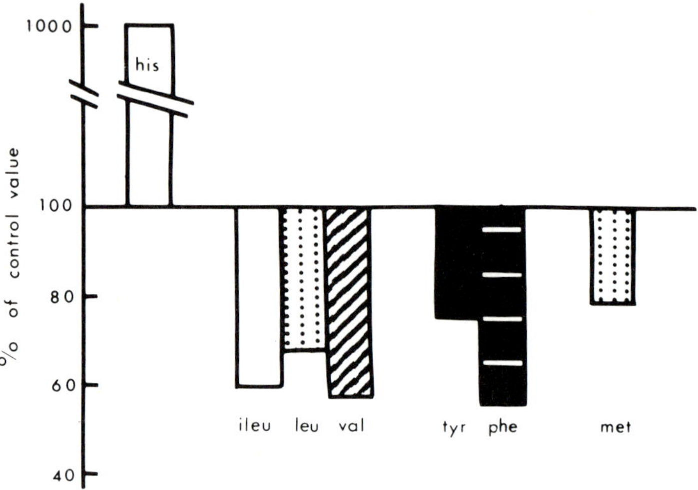

FIGURE 25.4 Changes in brain concentration of some amino acids 1 hour after an intraperitoneal injection of histidine in immature rats.

has been modified in recent years as results such as those presented here, and similar results obtained with phenylalanine (McKean *et al.*, 1968), seem to suggest that, in some respects, the immature brain has transport processes which are as highly selective as the mature brain.

One difference between the adult and the immature brain did emerge, however, when the time curves for the uptake of histidine were compared. Figure 25.5 shows that in the adult the maximum concentration of histidine occurred in the brain 15–20 minutes after the intraperitoneal injection and subsequently fell quite rapidly. In the immature animal (Figure 25.6) the time curve was parabolic, the initial rate of histidine uptake being far slower than in the adult, no fall in brain concentration

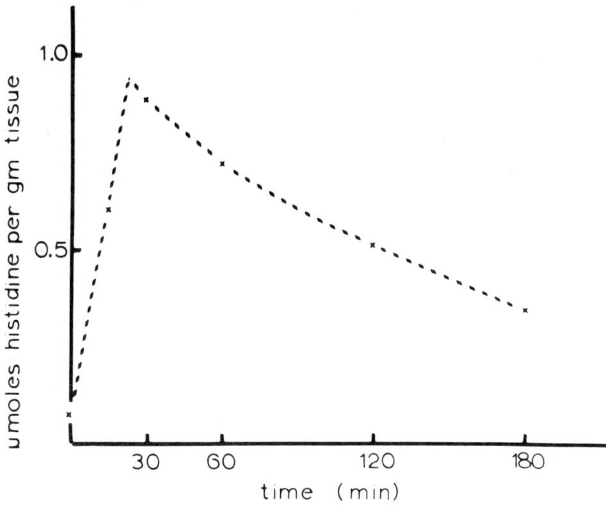

FIGURE 25.5 Changes in the cerebral histidine concentration following an intraperitoneal injection of histidine in an adult rat.

being observed even up to 2 hours after the injection. It was apparent that the ability to control brain histidine levels, which is the result not only of rate of uptake and efflux, but also of metabolism and utilisation of the amino acid, was less developed in the immature brain. It may be important to note that the age of 8 days was chosen for the experiments because it is a period of maximum brain growth in the rat (Davison and Dobbing, 1966) and that this corresponds to a period in the third trimester of pregnancy in man. Hence, this lack of control of histidine level could be significant in accounting for a prenatal susceptibility to histidinaemia.

The experiments in which histidine was administered intraperitoneally have revealed certain differences between mature and immature rats in the handling of histidine and an effect of histidine on the transport of amino acids into brain, but they do not simulate the long-term effects of the hyperhistidinaemia which occurs in the inherited condition. To attempt to produce these conditions rats were fed a diet supplemented with 7 g of histidine per 100 g of feed. Control rats were fed a diet which was reconstituted in an identical way, but without added histidine. Both groups of animals maintained their weight on their respective diets and they were sacrificed after 8 days. The plasma histidine was doubled in the test animals compared with

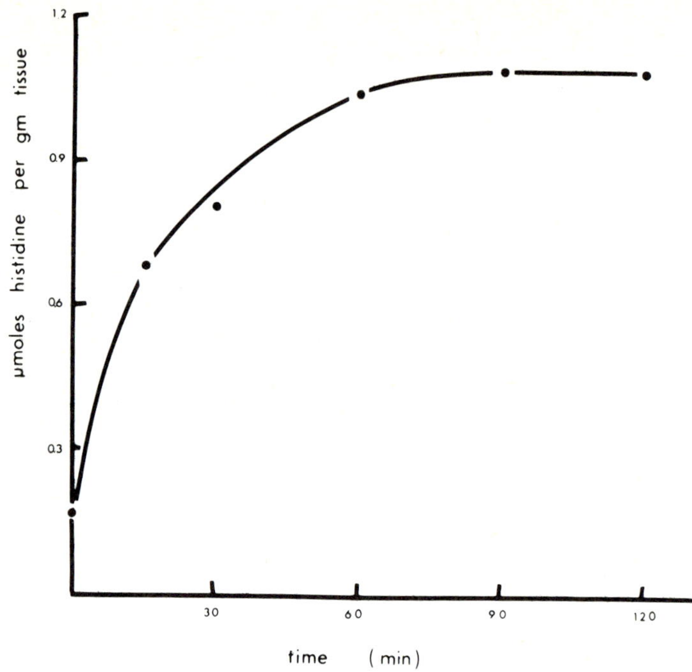

FIGURE 25.6 Changes in the cerebral histidine concentration following an intraperitoneal injection of histidine in an immature rat.

the controls, whilst the brain histidine was increased two and a half times. The histidinaemic animals excreted significant amounts of abnormal imidazole compounds but there was no alteration in the brain concentration of other amino acids. Hence, in the next experiment, the concentration of histidine in the diet was doubled to 14 g per 100 g of feed and animals were again kept on this regime for 8 days.

The results of feeding animals the higher histidine supplement are recorded in Figure 25.7. The plasma histidine was four times the control value, whilst the brain level was increased by seven times. Thus it was confirmed that, in these feeding experiments unlike the injection experiments, the brain level of histidine was maintained considerably higher than that of plasma. Also, there was a generalised increase in brain amino acids in this case and a reduction in the plasma levels of most amino acids.

To explain the widespread increase in brain amino acids it seems reasonable to postulate that there was some effect on the cerebral macromolecules in the histidinaemic animals. Preliminary experiments,

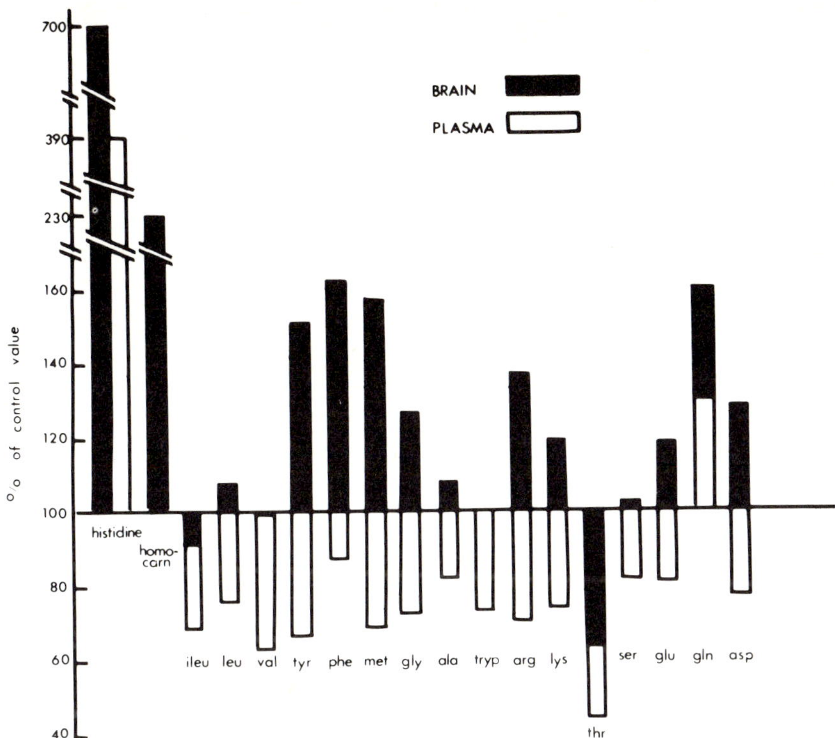

FIGURE 25.7 Brain and plasma amino acid concentrations in rats fed a high histidine diet for 8 days, compared with rats on a normal diet.

using ^{3}H-lysine have pointed to a reduction in cerebral protein synthesis, but further experiments will have to be done to provide more conclusive proof.

There are one or two particular changes in the feeding experiments which deserve some comment. Both brain and plasma levels of threonine fell significantly by 30–40% on both feeding regimes. The only apparent explanation for this is an increased metabolism of threonine to glycine, but changes in the glycine concentration did not support this.

The large increase in brain homocarnosine concentration in both feeding experiments was interesting, no similar changes being observed after the injection experiments although the histidine levels were much higher in the latter. It seems probable that homocarnosine synthetase activity increases in brain as an adaptive response to high histidine levels, but there would not be enough time for this to occur in the injection studies.

The work described indicates that histidine affected the transport of other amino acids into brain and also may have reduced the synthesis of cerebral protein in the long-term experiments. A difference in the control of histidine levels in the adult and the immature brain has been demonstrated. These changes may be invoked in explaining variations in the clinical expression of the defect in humans and this could be explored if a readily available source of cellular material which responded to a high histidine level could be found.

REFERENCES

AUERBACH, V. H., DI GEORGE, A. M. and CARPENTER, G. G. (1967). Histidinaemia, direct demonstration of absent histadase activity in liver and further observations of the histidinaemic disorder. In W. L. Nyham (ed.), *Amino Acid Metabolism and Genetic Variation*, p. 145. (New York : McGraw-Hill Book Company)

CLAYTON, B. E. (1974). Population screening. In D. N. Raine (ed.), *Molecular Variants in Disease*, p. 145. (London : J. Clin. Pathol.)

DAVISON, A. N. and DOBBING, J. (1966). Myelination as a vulnerable period in brain development. *Br. Med. Bull.*, **22**, 40

KACSER, H., BULFIELD, G. and WALLACE, M. E. (1973). Histidinaemic mutant in the mouse. *Nature*, **244**, 77

LYON, I. C. T., GARDNER, R. J. M. and VEALE, A. M. O. (1974). Maternal histidinaemia. *Arch. Dis. Child.*, **49**, 581

McKEAN, C. M., BOGGS, D. E. and PETERSON, N. A. (1968). The influence of high phenylalanine and tyrosine on the concentrations of essential amino acids in brain. *J. Neurochem.*, **15**, 235

MOHYUDDIN, F. and SCRIVER, C. R. (1970). Amino acid transport in mammalian kidney, multiple systems for amino acids and glycine in rat kidney. *Am. J. Physiol.*, **219**, 1

NEAME, K. D. (1964). Effect of amino acids on uptake of L-histidine by rat brain slices. *J. Nerochem.*, **11**, 67

NEVILLE, B. G. R., BENTOVIM, A., CLAYTON, B. E. and SHEPHERD, J. (1972). Histidinaemia: study of relation between clinical and biological findings in seven subjects. *Arch. Dis., Child.*, **47**, 190

NEVILLE, B. G. R., HARRIS, R. F., STERN, D. J. and STERN, J. (1971). Maternal histidinaemia. *Arch. Dis. Child.*, **46**, 119

POPKIN, J. S., CLOW, C. L., SCRIVER, C. R. and GROVE, J. (1974). Is hereditary histidinaemia harmful? *Lancet*, **i**, 721

STIFEL, F. B. and HERMAN, R. H. (1971). Histidine metabolism. *Am. J. Clin. Nutr.*, **24**, 207

26

Galactokinase deficiency in an Italian infant

F. Vecchio, F. Carnevale and G. Di Bitonto

Galactose, an aldose essential for the endogenous synthesis of cerebrosides and complex polysaccharides, is almost completely metabolised to UDP-glucose. The conversion of galactose to glucose involves three metabolic steps, each catalysed by a specific enzyme:

(a) Phosphorylation of galactose in the C_1-position by galactokinase:

$$\text{Galactose} + \text{ATP} \longrightarrow \text{galactose-1-P} + \text{ADP}$$

(b) Conversion of galactose-1-phosphate to UDP-galactose by transferase:

$$\text{UDP-glucose} + \text{galactose-1-P} \longleftrightarrow \text{UDP-galactose} + \text{glucose-1-P}$$

(c) Interconversion between UDP-galactose and UDP-glucose by UDP-galactose-4-epimerase:

$$\text{UDP-galactose} \longleftrightarrow \text{UDP-glucose.}$$

The deficiency or lack of these enzyme activities results in an accumulation of the metabolite(s) before the block in blood or in tissues, and alternative metabolic pathways become active. The major one is the reduction of galactose to its corresponding polyol (galactitol) operated through a NADP-dependent aldose reductase (Hayman and Kinoshita, 1965; Hayman *et al.*, 1966), or to a much lesser extent through an L-gluconate-NADP reductase (Mano *et al.*, 1961). Galactitol has in fact been found in tissues of laboratory animals fed galactose (Van Heyningen, 1959) as well as in tissues (Quan-Ma *et al.*, 1966; Gitzelmann *et al.*, 1967) and in urine of galactosaemic patients (Gitzelmann *et al.*, 1966; Cuatrecasas and Segal, 1966). Another secondary metabolic pathway is the direct oxidation of galactose, catalysed by a specific NAD-dependent dehydrogenase (Cuatrecasas and Segal, 1966), which results in galactonate formation. Urinary elimination of galactonate was observed after galactose administration both in galactosaemic patients with transferase deficiency (Bergren *et al.*, 1972) or with galactokinase deficiency (Gitzelmann *et al.*, 1974), and in normal subjects.

Case reports of galactokinase deficiency are still relatively scanty.

Galactokinase deficiency was discovered by Gitzelmann (1965) in a Swiss gypsy aged 44, who had previously been described by Fanconi (1933) as having a condition of 'galactose diabetes' or 'galactose intolerance' associated with neurofibromatosis at the age of 9 years.

We now describe a further example of galactokinase deficiency in an Italian infant coming from an Apulian family who live in the province of Bari.

Materials and methods

Total blood sugar was determined by a reduction method (potassium ferricyanide ⟶ potassium ferrocyanide) and true blood glucose with glucose oxidase (Boehringer). Galactokinase activity was assayed with [1-^{14}C]galactose as the substrate (Gitzelmann, 1967), urinary galactose and glucose with glucose oxidase and galactose dehydrogenase respectively (Boehringer), urinary galactitol by gas-liquid chromatography as described by Gitzelmann *et al.* (1966) and urine and serum aminoacids were examined by chromatography on thin layer pre-coated plates (Merck-test) and also by high-voltage electrophoresis.

Case report

P.V., a male infant, was born after a normal 40 weeks' gestational period. Birth and delivery were unremarkable. Birthweight 3·4 kg. He was the second child of apparently healthy, unrelated parents, with no known gypsy blood in the family. His 3-year-old sister was healthy. Neonatal jaundice was noticed by the parents on the 2nd day of life; it was said to have lasted a full week regressing very slowly. The baby was breast fed until the 7th month. There was no history of milk intolerance, no failure to thrive or vomiting. Failing vision was noted by the parents when the child was 3½ months old. Two months later they decided to ask for an opinion by an ophthalmologist. Bilateral nuclear total cataracts were diagnosed and the parents were advised that operative discision of the cataracts would be necessary.

He was brought to the Paediatric Clinic of Bari University when he was 7½ months old. Head circumference (44 cm); length (69 cm) and weight (8·8 kg) were on the 50th percentile. Physical examination, including a neurological examination, showed no abnormalities. In particular, no liver or spleen enlargement was present. Chest X-ray,

ECG and EEG were normal. Bilateral dense cataracts were evident, and a horizontal nystagmus was prominent on both eyes.

Serum transaminases (GOT, GPT), blood urea nitrogen, and serum electrolytes were normal. On repeated examinations, urinalysis revealed a marked increment of reducing substances (positive Benedict and Fehling reactions), but no glucose, as evidenced by a negative Clinistix test. The total blood sugar was 120 mg/100 ml but true blood glucose was 70 mg/100 ml. At that time, milk was removed from the patients' diet and replaced with a milk formula free of lactose. Urine and serum chromatography for amino acids revealed a normal pattern.

Heparinised blood specimens of the propositus and two controls were sent by air mail for galactokinase determination to Zurich. The diagnosis of galactokinase deficiency was established. Blood specimens from the remaining three members of the family and two frozen urine specimens of the propositus were also examined. The results are shown in Tables 26.1 and 26.2. The three family members are presumed heterozygotes. A urine specimen, collected at the age of 8 months, before the start of

Table 26.1 *Erythrocyte galactokinase activity/μmoles galactose phosphorylated/h/ml RBC) in a family with galactokinase deficiency*

Subject	*Age*	*Galactokinase activity*
Propositus	15 months	0·0
Sister	3 years	0·337
Father	33 years	0·328
Mother	27 years	0·235
Control 1	21 months	0·810
Control 2	34 years	0·490

Table 26.2 *Glucose, galactose, galactitol and creatinine levels (mg/100 ml) in two random urine specimens collected at ages of 8 and 12 months*

Age (months)	*Glucose*	*Galactose*	*Galactitol*	*Creatinine*
8	1	149	12	31
12	2	322	3	60

Table 26.3 *Eighteen cases of galactokinase deficiency*

Author	*Year of publication*	*Age when diagnosed*	*Sex*	*Cataracts*	*Associated findings*	*Family history*
Gitzelmann	1965	44 years	M	+	Neurofibromatosis, galactosuria	Gypsy; related parents
Gitzelmann	1967	64 years	F	+	Galactosuria	Sisters of the first patients
		62 years	F	+	Considered mentally retarded	
Thalhammer *et al.*	1968	17 days	F		Hypergalactosaemia, galactosuria, mild jaundice	Gypsy; unrelated parents
Linneweh *et al.*	1970	1 month	F	+	Hypergalactosaemia, galactosuria	Apparently gypsy; related parents
Dahlqvist *et al.*	1970	3 weeks	M	+	Hypergalactosaemia, galactosuria	Non-gypsy; unrelated parents
Vigneron *et al.*	1970	neonatal period	F		Transient deficit: it persisted until 6 months	Non-gypsy; unrelated parents

Cook *et al.*	1971	2 months	M	+	Galactosuria; neonatal jaundice	Non-gypsy; unrelated parents
Kerr *et al.*	1971	45 days	F	+	Galactosuria; neonatal jaundice	Non-gypsy; unrelated parents
Monteleone *et al.*	1971	9 years	F	+	Hypergalactosaemia, galactosuria	Non-gypsy; distantly related parents
McVie *et al.* (2 cases)	1971	neonatal period	F	+	Hypergalactosaemia; galactosuria; hernia in both	American-Mexican twins. Non-gypsy; unrelated parents
Levy *et al.*	1972	54 years	M	+		Brothers. Non-gypsy; related parents
		70 years	M	+		
Pickering *et al.*	1972	21 years	F	+	Galactosuria; severe recurrent seizures	Non-gypsy; unrelated parents
Kaloud *et al.*	1973	1 year	F	(+)	Hyperglactosaemia	Non-gypsy; unrelated parents
Beutler *et al.*	1973	13 years	F	+		
Vecchio *et al.* (present case)	1974	15 months	M	+	Galactosuria; neonatal jaundice	Non-gypsy; unrelated parents

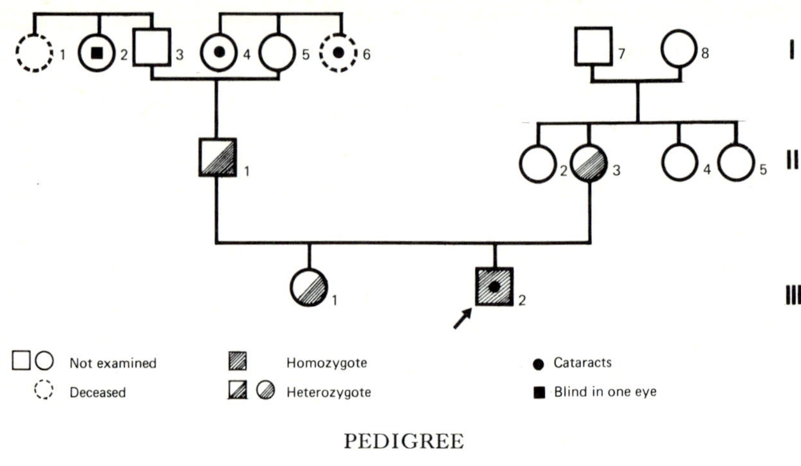

PEDIGREE

FIGURE 26.1

the diet, contained galactose at a considerable concentration and some galactitol. A second sample, at the age of 12 months, should not have contained any galactose as the patient was kept on a lactose-free diet: we suspect that the patient had been given some milk on that day.

Cataract discision was performed on the patient's left eye and his right eye will soon be operated on as well.

Discussion

The diagnosis was suspected because of total bilateral nuclear cataracts as an isolated sign in a healthy infant with no signs whatsoever, of liver, brain, or kidney damage. The suspicion was strengthened by the finding of a mellituria in the absence of glucose, and by the considerable difference between total blood sugar and true glucose levels.

This case appears to be the 18th in the medical literature (Table 26.3) and the first detected in Italy. The average frequency of galactokinase homozygotes would be approximately 1/46 000 individuals, according to the data collected by Mayes and Guthrie (1968) and by Gitzelmann (1967).

Galactokinase deficiency is monosymptomatic; this is in contrast to galactosaemia, i.e. transferase deficiency, where a dramatic course of the disease is common, starting in the first days of life. The different location of the biochemical lesion accounts for the difference in toxic symptoms. In transferase deficiency there is an accumulation not only of galactose and galactitol, but also of galactose-1-phosphate which is thought to be the prime toxic agent within the cells.

Cataract formation is common to both disorders. It is caused by the excessive accumulation of galactitol in the lens fibres leading to hyperosmotic swelling and eventual disintegration of the osmotic barrier, i.e. the cell membrane, resulting in the irreversible denaturation of lens proteins.

Neonatal jaundice with slight enlargement of liver and spleen has been reported in some cases of galactokinase deficiency (Thalhammer *et al.*, 1968; Cook *et al.*, 1971; Kerr *et al.*, 1971). Thalhammer *et al.* (1968) suggest a possible causal relationship between galactokinase deficiency and neonatal hyperbilirubinaemia. Neonatal jaundice which lasted approximately 1 week was observed in our patient. However, the occurrence of both kinase deficiency and jaundice, may well have been coincidental as prolonged neonatal hyperbilirubinaemia without discernible cause is quite frequent in the Apulian region.

The lactose-free formula, supplemented with vitamins and minerals has been well tolerated and fully compatible with normal growth and development in our patient to date. Clearly, the strict lack of exogenous galactose is counterbalanced by the action of epimerase providing for the endogenous production of galactose from glucose. Dietetic control, however, could not induce regression of the cataract; discision on the right eye must follow the antecedent discision of the left one.

Previous experience (Thalhammer *et al.*, 1968; Dahlqvist, *et al.*, 1970; Cook *et al.*, 1971) showed that the effect of dietary management on the regression of cataracts depends on its early introduction. For this reason early detection through newborn mass screening must be advocated.

Acknowledgement

The help of Professor Richard Gitzelmann who provided the biochemical data in Tables 26.1 and 26.2 is greatly appreciated.

REFERENCES

Bergren, W. R., Ng, W. G., Donnell, G. H. and Markey, S. P. (1972). Galactonic acid in galactosemia: identification in the urine. *Science*, **176**, 683

Beutler, E., Matsumoto, F., Kuhl, W., Krill, A., Levy, N., Sparkes, S. R. and Degnan, M. (1973). Galactokinase deficiency as a cause of cataracts. *New Engl. J. Med.*, **288**, 1203

Cook, J. G. H., Don, N. A. and Mann, T. P. (1971). Hereditary galactokinase deficiency. *Arch. Dis. Child.*, **46**, 465

Cuatrecasas, P. and Segal, S. (1966). Galactose conversion to D-xylulose: an alternate route of galactose metabolism. *Science*, **153**, 549

Dahlqvist, A., Gamstorp, I. and Madsen, H. (1970). A patient with hereditary galactokinase deficiency. *Acta Paediatr. Scand.*, **59**, 669

Fanconi, G. (1933). Hochgradige Galaktose-Intoleranz (Galaktose-Diabetes) bei einem Kinde mit Neurofibromatosis Recklinghausen. *Jahrbuch Kinderheilkd.*, **138**, 1

Gitzelmann, R. (1965). Deficiency of erythrocyte galactokinase in a patient with galactose diabetes. *Lancet*, **ii**, 670

Gitzelmann, R., Curtius, H. C. and Müller, M. (1966). Galactitol excretion in the urine of a galactokinase-deficient man. *Biochem. Biophys. Res. Commun.*, **22**, 437

Gitzelmann, R. (1967). Hereditary galactokinase deficiency, a newly recognized cause of juvenile cataracts. *Pediatr. Res.*, **1**, 14

Gitzelmann, R., Curtius, H. C. and Schneller, I. (1967). Galactitol and galactose-1-phosphate in the lens of a galactosemic infant. *Exp. Eye Res.*, **6**, 1

Gitzelmann, R., Wells, H. I. and Segal, S. (1974). Galactose metabolism in a patient with hereditary galactokinase deficiency. *Eur. J. Clin. Invest*, **4**, 79

Hayman, S. and Kinoshita, J. H. (1965). Isolation and properties of lens aldolase reductase. *J. Biol. Chem.*, **240**, 877

Hayman, S., Lou, M. F., Merola, L. O. and Kinoshita, J. H. (1966). Aldoso-reductase activity in lens and other tissues. *Biochim. Biophys. Acta*, **128**, 474

Kaloud, H., Sitzmann, F. C., Mayer, R. and Paltauf, F. (1973). Klinische und biochemische Befunde bei einem Kleinkind mit Galaktokinase-Defekt. *Klin. Pädiatr.*, **185**, 18

Kerr, M., Logan, R. W., Cant, J. S. and Hutchison, J. H. (1971). Galactokinase deficiency in a newborn infant. *Arch. Dis. Child.*, **46**, 864

Levy, N. S., Krill, A. E. and Beutler, E. (1972). Galactokinase deficiency and cataracts. *Am. J. Ophthalmol.*, **74**, 41

Linneweh, F., Schaumloffel, E. and Vetrella, M. (1970). Galaktokinase-Defekt bei einem Neugeborenen. *Klin. Wochenschr.*, **48**, 31

McVie, R., Deutsche, M. A., Olambiwonnu, N. O., Frasier, S. D. and Donnell, G. N. (1971). Galactokinase deficiency: clinical and biochemical studies in identical twins. *Clin. Res.*, **19**, 216

Mano, Y., Suzuki, K., Yamata, K. and Schimazono, N. (1961). Enzymic studies on TPN L-hexonate dehydrogenase from rat liver. *J. Biochem.* (*Tokyo*), **49**, 618

Mayes, J. S. and Guthrie, R. (1968). Detection of heterozygotes for galactokinase deficiency in a human population. *Biochem. Genet.*, **2**, 219

Monteleone, J. A., Beutler, E., Monteleone, P. L., Utz, C. L. and Casey, E. C. (1971). Cataracts, galactosuria and hypergalactosemia due to galactokinase deficiency in a child. *Am. J. Med.*, **50**, 403

Pickering, R. W. and Howell, R. R. (1972). Galactokinase deficiency: clinical and biochemical findings in a new kindred. *J. Pediatr.*, **81**, 50

Quan-Ma, R., Wells, H. I., Wells, W. W., Sherman, E. F. and Egan, T. J. (1966). Galactitol in the tissues of a galactosemic child. *Am. J. Dis. of Child.*, **112**, 477

Thalhammer, O., Gitzelmann, R. and Pantlitschko (1968). Hypergalactosemia and galactosuria due to galactokinase deficiency in a newborn. *Pediatrics*, **42**, 441

van Heyningen, R. (1959). Formation of polyols by the lens of the rat with 'sugar' cataracts. *Nature*, **184**, 194

Vigneron, C., Marchal, G. and Deifts, C. (1970). Deficit partiel et transitoire en galactokinase erythrocytaire chez un nouveau-né. *Arch. Fr. Pediatr.*, **27**, 523

Wells, W. W., Pittman, T. A. and Egan, T. J. (1964). The isolation and identification of galactitol from the urine of patients with galactosemia. *J. Biol. Chem.*, **239**, 3192

27

Homocystinuria : Cyst(e)ine levels in the plasma

I. B. Sardharwalla, B. Fowler and G. M. Komrower

The levels of cyst(e)ine in the plasma of untreated patients with homocystinuria are usually very low. It is difficult to postulate that this might be due solely to lack of methionine conversion to cysteine when a normal diet contains a generous amount of cystine. Furthermore, in spite of low plasma cyst(e)ine, the nutrition of the patients is not adversely affected, indicating that the intracellular concentration of cyst(e)ine is adequate. In an attempt to find a more satisfactory explanation, we have carried out studies on two patients with homocystinuria, and the results are presented here.

In the case of the first, a 7-year-old patient, the study was divided into three parts. During Phase I, the patient was placed on a low methionine diet, as a result of which plasma methionine and cyst(e)ine were near normal while homocyst(e)ine was significantly reduced. When 800 mg of L-methionine/day was added to this basic diet (Phase II) there was a rise in plasma methionine and homocyst(e)ine *but a marked fall in cyst(e)ine was observed.* In Phase III, betaine was added to this high methionine diet with the result that plasma methionine rose further, homocyst(e)ine almost disappeared *but the concentration of cyst(e)ine increased to normal. It should be emphasised that the dietary cyst(e)ine was kept constant throughout the study.* The results showed that there was a reciprocal relationship between plasma levels of homocyst(e)ine and cyst(e)ine.

In the second study, two cysteine loads (100 mg/kg of free base) were administered to a 21-year-old patient; (1) before and (2) during betaine therapy, while the patient was on a *constant* normal diet so that he received a constant amount of protein, methionine and cystine throughout the study. The amino acids in plasma and urine obtained during the first 6 hours after the load were measured by ion-exchange chromatography. In addition the urine was also examined for idioplatinate-reacting sulphur compounds by both column chromatography (Fowler and Robins, 1972) and by paper chromatography.

On a fixed normal diet, the results following cysteine loading showed that (1) the plasma levels of homocysteine-cysteine-disulphide increased significantly, (2) the level of homocyst(e)ine decreased and (3) there was a considerable increase in the excretion of certain unidentified idioplatinate-reacting compounds in the first 6 hours.

When betaine was added to the normal diet so that plasma homocyst(e)ine virtually disappeared, the levels of cyst(e)ine after the load were significantly higher than those when plasma homocyst(e)ine was high. The number of unidentified idioplatinate-reacting sulphur compounds was reduced.

The conclusions to be drawn are: (1) when plasma homocyst(e)ine is raised the low level of cyst(e)ine is due to the incorporation of a very significant proportion of dietary cyst(e)ine into homocysteine-cysteine-disulphide and into other unidentified sulphur compounds which, in part, may be derived from this mixed disulphide; (2) reduction in the level of homocyst(e)ine causes less removal of cysteine by binding, thereby resulting in a rise in its concentration in the plasma; (3) So long as plasma homocyst(e)ine is elevated, addition of cyst(e)ine to the diet has little effect on the plasma concentration of cyst(e)ine which remains low. Therefore, if a satisfactory rise in cyst(e)ine is to be expected with treatment, plasma homocyst(e)ine should be appreciably reduced or eliminated.

REFERENCE

Fowler, B. and Robins, A. J. (1972). Methods for the quantitative determination of sulphur containing compounds in physiological fluids. *J. Chromatogr.*, **72**, 105

DISCUSSION ON PAPER 1

Dr Winokur asked if the toxity of $1,25(OH)_2D_3$ had been compared to that of other vitamin D compounds. If less toxic, could its use be recommended in the prevention of rickets and osteomalacia in patients on anticonvulsant drugs.

Dr Moore noted that throughout Professor DeLuca's paper no distinction had been made between total and ionised serum calcium. Had any work been done to distinguish between ionic and total calcium, for example, in severe acidosis or alkalosis. Dr Moore also asked if there was any function for calcitonin in the scheme which had been presented.

Professor Teller enquired about the influence of vitamin D derived hormones on the level and activity of the calcium binding hormone in the gut. In certain disease states such as vitamin D deficiency and chronic uraemia, Ca-binding protein activity seemed to vary.

Professor Brodehl wanted to know why Professor DeLuca did not think that vitamin D had an effect on tubular phosphate reabsorption as had been shown by micropuncture studies. How would Professor DeLuca explain vitamin D metabolism in chronic renal insufficiency since he had shown that in acute uraemia the hydroxylation to $1,25(OH)_2D_3$ was still very active.

Professor MacIntyre wondered if the lack of effect of 3-deoxy $1\alpha(OH)D_3$ on phosphate was due to the transience of its effect. What happened if the compound was given in divided doses? Had anyone looked for an abnormality of the $25(OH)D_3$ binding protein in the kidney of patients with vitamin D dependent rickets? Did the widespread occurrence of the $25(OH)D_3$ cytosol receptor mean that vitamin D acts on many or all tissues? How could recent results be explained in which adaptation of rats to varying calcium intakes was demonstrated despite thyroparathyroidectomy?

Professor Dent asked how a good response to high doses of cholecalciferol in vitamin D dependency rickets could be explained if the patients lacked the enzyme to dihydroxylate $25(OH)D_3$.

Professor Bickel asked what happened to $25(OH)D_3$ and $1,25(OH)_2D_3$ in severe liver damage. How severe had this to be to reduce the production of these metabolites.

Dr Scriver pointed out that mutation could result in an abnormal enzyme with altered (raised) K_m value for substrate. In these circumstances a higher concentration of substrate was required to achieve product formation; hence, presumably the need for pharmacological doses of prohormones in vitamin D dependency. In this 'Garrodian' situation, one anticipated substrate accumulation, and the finding of elevated 25-OH vitamin D levels in two patients with the dependency syndrome who were not on D_2 therapy and who had symptoms of the disease phenotype, fitted this hypothesis. Finally, one could anticipate different forms of D-dependency with defects at different levels of biosynthesis or hormone utilisation.

Professor DeLuca replied that $1,25(OH)_2D_3$ had not yet been compared to vitamin D_3 in regards to toxicity but would be expected to be much more toxic since it is not subject to feed back regulation. However, recovery from toxicity would also be more rapid since $1,25(OH) D_3$ is cleared from the body more rapidly.

As to the points raised by Dr Moore, none of the work described in his report involves measurement of ionised calcium nor was he familiar with the effects of acidosis or alkalosis on vitamin D metabolism. In his view calcitonin played no role in the regulation of vitamin D metabolism despite an earlier report from Professor MacIntyre's laboratory. The effect of calcitonin was due to a secondary response of the parathyroid glands.

Professor DeLuca explained that vitamin D metabolites stimulate the appearance of calcium binding protein in the gut, $1,25(HO)_2D_3$ being most active. However, calcium binding protein had not been measured in chronic uraemia in man, nor in vitamin D dependency disease in relation to treatment with vitamin D metabolites.

The question whether vitamin D or one of its metabolites has a direct effect on tubular phosphate reabsorption remained to be settled. Micropuncture studies certainly gave support to the idea that vitamin D does influence phosphate reabsorption. However, experiments were required with vitamin D deficient animals which were thyroparathyroidectomised before this phenomenon could be considered established. In acute uraemia brought about by ureteric ligation, it had to be borne in mind that the kidney tissue was exposed to the uraemic state for only a few hours. Thus the enzyme for hydroxylation had not yet been switched off. If the uraemic state could be prolonged to several days, he was certain the hydroxylation reaction would have been switched off.

Professor DeLuca suggested in reply to Professor MacIntyre that the lack of effect of 3-deoxy-1α(OH)D_3 was not due to the transience of its effect since they had studied the time course of response to the 3-deoxy compound. However, one could obtain responses if large doses of 3-deoxy-1α(OH)D_3 were used. As far as he knew no one had looked for an abnormality in the plasma binding protein for 25(OH)D_3 in the vitamin D dependency disease. The widespread occurrence of the 25(OH) D_3 binding protein in the supernatant fraction of many tissues did not mean that vitamin D acts in many tissues, since it was not clear that this protein is in fact a receptor. The idea that adaptation of calcium absorption to low calcium diets was not related to parathyroid secretion and 1,25$(OH)_2D_3$. Synthesis was in his view not established by experiments with thyroparathyroidectomised animals. In these experiments only survivors of the surgery were used and these were likely to have residual parathyroid tissue, which made possible their survival. They had done experiments in which thyroparathyroidectomised animals were given constant exogenous sources of parathyroid hormone. These animals had identical rates of intestinal calcium transport regardless of dietary calcium level. Thus, in his view, the parathyroids are included in this adaptation phenomenon.

Professor DeLuca surmised in reply to Professor Dent that patients with vitamin D dependency probably do not lack the 25(OH)D_3-1-hydroxylase but instead possess a defective enzyme with a large Michaelis constant for substrate. Thus, large amounts of 25(OH)D_3 would be needed to effect a reasonable reaction rate. Alternatively, it was possible that large amounts of 25(OH)D_3 can substitute for 1,25$(OH)_2D_3$ in the target tissue because of the limited discretion afforded by the receptors in those target tissues.

There was some evidence that rickets can be associated with hepatic damage. Diseases such as biliary atresia could be more than a lack of absorption of vitamin D. However, deranged metabolism of vitamin D due to hepatic disorder was likely to be rare since liver disease was often fatal because of more critical physiological failure than that due to defects in skeleton and vitamin D metabolism resulting from hepatic failure.

DISCUSSION ON PAPER 2

Professor DeLuca did not want to leave the impression that 1,25$(OH)_2D_3$ is the sole regulator of intestinal calcium absorption, other factors were also involved. It was important in correlation experiments to bear in mind that other hydroxylated vitamin D compounds might also function in the intestine. He had not found a correlation between growth and intestinal calcium absorption in rats given $1,25(OH)_2D_3$. He believed that $1,25(OH)_2D_3$ is at least part of the Nicolaysen endogenous factor.

Dr Scriver asked if the 'X-linked patients' had been unequivocally of the X-linked genotype. In the literature there was also an autosomal dominant form of hypophosphataemia and some believed there also was an autosomal recessive form. These were different mutations and would, therefore, affect visceral metabolism differently from the X-linked form. It was essential that the important findings for calcium absorption were unequivocally valid for the X-linked phenotype.

Professor MacIntyre wondered why the level of $1,25(OH)_2D_3$ had not been elevated in the case of primary hyperparathyroidism.

Professor DeLuca agreed that the relationship between parathyroid hormone and $1,25(OH)_2D_3$ need not be linear. His colleague Dr Haussler had reported high levels of $1,25(OH)_2D_3$ in hyperparathyroid patients.

Professor Stanbury, in reply, agreed that the demonstrated linear relationship between serum iPTH and serum labelled $1,25(OH)_2D_3$ in the control subjects was most unlikely to be invariably applicable. In fact, if all the available control data are aggregated with those from the cases of primary hyperparathyroidism, the relationship between serum iPTH and $1,25(OH)_2D_3$ in the combined data is best described by a log-linear function. It was not certainly known why the serum concentration of labelled $1,25(OH)_2D_3$ was not found to be elevated in their cases of primary hyperparathyroidism. One possibly relevant factor was that the group of patients studied with this disease had evidence of mild secondary renal impairment (creatinine clearance, mean 63 ml/min, SD 25·5. This might suggest that the formation of $1,25(OH)_2D_3$ was relatively high per unit mass of renal tissue. But there was no significant correlation between the creatinine clearance and the serum $1,25(OH)_2D_3$ and, despite this evidence of renal impairment, the other renal metabolite, $24,25(OH)_2D_3$ was formed in amounts greater than in the controls.

In answer to Dr Scriver, he said that some of the hypophosphataemic patients studied came from unquestionably X-linked pedigrees; others were sporadic cases. All shared a common phenotype, including the bizarre skeletal features developing in adults with the X-linked syndrome. Since other modes of inheritance are exceptionally rare, it was considered that the patients studied could be regarded as a homogeneous group.

DISCUSSION ON PAPERS 3 and 4

Professor Teller presumed that the hPTH had been extracted from an adenoma. All parathyroid adenomata should perhaps be collected by the European Parathyroid Study Group. A point of reference for obtaining hPTH for immunisation would be desirable.

Professor MacIntyre wondered if the hPTH(1–34) sequence of Potts had been used in Dr Fischer's studies. If not, it would be of interest to obtain for comparison some of this material from the Boston Group.

Professor Stanbury pointed out that it might be necessary to consider separately hormonal release and hormonal synthesis when considering the lag in the correction of hypocalcaemic rickets due to the restoration of serum iPTH to normal levels on treatment with vitamin D. In immigrant Asians with chronic vitamin D deficiency, very high serum levels of iPTH could be associated with normal or even moderately elevated levels of serum calcium. Yet in such patients as in patients with hypocalcaemic rickets the most trivial further acute elevation of the serum calcium (by less than 1 mg/100 ml) could reduce serum hormone levels by 80–85%; and the rapid restoration of control hormonal values suggested that raising the serum calcium level arrested hormonal release but not hormonal synthesis (cf. Lumb and Stanbury, *Am.J.Med.*, **56**, 833, 1974). Parathyroid hyperplasia might also contribute to the lag referred to. The situation was in many ways analogous to that in chronic renal failure in which a physiological reaction to hypocalcaemia could sometimes lead to overreaction and the production of hypercalcaemia.

Dr Buist had studied familial hypoparathyroidism in seven subjects in three generations with a dominant mode of transmission. They had classical idiopathic PTH sensitive hypoparathyroidism and responded to exogenous PTH with increased urinary excretion of cyclic AMP and phosphate. PTH levels were undetectable but thyrocalcitonin levels were elevated. What mechanism would permit the dominant transmission of such a trait? The primary defect might not be in the synthesis of the hormone.

Dr Scriver said that the progression of repair in serum iPTH, calcium and phosphorus levels in the patient with pseudo-deficiency rickets was compatible with transition from stage-3 to stage-2 vitamin D deficiency according to the classification of Fraser, Kook and Scriver (*Pediatr. Res.*, **1**, 426, 1967). Of interest was the anomalous (high) iPTH level in relation to the normal serum calcium in stage-2 of the syndrome, and we had to explain this finding. He believed it to be compatible with low cytosol calcium in parathyroid gland cells—low because vitamin D repletion was insufficient to maintain the normal distribution of cellular calcium. Presumably, parathyroid adenylcyclase remained 'activated' when cytosal Ca^{2+} was low.

Professor Brodehl asked how long it took for PTH in serum to normalise in vitamin D deficiency after treatment with vitamin D. How did the plasma phosphate level in the newborn with hypophosphataemic rickets develop in the period after birth.

Dr Steendijk referred to the authors' finding of a low serum phosphate in the cord blood of a baby with hypophosphataemic rickets. He thought observations by Tracy *et al.* (*Oral Surg.*, **32**, 38, 1971) were important. *Prenatal* dental lesions (intraglobular dentine) only occurred in the patient when the mother was hypocalcaemic during pregnancy. Intraglobular dentine occurred only *after birth* when the serum phosphate in the mother during pregnancy was normal. This implied that the prenatal serum phosphate level in the fetus reflected the level of the mother.

Professor Spranger asked if the authors had observed a conversion from pseudohypoparathyroidism to pseudopseudohypoparathyroidism. If this change occurred, did the PTH levels come down to normal?

Professor Fanconi replied to Professor Brodehl that he had insufficient data to answer the first question. He would guess that serum PTH needs at least a few days of vitamin D treatment to become normal. After 3 weeks it was within the normal range in all the cases examined.

In the newborn baby with hypophosphataemic rickets the serum phosphorus concentration was 4·7 mg/100 ml at birth and 3·6–4·6 mg/100 ml in the first 3 months.

As to Professor Spranger's question, they did not observe a conversion from pseudo- to pseudopseudohypoparathyroidism, using hypocalcaemia and lack of response of urinary cyclic AMP to parathyroid extract as diagnostic criteria for psuedohypoparathyroidism. However, both conditions have occurred in the same family.

DISCUSSION ON PAPER 5

Dr Scriver asked if the iPTH assay sensed high levels of hormone and hormone residues reliably. This would be important for the interpretation of the data on some of the hypocalcaemic patients. Was the assay a consistent and appropriate discriminant of circulating PTH?

Dr Steendijk referred to the children with celiac disease and hypocalcaemia who had surprisingly low levels of PTH in serum, and asked if the patients had evidence of rickets on X-ray examination.

Professor Stanbury suggested that the 'usually low' but sometimes 'normal' levels of immunoreactive parathyroid hormone in children with idiopathic hypercalcaemia implied some abnormal reactivity of the parathyroid gland in this syndrome. Measurable values ('low' or 'normal') in the presence of hypercalcaemia surely indicated inappropriate secretion of parathyroid hormone.

Professor Clayton in reply to Professor Stanbury agreed that the findings of 'low' or 'normal' concentrations of iPTH in idiopathic hypercalcaemia would appear to indicate inappropriate secretion. Since the measurement also depends on which circulating fragments are recognised by the anti-serum, it was possible, in addition, that the peripheral degradation of the hormone was altered.

The assay was satisfactory and high concentrations had been found on numerous occasions. The anti-serum was one used by many adult centres in the UK. They had studied many adults with hyperparathyroidism who had values ranging from 940 pg/ml to 6·2 ng/ml. Amongst children they had studied a 9-year-old girl with pseudohypoparathyroidism who had a concentration of 2·05 ng/ml. In contrast, four children aged 1, 2, 4 and 16 years with hypoparathyroidism had concentrations of 100, 40, 50 and <40 pg/ml respectively, and an 11-year-old boy with pseudopseudohypoparathyroidism had a concentration of 207 pg/ml.

A particularly interesting family with the sex-linked dominant form of Albright's hereditary osteodystrophy gave the following results: Father (normal): iPTH, 345 pg/100 ml; Ca, 9·7 mg/100 ml; phosphorus, 3·3 mg/100 ml. Mother (pseudopseudohypoparathyroidism): iPTH, 353 pg/ml; Ca, 9·3 mg/100 ml; phosphorus, 3·5 mg/100 ml. Girl (pseudopseudohypoparathyroidism, 6 years): iPTH, 416 pg/ml; Ca, 9·2 mg/100 ml. phosphorus, 4·9 mg/100 ml. Boy (pseudohypoparathyroidism, 8 years): iPTH, 1·8 mg/ml; Ca, 8·7 mg/100 ml; phosphorus, 5·6 mg/100 ml.

With regard to the patients with celiac disease, the girl aged 4 months presented with rickets, but the infant of 5 months had no evidence of rickets either clinically or on X-ray examination in spite of the hypocalcaemia.

DISCUSSION ON PAPER 6

Professor MacIntyre thought that it was unnecessary to assume that, because 1 μg of $1,25(OH)_2D_3$ was effective in hypoparathyroidism, endogenous production was nil, since 1 μg of $1,25(OH)_2D_3$ was effective in normal volunteers.

Professor Stanbury reported that he had studied the metabolism of labelled vitamin D_3 in two patients with hypoparathyroidism complicating thyroid surgery. He had been unable to detect the formation of $1,25(OH)_2D_3$.

Dr Smith commented that although the effect of $1,25(OH)_2D_3$ in hypoparathyroidism suggested that this metabolite was deficient, it did not prove it. If there was a deficiency of $1,25(OH)_2D_3$ this could be due to the high plasma phosphate and lowering the plasma phosphate should have increased the plasma calcium and calcium absorption in their patients. They had been unable to demonstrate this. The source of added calcium was of interest when $1,25(OH)_2D_3$ was given. It was mainly the result of increased absorption, although an increase in fasting calcium/creatinine ratios in the urine might suggest increased bone resorption. He did not know why such patients with presumed $1.25(OH)_2D_3$ deficiency did not develop rickets (cf. also Russell *et al.*, *Lancet*, **ii**, 14, 1974).

Professor DeLuca had supplied $1,25(OH)_2D_3$ and $1\alpha(OH)D_3$ to several clinical groups and some had reported responsiveness of pseudohypoparathyroid patients. He agreed that response to 1 μg of $1,25(OH)_2D_3$ did not constitute proof that synthesis of the metabolite was absent, but results from measurement of $1,25(OH)_2D_3$ in hypoparathyroidism was supportive of this view. Hypoparathyroid rats did not make $1,25(OH)_2D_3$ provided they were not hypophosphataemic. Similar results could be obtained with chicks.

Professor Brodehl asked whether the urinary excretion of phosphate was increased.

Professor Teller asked why $25(OH)D_3$ had also been used. The amount given was apparently insufficient. Was a higher dose tried? Did the authors assume that in hypoparathyroid patients there is also a blockade in the transformation of $25(OH)D_3$ to $1,25(OH)_2D_3$?

Professor Wolf wondered if it was possible for the 1-hydroxylation to be blocked by the high blood phosphate levels in hypoparathyroidism.

Dr Kind replied to Professors Brodehl, Teller and Wolf that urinary excretion of phosphate was not measured. $25(OH)D_3$ was used to compare the dose requirement with that of $1,25(OH)_2D_3$. The doses of $25(OH)\ D_3$ used were ineffective. Impaired conversion of $25(OH)D_3$ to $1,25(OH)_2D_3$, possibly induced by high phosphate levels, caused by the absence of PTH in the case of hypoparathyroidism, is certainly the most likely explanation for the differences in response to the two metabolites.

DISCUSSION ON PAPER 7

Professor Dent asked if in patients given calcitonin for long periods of time biopsy studies indicated any possible effect on normal skeletal bone, in contrast to the clear cut known effects of acute administration.

Professor DeLuca asked for evidence in support of the statement that calcitonin acts only on osteoclasts. In the experiments on adaptation of parathyroidectomised rats to dietary calcium levels, was there a possibility that extra parathyroid tissue existed in these animals. How did the parathyroidectomised rats survive on a low calcium diet.

Dr Scriver wondered if the hypothesis that calcitonin enhances calcium flux into mitochondria thus depleting cytosol of calcium and further enhancing the asymmetry of intracellular calcium distribution played an integral part in the speaker's view of the calcitonin effect on bone. What was the proof for calcitonin having its effect on bone only as an inhibitor of calcium flux out of bone—or a possible effect as an augmentor of calcium influx from the extracellular fluid into bone tissue. Did calcitonin play an important physiological role in man? Was it perhaps a vestigial hormone since its deficiency was perhaps unimportant and a chronic excess was probably benign. If it was vestigial what role did it really play in fish, for example, or in early land animals. Could the extraordinary increase in blood calcitonin in salmon at spawning time tell us anything?

Dr Winokur asked about the value of calcitonin in the treatment of adult Paget's disease or any disease other than Paget's.

Dr Carter was curious how the effect of whisky in raising calcitonin in those carrying the gene responsible for thyroid medullary carcinoma had been discovered.

Dr Stamp asked if the speaker regarded it as a paradox that while osteoclastic activity was necessary for bone remodelling, it was inhibited by calcitonin which none the less had been shown to improve bone remodelling in juvenile hyperphosphatasia.

Dr Steendijk observed that porcine calcitonin had no effect whatsoever in a very severe case of polyostotic fibrous dysplasia. Like juvenile Paget's disease this was a high turnover bone disease but bone structure was abnormal. In spite of the fact that the number of osteoclasts was increased they did not seem to react to long term treatment with calcitonin in high doses. The reason for the difference in response between polyostotic fibrous dysplasia and Paget's disease was obscure.

Professor Spranger said that osteoclasia with macrocranism (juvenile hyperphosphatasia) probably should not be called juvenile Paget's disease since this would imply an identical pathogenesis of (dominant) Paget's disease and (recessive) hyperphosphatasia. This had not been proven. Had any calcitonin assays been done in osteoclasia before treatment?

Dr Smith remarked that if calcitonin had an effect on bone remodelling one would expect to find elevated values in the hyperostoses such as marble bones disease, Engelman's disease, etc.

Dr Mehls pointed out that serum calcitonin levels are not increased in patients with renal osteodystrophy even in states of hypocalcaemia.

Dr Winokur enquired if calcitonin has a selective action only on those osteoclasts which are in a pathological environment (as in juvenile Paget's disease) or if it acts equally on all osteoclasts throughout the body.

Dr Buist referred to a family with hypoparathyroidism already mentioned in the course of this symposium. The thyrocalcitonin levels were elevated, and he asked Professor MacIntyre to speculate about the mechanism.

Professor MacIntyre in reply noted that histological changes had not been observed on normal bone in those patients given calcitonin for long periods for Paget's disease. As for Professor DeLuca's statement, he did not believe that calcitonin acts only on osteoclasts. It had a major effect on osteocytes and this was perhaps most clearly shown in cases of hyperphosphatasia given human calcitonin (Horwith *et al. Proc. 5th Intern. Symp. Endocrinol.*, 1976, in the press).

The hypothesis that calcitonin involves enhanced mitochondrial uptake of calcium with a consequent depression of cytosolic calcium levels was, at the moment, only a theory without full experimental support, although some of Borle's work agreed with this idea.

The effect of whisky in raising calcitonin levels in medullary carcinoma was first suggested from an observation of Cohen *et al.*, *Lancet*, **ii**, 1172, 1973 the mechanism was still not clear.

Professor MacIntyre agreed with Dr Stamp that there was an apparent paradox in that calcitonin improves bone remodelling in hyperphosphatasia but nevertheless inhibits osteolysis. Perhaps this merely meant that excessive rates of bone resorption prevent normal modelling and that calcitonin merely slows down osteolysis to more nearly physiological levels. He agreed with Professor Spranger that they should not call their cases juvenile Paget's disease. On reflection they should have used the term 'hyperphosphatasia' since this did not imply identity with the adult disease.

DISCUSSION ON PAPER 8

Professor Harris reported two examples of X-linked hypophosphataemic rickets in both mother and son and in both instances the mother was more severely affected by skeletal deformity than the son. The question was if orthopaedic surgery was ever indicated before puberty or even after puberty. How were these patients to be managed if surgery was undertaken.

Dr Balsan had not observed catch-up growth in a group of patients with familial hypophosphataemic rickets. At the beginning of therapy the impression of catch-up growth was sometimes given by the appearance of the growth curve, but this was secondary to correction of bone incurvations. They had never seen sudden catch-up growth in the late stages of treatment of their patients.

Professor Bickel described a patient with typical vitamin D refractory rickets now of school age who was at the 50th percentile for height and had grown normally from his second year of life. He needed high doses of vitamin D_3 (100 000 to 200 000 IU daily) and for the past 2 years he had also been given phosphate salts. The boy was well monitored by highly intelligent parents and had never shown signs of overdosage of D_3. His plasma phosphate levels always remained low, between 3–4 mg/100 ml.

Dr Brenton asked for the evidence that the plasma concentration of the various vitamin D metabolites went on increasing with the dose of vitamin D even when very big doses were used. Since the disease was referred to as 'resistant' rickets he wondered if the patients were resistant to the hypercalcaemic effects of the vitamin, and if so, what the basis was of this resistance.

Dr Balsan referred to measurement of serum 25(OH) D_3 levels by Dr Belsey (Boston) in some of her patients treated for several years with vitamin D_3. Elevated levels were found ($>$250 ng/ml.) As for the problem of 'resistance to vitamin D' in these patients with hypophosphataemic rickets, some of the first patients described in the literature had been given large amounts of vitamin D_2 (5–10 mg/day) for months without showing hypercalcaemia. On the other hand, in paediatric departments, luckily quite rarely, children were seen who had been given 5 mg/day of vitamin D for a much shorter period who were severely ill with serum calcium concentrations of up to 16 or 18 mg/100 ml.

Professor DeLuca explained that the regulation of 25-hydroxylation was not absolute. There was some increase in serum 25(OH)D_3 with high dosage of D_3. For example, a 1000-fold increase in D_3 dosage increased serum 25(OH)D_3 twofold in contrast to DHT_3 in which a 1000-fold increase in dose gave a 1000-fold increase in 25(OH)DHT_3 in serum. It should be noted that huge amounts of vitamin D could do everything that 1,25$(OH)_2D_3$ did even in nephrectomised animals. It was uncertain whether D_3 itself was a poor substitute for 1,25$(OH)_2D_3$ or whether its activity was due to a contaminant such as 5,6 trans vitamin D_3.

Dr Stamp said that jointly with Dr Haddad they had published full dose-response curves for plasma 25(OH)D_3 and oral vitamin D (*Am. J. Med.*, **57**, 57, 1974). There was no difference in dose response between patients with primary hypophosphataemia and those with hypoparathyroidism. In support of Professor DeLuca's data they had shown a striking relationship between plasma $25(OH)D_3$ response to intravenous D_3 and initial levels; there was very little response in the D-replete individual but a clear response in the deficient patient.

Professor Stanbury wondered if Dr Steendijk regarded the lesion he described in bone as specific for X-linked hypophosphataemia. How early in life was this osteolytic abnormality detected? Since a popular hypothesis held that the bone disease was secondary to renal phosphaturia and hypophosphataemia, one might expect similar osteolytic lesions in other types of hypophosphataemic osteomalacia such as the Fanconi syndrome or vitamin D deficiency, if this hypothesis was correct. Had similar observations been made in other hypophosphataemic states?

Dr Buist asked what therapy could be offered to adults with vitamin D 'resistant' rickets.

Professor Dent replied that he did not treat asymptomatic hypophosphataemic adults. He followed them 6-monthly, and X-rayed them if they had bone pain. If he saw Looser zones he started them on high dosage vitamin D; sometimes he treated them on symptoms only, usually backache. The alkaline phosphatase did not always rise in the early stages and a normal value should not deny treatment if indicated on other grounds. He expected most adults to go into a phase of remission at 20–50 years of age: later they often relapsed. In pubertal children he stopped vitamin D when growth in stature ceased. If the phosphatase was still a little raised, this usually continued to fall without treatment. Severely affected males sometimes recurred quickly and had to be kept on vitamin D all their lives.

Dr Visakorpi asked about the incidence of hypophosphataemia, which was described as the 'commonest form of dwarfism'.

Professor DeLuca could not yet tell if it was necessary for $1\alpha(OH)D_3$ to be converted to $1,25(OH)_2D_3$ before it functioned. Haussler had published evidence that it was. However, the kinetics of function of the $1\alpha(OH)D_3$ compound suggested that it need not be so converted to work on intestine, but had to be hydroxylated before it worked on bone. They were preparing tritiated $1\alpha(OH)D_3$ to study this problem.

Dr Steendijk replied that it was indeed possible that within any one family women could be more severely afflicted than men. Individual variation in factors which affect the strength and structure of bone, such as nutrition, bone turnover and other aspects of calcium and phosphate metabolism might explain this observation. On the basis of the genetics of the disease, however, men should be more severely afflicted than women; and this was generally found.

Surgery before puberty was only indicated when the deformities were so bad that permanent damage to the knee- or ankle-joints would result if surgery was postponed. After puberty the more severe and conspicuous deformities of the legs should be corrected. This had to be done with the utmost care, since insufficient correction could lead to recurrence of the deformities a number of years later.

Whether vitamin D should be given to adults with this disease was a question Dr Steendijk could not answer at this stage. Not enough experience had been gathered during long term follow-up of adults to be certain about the pros and cons of this form of treatment.

As to catch-up growth, this was very rare indeed and it probably only happened in the least affected patients. Perhaps the advent of phosphate-therapy would change this for the better.

The question of the resistance to the hypercalcaemic effect of vitamin D was an important one. There was no doubt that serum calcium rose to values above the normal range if one went on increasing the dose of vitamin D. Some patients got hypercalcaemia on a relatively low dose of perhaps 1–1·5 mg/day. As mentioned by Dr Balsan, others did not become hypercalcaemic even when 5 mg/day was given for a long period of time. Apparently, sensitivity to the toxic effects of vitamin D was highly variable. The trouble was that—for obvious reasons—we did not have enough data on this variability in normal people.

Dr Steendijk pointed out that the lesion in the bone was not a pathognomonic feature of X-linked hypophosphataemia or sporadically occurring hypophosphataemic rickets. It did occur in the two conditions he had mentioned which were not characterised by hypophosphataemia. Whether it was present in other hypophosphataemic conditions, such as Fanconi syndrome, he did not know. He did not think this point had been examined.

Finally as to the incidence of the disease a reliable estimate was difficult to make since a number of people who carried the gene were asymptomatic except perhaps for some reduction in stature (Winters *et al.*, *Medicine*, **37**, 97, 1958). According to Burnett, Dent, Harper and Warland (*Am. J. Med.*, **36**, 222, 1964), however, the incidence was 1 : 20 000.

DISCUSSION ON PAPER 9

Professor MacIntyre wondered if there might not be an alternative explanation for pseudo-D-deficiency, such as an abnormality in either or both the plasma and kidney of 25-OH-binding protein.

Dr Scriver observed that an important message from vitamin D dependency was that the fetus is well provided as to calcium despite his inborn error of vitamin D hormone biosynthesis. He asked if anything was known about the mechanism by which the fetus receives calcium across the placenta.

Professor DeLuca pointed out that DHT was an analogue of $1,25(OH)_2D_3$ inasmuch as it functioned on intestine just as well without kidney as with kidney. However, large amounts were required for its effect relative to $1,25(OH)_2D_3$. DHT had poor calcification properties relative to vitamin D itself. Thus, DHT might be a reasonable substitute for some functions of $1,25(OH)_2D_3$ and a poor one for others.

Professor Brodehl wondered if the biochemical abnormalities in pseudo-deficiency rickets were really exactly the same as in deficiency rickets. The serum phosphate level had stayed quite normal throughout the first year of life of Professor Prader's first patients and this could be explained by the fact that in deficiency rickets all metabolites of vitamin D are missing, while in pseudo-deficiency rickets $1,25(OH)_2D_3$ alone is missing, since normal doses of vitamin D were given in this case.

Dr Smith asked if severe myopathy was a feature of the disease in children. Why did this not return in adults when vitamin D therapy was stopped and osteomalacia recurred. One could suggest that histological osteomalacia did not recur because growth had stopped, but was it not peculiar that the myopathy did not recur in the presumed absence of $1,25(OH)_2D_3$.

Professor Prader replied by pointing out that the questions concerned aspects of pseudo-D-deficiency which are not yet fully understood. There is only indirect evidence for an enzymatic defect, and one has certainly also to consider a defect of a binding protein in the plasma or the kidney. The reasons why the fetus is protected are not known. He assumed that it is due to a placental transfer of maternal D-metabolites, but it may also simply be due to the placental transfer of calcium which is regulated by unknown mechanisms. He was not sure whether the plasma phosphorus is significantly different from that seen in deficiency rickets. Finally, he did not know why muscular hypotonia is severe in the affected infant and absent in the affected adult.

DISCUSSION ON PAPER 10

Professor DeLuca asked if the phosphate diuresis produced by excess parathyroid hormone in primary hyperparathyroidism was a contributor to the rickets occasionally seen in this disease.

Professor MacIntyre felt that in the osteomalacia sometimes seen in primary hyperparathyroidism phosphate depletion was not a likely explanation. He thought that there probably was an impairment in vitamin D metabolism, perhaps in the conversion of $25(OH)D_3$ to $1,25(OH)_2D_3$ similar to that produced experimentally in the rat on a high calcium diet when given parathyroid extract.

Dr Steendijk stressed the importance of the bone turnover rate in the relation between rickets, hyperparathyroidism and serum phosphate. Serum phosphate in babies was 6 mg/100 ml, in adults just over 3 mg/100 ml. Babies with a serum phosphate of 3 mg/100 ml had rickets, adults had no osteomalacia with this serum phosphate level. This was perhaps related to the fact that bone turnover in the first year of life was 50% per year, in adults it was only 5% per year. Apparently a high serum phosphate is required for normal mineralisation when turnover is high. The rickets encountered in primary hyperparathyroidism in children might therefore be related to the increased bone turnover which is a feature of this disease.

Dr Smith described a family in which there appeared to be a dominantly inherited renal tubular osteomalacia presenting in adult life. The patient, in her early twenties, presented with osteomalacia, muscle weakness, hypophosphataemia, Looser zones, renal glycosuria and systemic acidosis. Her adult sister had hypophosphataemia and renal glycosuria, her father renal glycosuria and osteomalacia and hypophosphotaemia. He later died in diabetic coma. One of his brothers also died of diabetic coma in early life and his father had diabetes and 'bone disease'. Dr Smith asked if other such kindred had been described.

Dr Scriver reviewed the requirements in man for calcium and vitamin D. He referred to a patient (cf. *Pediatrics*, **46**, 865,1970) with pure calcium deprivation rickets. This case demonstrated a minimum requirement for calcium, in general, the picture of minimum and maximum requirements for calcium at various ages and phosphate intakes remained confused. With regard to vitamin D requirements the Nutrition Canada survey had revealed that the median nutritional intake of vitamin D in rapidly growing adolescents was in the vicinity of 200 IU/day, not one patient with nutritional deficiency was found in the survey. An allowance of 400 IU might be erroneously high for a few adolescents. What was the true need for vitamin D?

Dr Steendijk confirmed that when the most recent recommendations on vitamin D intake were used by the World Health Organisation it was already suspected that the recommended daily intake might be too high. However, due to uncertainties about the amount of vitamin D derived from irradiation by the sun it was not deemed advisable to reduce the recommended intake.

Dr Blau asked about the status of the theory that cystinosis was a defect of lysosomal cystine transport, and that cystine could be mobilised by passive efflux as cysteine after reduction with dithiothreitol.

Dr Scriver recalled that this idea that dithiothreitol (DTT) could deplete cystinotic cells of cystine had been originated by Goldman *et al.* (*Lancet*, **i**, 811, 1970). They had treated two patients with infantile nephropathic cystinosis for 8 months with DTT (25 mg/kg/8 h) given in capsules by mouth. In both patients leucocyte cystine fell steadily from homozygous to heterozygous levels and the glomerular nephropathy stabilised. When DTT was stopped cystine re-accumulated in the leucocytes and steady deterioration of renal function reappeared. These preliminary observations suggested that DTT was tolerated, could partially alleviate cystine storage and perhaps attenuate the progress of the disease.

Professor Bickel referred to recent work by Schneider and colleagues in San Diego who had investigated a cystinotic fetus after termination of pregnancy at the 18th week. In most tissues the cystine concentration was already increased 50–100-fold. A noteworthy exception were the adrenals which even showed subnormal cystine levels. This was perhaps due to the high ascorbic acid concentration in this organ. Fibroblast cultures of cystinotic patients reduced their cystine concentration considerably under the influence of ascorbic acid added to the medium. Therapeutic trials with ascorbic acid (3 g/day or more) were now under way in San Diego and one patient was being treated in Heidelberg.

Dr Buist pointed out that when children with cystinosis received renal transplants the rickets disappeared as did all requirements for extra vitamin D.

Dr Carton asked if thyroid studies had been performed in cystinotic children who were known to be prone to the development of hypothyroidism in the later stages of the disease.

DISCUSSION ON PAPER 11

Professor MacIntyre suggested that the elevated level of $25(OH)D_3$ found in D-dependent rickets could not be due to a block in the metabolism of that compound because it was not seen in nephrectomised subjects in whom there is, of course, no metabolism of $25(OH)D_3$ to $1,25(OH)_2D_3$. Nor was there elevation of $25(OH)D_3$ in renal osteodystrophy where impaired conversion to $1,25(OH)_2D_3$ is present. Another mechanism had to be invoked to explain Dr Scriver's findings in D-dependent rickets. He thought it unlikely that dialysis could remove much $25(OH)D_3$ in nephrectomised patients.

Dr Steendijk wondered if there was not a hazard of hypercalcaemia if one gave phosphate to patients with X-linked hypophosphataemia in conjunction with vitamin D if the patients stopped taking the phosphate but continued taking the vitamin.

Dr Smith referred to the evidence presented that the concentration of inorganic phosphate within the red cell is mainly determined by that in the plasma, and the implication that the same occurs in other cells of the body. Did this apply to the renal tubular cells, and if the inorganic phosphate was low in the renal tubule cell in type-1 rickets, why did this not stimulate production of $1,25(OH)_2D_3$ and cause over-absorption as Professor Dent had suggested in his case of aludrox-induced hypophosphataemic osteomalacia. Dr Smith suggested that the concentration of phosphate in the renal tubular cell is probably normal in type-1 rickets.

Dr Buist reported a girl with vitamin D resistant rickets who developed hyperparathyroidism, and a patient with cystinosis who did likewise—both had adenomata. The diagnosis was difficult since the elevated Ca^{2+} level was attributed to overdose of vitamin D. During the post-operative period the % TRP rose to normal for a day or two but within 2 weeks the tubular defects were as bad as they had always been in the past.

Professor Brodehl replied to a query about a breed of pigs with vitamin D dependency presumably caused by a mutation not unlike that found in man. The animals had been studied at the Veterinary School in Hanover. Unfortunately, he could report no new data on these rachitic pigs. There were difficulties in working with and anaesthetising these animals.

Dr Watts urged caution in transferring findings in, and arguments developed from the study of animals with mutant enzymes to the human species. The well known problems of genetic heterogeneity within the human species were increased by crossing from one species to another. Also, caution was necessary in interpreting the results of electrolyte analysis on whole tissue (kidney) because we were looking at parenchymal cells, interstitial fluid and renal tubular fluid, all at once. These compartments were differently affected by the hormones concerned.

Dr Scriver, in reply to Professor MacIntyre, agreed that the assumption was that 25-hydroxylation itself was not impaired by the metabolic events of renal failure, and he supposed also that other phenomena, such as the prior intake of vitamin D_2 besides a block in vitamin D hormone biosynthesis, could explain the high 25-OH vitamin D levels in the Vitamin D dependency state.

Dr Scriver agreed with Dr Steendijk that hypercalcaemia is a hazard of treatment in XLH as it always is when supranormal doses of vitamin D are prescribed. But the hazard was probably less at vitamin D doses of 50 000 units per day and less—the dose range used in conjunction with phosphate treatment—than it would have been if the vitamin D dose greatly exceeded 50 000 units daily, as it usually does in clinics using vitamin D alone for the treatment of XLH. But data speak better than speculation. They had experienced only a few days of mild hypercalcaemia among over 20 000 patient-treatment days. Was this bad or good? Of course there were risks, but Mrs Reade in their group kept the risks to a minimum.

He agreed with Dr Smith that renal parenchymal phosphate concentration is probably normal in XLH. It appeared to be so in the mouse, as mentioned in the paper, and he had offered supportive reasoning in this same vein regarding the human disease (Scriver, 1971).

Dr Scriver was delighted that Dr Buist's information corroborated their own findings about the lack of benefit from parathyroidectomy in

XLH. He hoped that some day we would know just what the problem was in the famous pigs who seemed to have a hereditary defect of vitamin D metabolism analogous to vitamin D dependency. Once we knew that, we should be able to decide whether the porcine disease is an event in convergent or divergent evolution, in relation to the human disease.

DISCUSSION ON PAPER 12

Professor MacIntyre pointed out that both $1\alpha(OH)D_3$ and $1\alpha,25(OH)_2D_3$ were unstable on exposure to light and air, as were other vitamin D compounds. The very small doses made such deterioration more obvious than with the less potent compounds. He wondered if the continued potency of the compounds had been checked. He had found high speed liquid chromatography a useful method for this purpose.

Professor DeLuca said that the problem of $1\alpha(OH)D_3$ stability applied to all forms of vitamin D, namely oxidation of the cis triene structure and photoisomerisation. There were no special problems with $1\alpha(OH)D_3$ or $1,25(OH)_2D_3$ except for the elimination of the 1α-hydroxyl group at high temperatures as experienced in gas–liquid chromatography.

Dr Brodehl wanted to learn more about the case of cystinosis combined with glycogen storage disease. He agreed that % TRP was a bad parameter for the estimation of tubular phosphate reabsorption. It was dependent on phosphate load and varied therefore, enormously. One should use T_p or T_p/C_{In}.

Dr Carter said it was possible to have two independent recessive conditions in one child but this was unlikely to occur unless the parents were consanguineous, and wondered if there was any information on this point.

Dr Moore knew of several itinerant families in Ireland with unusual inborn errors of metabolism whom they could not investigate properly. In Scotland there was an itinerant family of 30, 40 or 50 persons with a hereditary thyroid disorder who had also proved difficult to study. Dr Balsau's problem was thus shared by others, but that was but poor consolation.

Dr Balsan, in reply, confirmed that the activity of $1,25(OH)_2D_3$ and $1\alpha(OH)D_3$ had been checked on experimental animals all through her study. As to Dr Scriver's question, the D deficient child was in fact much younger, i.e. 16 months, than the child with 'pseudo-deficiency rickets' who was 7 years. Yet she was not sure that this difference in body mass could wholly explain the difference in sensitivity to $1\alpha(OH)D_2$ therapy of these two subjects. In fact, in another family with three affected children with 'pseudo-deficiency rickets' the active dose of $1{,}25(OH)_2D_3$ and $1\alpha(OH)D_3$ were 2 μg/day and 4 μg/day for a 12-year-old child; the doses being 4 μg/day of $1{,}25(OH)_2D_3$ and 8 μg/day of $1\alpha(OH)D_3$ for her 8-year-old sister.

DISCUSSION ON PAPER 13

Dr Scriver stressed the need for a continuing search for toxic metabolites in the idiopathic Fanconi Syndrome (FS). They had used gas chromatography mass spectrometry in two patients but without success. With regard to the pathogenesis of the tubular leak Dr Scriver reminded the meeting that the FS had been absent in a hypoparathyroid patient with hereditary fructosaemia; the tubulopathy appeared only when PTH was given to the patient. This and other observations implied that cellular ATP played a key part in the pathogenesis of the FS. This meant that an 'energy coupling' defect was important, whereas transport sites and membranes could remain intact. They had shown by proline infusion studies in two patients with the idiopathic FS that the relevant transport sites were intact, but the ability to transport solute against a gradient from urine into the cell was diminished and in fact negative reabsorption of proline occurred at high loads. This finding was compatible with *in vitro* data of Rosenberg's group showing non-competitive inhibition of uptake by kidney slices by FS producing agents, and the *in vivo* data by Bergeron's group showing increased flux of solute from blood across tubule epithelium to urine in the maleic acid induced FS in the rat.

Professor Fanconi pointed out that in patients with cystinosis PTH was found to be normal as long as glomerular filtration was not impaired. When glomerular failure developed PTH, as expected, was raised. In an 18-year-old girl with idiopathic FS and a glomerular filtration rate near the lower limit of normal, PTH levels were near the upper limit of normal even in the presence of rickets. PTH levels were, therefore, as in familial hypophosphataemia.

Professor Tada reported that he had studied 17 cases of the so-called

Fanconi Syndrome. Of these, three cases had been idiopathic and no underlying metabolic abnormality could be detected. In the remaining 14 cases primary lesions could be found as follows: cystinosis—two cases, Lowe's syndrome—three cases, tyrosinosis—one case, galactosaemia—one case, glycogen storage disease (type I)—one case, Wilson's disease—four cases and homocystinuria—two cases. Homocystinuria had so far not been described amongst the disorders responsible for the FS. In all, Professor Tada had seen 10 cases of homocystinuria and two of these had the typical features of the FS: rickets, hypophosphataemia, generalised aminoaciduria, proteinuria or glycosuria. However, amino acid analysis revealed elevation of homocystine and methionine in blood and urine, and the diagnosis was confirmed by the absence of cystathionine synthetase in liver. Professor Tada thought that the FS was caused by many heterogeneous disorders, and that an unknown metabolic error might also underlie the idiopathic form. He then asked about the earliest biochemical signs of the FS in its idiopathic form. This was important for the early and possibly prenatal diagnosis.

Dr Scriver reported that he had seen the onset of the tubulopathy in cystinosis in the fourth month after birth in a sibship. He had not observed the idiopathic FS from birth although one of his current patients had come to medical attention with advanced sequelae of the FS tubulopathy at one year of age suggesting post-natal evolution of the manifestations by mid-first year.

Dr Balsan asked why hypercalciuria had not been mentioned as one of the possible symptoms of the de Toni–Dabré–Fanconi syndrome. In some patients with cystinosis they had observed a very high urinary output of calcium when no vitamin D therapy was given and when the acidosis had been corrected. Calcium output was further increased when these patients were treated with vitamin D making management of their bone disease quite difficult.

Professor Bickel said that in his experience hypercalciuria was not present in cystinosis but was seen in other types of the FS, e.g. in two siblings with an unexplained hepato-renal syndrome (*not* tyrosinosis, *nor* fructose intolerance). He did not understand why some cases of the FS showed hypercalciuria and others did not. The term 'Fanconi Syndrome' implied too much uniformity considering the many known causes of the syndrome, so when using the term one should add the form of the syndrome, such as 'FS with cystinosis', 'idiopathic FS'—whatever that meant. He wondered if Dr Brodehl considered the renal disorder in cystinosis to be primary. Could it not just as well represent secondary progressive renal damage due to a still unknown prerenal metabolite or mechanism.

Dr Blau thought that the energy depletion suggestion of Dr Scriver tied in with the syndromes listed by Professor Tada, all of which could be plausibly linked with a functional loss of precursors of ATP. For example, in galactosaemia and hereditary fructose intolerance there was well-documented depletion of phosphate, and in homocystinuria ATP was immobilised as S-adenosyl homocysteine. Since renal tubular reabsorption was an energy-linked process, a depletion of the energy charge of the renal tubular cells could well be involved in the Fanconi-type syndrome.

Dr Wolf asked if the association of glycogenosis and FS was only possible in cases with a distinct enzyme defect such as glucose-6-phosphatase deficiency, debranching enzyme deficiency or phosphorylase deficiency.

Dr Baerlocher wondered if it was correct to include fructosaemia solely in the group of Fanconi Syndromes of prerenal origin. In fructosaemia, the enzyme defect was also present in the kidney cortex leading to an accumulation of fructose-1-phosphate, probably a toxic metabolite.

Dr Blom described two brothers, one of whom developed the nephrotic syndrome and died. The other boy also developed the nephrotic syndrome but in addition a classical Fanconi Syndrome. The cause of this renal failure was probably an autoimmune reaction against the tubular cells.

Dr Watts enquired if any cases of the 'idiopathic Fanconi Syndrome' arose from prenatal damage to the fetus. A toxic metabolite acting at this time could be as important as one acting post-natally.

Professor Brodehl in reply to Dr Scriver pointed out that in patients with the FS without glomerular insufficiency there is no evidence of hyperparathyroidism. This had just been confirmed by Professor Fanconi, and was so in his experience also. He agreed that parathormone endogenously or exogenously applied was capable of enhancing the tubular defect, especially the hyperaminoaciduria, as they had found in vitamin D deficiency rickets (Brodehl *et al.*, *Pediatr. Res.*, **5**, 591, 1967).

He was interested in Professor Tada's comments. They had never seen the FS in homocystinurics and to his knowledge it had so far not been described in the literature.

The earliest biochemical disturbances amongst their cases were noted at 5 months in a boy with cystinosis. Very recently, Garty *et al.* (*J. Pediatr.* **85**, 821, 1974) noted the appearance of the FS in a child with glycogenosis as early as 1½ months of age.

Hypercalciuria, as stated by Dr Balsan, was not regularly found in their cases with FS, especially not in those with cystinosis. In his view it reflected that state of bone mineralisation and demineralisation, and seemed to decrease when the blood phosphate level could be raised.

In reply to Professor Bickel, Professor Brodehl suggested that in cystinosis there must be a cellular defect in addition to the systemic prerenal defect. The strongest indication for this was the experience with patients with cystinosis who had transplants, and who did not develop a FS, in spite of the fact that cystine again accumulated in the transplanted kidney.

The combination of the FS with glycogenosis was very rare and in none of the cases described could an enzymatic defect be identified beyond doubt. Conversely, in those cases of glycogenosis with distinct enzymatic defects, a FS had never been described. He therefore concluded that this combination was of a special type in which the enzymatic defect still had to be identified.

Dr Baerlocher was right in his comment concerning fructose-1-phosphate aldolase, which was exclusively found in the proximal tubular convolution (Kranhold *et al.*, *Science*, **165**, 402, 1969). The combination of the nephrotic syndrome with the FS was also very rare, it too probably represented a special entity (Royer *et al.*, *Ann. Pediatr.*, **39**, 583, 1963).

Professor Brodehl did not think it was likely that prenatal toxic substances might be responsible for the idiopathic types of FS since the biochemical defects usually started later, post-natally and could reappear in transplanted kidneys (Briggs *et al.*, *N. Engl. J. Med.*, **286**, 25, 1972).

DISCUSSION ON PAPER 14

Dr Smith observed that severe abnormalities of the eyes as described by Dr Carter were not usually seen in osteogenesis imperfecta. Corneal abnormalities did, however, occur in the recessively inherited hydroxylysine deficiency collagen disease, which in some respects could resemble osteogenesis imperfecta.

Dr Griffiths had seen four patients including two siblings, all blind from congenital abnormalities of the eye who were also suffering from osteogenesis imperfecta, diagnosed radiologically, and wondered if this association had been described.

Dr Smith reported that in the severe form of osteogenesis imperfecta with long bone deformity, severe scoliosis, often white sclerae and only occasional family history, the stability of the polymeric collagen of the skin was reduced, suggesting a defect of cross linking. There were many possibilities for inborn biochemical defects in collagen, and a defect in the formation of the α_1(I) chain of collagen had been described in osteogenesis imperfecta.

Dr Scriver said that he and his colleagues had studied the blue-eyed, antosomal dominant osteogenesis imperfecta phenotype in cultured skin fibroblasts. As predicted, hydroxylating enzymes, glycosylating enzymes and cross linking reactions were normal. This led them to look at collagen chain synthesis rates. The expected ratio of 2 : 1 was found for a $\alpha_1 : \alpha_2$ chains in OI fibroblasts. Of great interest was the discovery of a constant morphological defect in OI fibroblasts in early and late phase culture. Packing was poor and surface outline was not spindle-shaped in OI cells.

Professor Spranger recalled that in patients with metaphyseal chondrodysplasia and immunodeficiency a decreased activity of adenosine deaminase had been observed. In one of his patients, a marfanoid habitus, multiple spontaneous fractures and enchondromatous bone lesions were associated with a complete failure of cultured fibroblasts to produce α_2 collagen chains. In both cases the biochemical abnormality could be causally related to the phenotypic aberration demonstrating the range of metabolic pathways to be investigated in the study of bone dysplasias.

DISCUSSION ON PAPER 15

Dr Buist asked if the anatomic abnormalities (of collapsed vertebrae) recovered with the aid of orthopaedics.

Dr Blau wanted to know how this kind of osteoporosis related to that in astronauts exposed to weightlessness or indeed to that which occurred in sleep.

Mr Griffiths enquired if the teeth were affected.

Dr Scriver asked if there were any abnormal urinary peptides in idiopathic juvenile osteoporosis and if cultured skin fibroblasts could provide an insight into pathogenesis.

Professor Teller observed that sodium fluoride had been used in the treatment of osteoporosis with apparently unsatisfactory results. Did Dr Brenton have any experience of this treatment.

Dr Batstone thought it important to exclude other causes when looking at osteoporosis in this age group. He had seen two cases who, whilst not showing other features of Cushing's disease, or high plasma or urinary steroids, had high cortisol secretion rates.

Dr Kind wanted to know the reasons for the use of any drug therapy for a disease in which eventually there was full spontaneous recovery. Did Dr Brenton have data showing that treatment improved the condition of the patient and shortened the course of the disease.

Professor Clayton explained that the cortisol production rate (CPR) on Dr Brenton's severely affected patient Rita had been performed some years ago in her laboratories. It was certain that the CPR was raised. Apart from Cushing's syndrome which the child definitely did not have she had seen similar values in some very obese children, and she did not recall that the patient was overweight.

Dr Brenton in reply said that collapsed vertebrae did show increasing height during recovery in the milder cases (as illustrated) without any form of orthopaedic treatment but in the very severest cases with little recovery the vertebrae remain collapsed. He considered that weightlessness was a form of disuse and disuse and immobilisation aggravates all forms of osteoporosis. He had never noticed any dental abnormalities and had not deliberately looked for abnormal urinary peptides. In general, total hydroxyproline excretion in the urine was normal. However Dr Roger Smith (Oxford) had some unpublished studies on skin collagen suggesting that there might be some underlying collagen defect in idiopathic juvenile osteoporosis.

In reply to Professor Teller Dr Brenton said that sodium fluoride had not been used in any of their patients with IJO. Since the natural history of idiopathic juvenile osteoporosis was variable there could be no simple way of proving that the treatment regimes tried affect the outcome. However the improved calcium balances in some patients had been taken as an indication of a beneficial effect. The interesting comments of Dr Batstone and Professor Clayton provided perhaps indications for further investigations of adrenal cortical function.

DISCUSSION ON PAPER 16

Professor Stanbury explained that in the rat and chick high doses (40 mg/kg) of EHDP cause impaired intestinal transport of calcium and inhibition of $1,25(OH)_2D_3$ synthesis. According to Fleisch smaller doses (1 mg/kg) could actually stimulate calcium absorption and perhaps also formation of $1,25(OH)_2D_3$. These results were not relevant to clinical use, and his own observations on the effect of the drug in man as yet incomplete. As to the therapeutic use of the drug, Professor Stanbury thought that the unpredictable natural history of dermatomyositis made it virtually impossible to assess results. This experience in dermatomyositis, other forms of calcinosis and myositis ossificans suggested that conventional dosage (20 mg/kg) was completely without beneficial effect. On the other hand, the deleterious effects were clear. All chronically treated patients developed defective mineralisation with a form of osteomalacia, which was symptomatic in several patients and produced a fracture in one. Equally impressive was the development of proximal muscular weakness similar to that in vitamin D deficiency osteomalacia, which had led several patients to stop treatment spontaneously. In myositis ossificans the drug prevented calcification of the dystrophic bone but had no effect on the new formation of this dystrophic tissue. Thus evidence of a reduction in the radiographically evident dystrophic bone was illusory as an index of improvement since an actual increase of unmineralised new bone might occur during treatment with EHDP.

Professor DeLuca said that they had studied the effects of EHDP on vitamin D metabolism in the rat and chick. Prolonged doses of 20 mg/kg a day were required to block vitamin D metabolism. An oral dose of 20 mg/kg a day was equivalent to 1 mg/kg a day as not more than 5% was absorbed. This amount was unlikely to inhibit vitamin D metabolism unless man was surprisingly more sensitive than the chick and rat.

Dr Smith reported that in Oxford they had extensive experience of the use of EHDP in Paget's disease. They had also used it in dermatomyositis with calcinosis but in this condition the results were very difficult to assess because the calcification could regress spontaneously. He agreed with Professor Stanbury that in growing children on EHDP defective mineralisation and proximal myopathy could occur, but the mechanism was uncertain. In myositis ossificans progressiva he did not think the situation was as gloomy as it had been described.

Dr Steendijk recommended that patients treated with EHDP to remove ectopic bone should not be given corticosteroids or ACTH as these agents diminished bone turnover which was necessary for the effects of EHDP to materialise.

Dr Belton recognised that the comments made by Professor Stanbury and Professor DeLuca about the effects of EHDP on vitamin D and calcium metabolism were of importance. However, it was always difficult to compare animal studies with human data. In addition, the animal studies of Morgan *et al.* (1971) and of Hill and his co-workers (1973) were of relatively short duration, 7 and 14 days respectively. The production of negative calcium balance and the increase in faecal calcium in their patients were all shown after at least 3 months' EHDP administration. Russell (*Br. J. Hosp. Med.*, **14**, 297, 1975) suggested that the half-life of EHDP in bone in the rat was about 2–4 weeks so that accumulation of EHDP may build up in the body during long-term therapy. The conclusions of Bonjour *et al.* (1972) were of importance also. They found that *in vivo* intestinal perfusion in the rat revealed a decrease in net calcium absorption in EHDP treated rats and that the calcium-binding protein content of the duodenal mucosa as well as the duodenal brush border activities of Ca^{2+}ATPase and alkaline phosphatase were also decreased. They suggested that a specific mechanism was involved which adjusted calcium absorption when EHDP inhibited bone mineralisation. Thus low calcium absorption may be an example of adaptation in response to the decreased needs of the organism due to the incapacity of bone to utilise calcium.

Dr Belton agreed with Dr Smith that in dermatomyositis with calcinosis, results were difficult to assess. However, the X-rays (Figures 16.5 and 16.6) indicated the very marked reduction in ectopic calcification in case 2 which occurred during EHDP therapy.

In reply to Dr Steendijk, Dr Belton contended that as steroids are the prime form of management for the myopathy in dermatomyositis, it was not always clinically feasible to withhold steroids, even though it might be undesirable to give corticosteroids or ACTH when EHDP is being administered.

DISCUSSION ON PAPER 17

Dr Scriver asked if Dr Pennock had a marker to identify hypophosphatasia in his patients. The urine should contain phosphoethanolamine in the 'classical' and 'pseudohypophosphatasia' types. Hydroxyproline—in urine at least—was not elevated in osteogenesis imperfecta as had been originally reported.

Dr Buist wondered if delay in removal of the tissue after death affected its chemistry.

Professor Spranger explained that the chemistry of cartilage depends on the site of biopsy. Epiphyseal cartilage might differ in biochemical composition from metaphyseal cartilage. Since even the different cartilage layers of the growth plate may differ, a comparison of normal and patient data might be difficult. A correct clinical diagnosis appeared essential in the interpretation of the biochemical data.

Dr Pennock, in reply to Dr Scriver, stated that he had not had an opportunity to measure urinary phosphoethanolamine, as he had only received tissues post-mortem. However, he was certain that the label 'hypophosphatasia' was incorrect in this case, which lent support to Professor Spranger's comment about correct diagnosis being essential. The latter was likely to be extremely difficult in many bone dysplasias, since, in most cases, diagnosis was based on clinical and radiological description.

In reply to Dr Buist, he said that there were insufficient data in the present study to pass comment but he felt that, provided that the sample was collected and processed soon after post-mortem, there should be no difficulty.

DISCUSSION ON PAPER 18

Professor Harris asked if Dr Stamp had any data on plasma levels of phenobarbitone and phenytoin in the affected patients.

Professor Bickel recalled that one of Dr Stamp's patients needed 10 000 IU of D_3 daily to control his osteomalacia. In his experience, patients needed less D_3, about the same as in ordinary rickets. Variable requirements introduced problems into the prophylactic treatment as proposed. Would it suffice to treat only those patients who when attending as outpatients had abnormalities in calcium, phosphate and alkaline phosphatase.

Dr Brenton asked about parathyroid hormone levels in these patients. Raised levels in Dr Stamp's patient with the parathyroid adenoma suggested that such levels might be common, and the action of the hormone prevented by the drugs, as indicated in bone culture studies. This would perpetuate the hypocalcaemia and result in a bigger stimulus to PTH excretion.

Dr Steendijk wondered if the higher incidence of anticonvulsant induced osteomalacia and rickets in Great Britain compared to the Continent was related to vitamin D nutrition which in Britain was sub-optimal.

Dr Scheffner said that in his experience there were patients who responded to vitamin D and some (a minority amongst children) who did not. He suggested a genetic basis for the variability in response and asked if there was a relationship between vitamin D deficiency and the frequency of fits. Dr Scheffner referred to two patients of Professor Clayton with low calcium but normal PTH levels and wondered how often PTH levels were in fact altered in epileptic patients who developed rickets under treatment with anticonvulsant drugs.

Professor Clayton confirmed that she had seen two young patients with much reduced calcium levels and PTH concentrations which were low. These patients were found when a biochemical profile was performed on admission, hypocalcaemia had not been suspected by the clinicians.

Dr Stamp replied that plasma levels of phenobarbitone and phenytoin were rather poorly correlated either with dosage or with indices of enzyme induction such as serum glutamyl transferase or urinary D-glucaric acid. They were analysing extensive data from a survey of 47 patients.

They had not done a systematic comparison of vitamin D_2 and vitamin D_3 in their patients except in a few cases. Resistance to treatment seemed equally marked.

The parathyroid assay was probably not sensitive enough to detect minor elevations of circulating immunoreactive hormone. He was not aware of any reports of raised PTH levels amongst these patients.

Dr Stamp thought it necessary to differentiate anticonvulsant induced osteomalacia and rickets in Great Britain from classical vitamin D deficiency. The latter was a danger amongst patients whose out-door activity was curtailed especially if they were institutionalised. Dietary intake of vitamin D could be low since there was no systematic fortification of foods. It was very difficult to be certain that drugs were responsible for the disease unless some degree of resistance to treatment could be demonstrated.

An anticonvulsant action of vitamin D in epileptic patients had been claimed by Christiansen *et al.* (*Br. Med. J.*, **2**, 258, 1974). One of his patients certainly required much less anticonvulsant therapy when his rickets was cured.

DISCUSSION ON PAPERS 19 AND 20

Dr Wadman asked if any increase in saccharopine had been observed after loading with lysine, and if the patients had metabolic acidosis.

Dr Gompertz wondered about the extractibility of α-ketoadipic acid into organic solvents, and the derivative formed with diazomethane. He agreed with Dr Gerritsen that a mutation affecting the active site for α-aminoadipic acid in the transamination was unlikely. He felt that as the SD of the Stanford Binet Test was 15 to 16 points an IQ of 86 should not be regarded as subnormal.

Dr Watts said that α-ketoadipic acid was extracted on to DEAE Sephadex.

Dr Winokur wanted to know what had prompted Dr Gerritsen to look for α-aminoadipic acid in the urine, and what the clinical features of the patient had been.

Professor Bickel asked if either of Dr Gerritsen's patients had evidence of minimal or moderate brain damage, as Dr Bremer's patient was retarded.

Professor Clayton asked if Dr Bremer's patient always had a positive DNP test. If this test was only periodically positive, were there any precipitating factors.

Professor Tada enquired about the level of the metabolites in the CSF. Blood levels essentially reflected disturbance of liver metabolism. In his case of hyperpyruvic acidaemia with severe mental defect the levels of lactic and pyruvic acids in CSF were found to be higher than in blood. The relationship of CSF levels and clinical symptoms was of interest.

Dr Scriver was impressed by the fact that Dr Bremer had identified his patient by the simple DNP screening test. He would be surprised if basal lysine and saccharopine levels were elevated since the enzyme in the pathway saccharopine to α-aminoadipate does not function significantly in the reverse direction in human tissues. Bonner's work with neurospora tryptophan pyrnolase showed that binding of pyridoxal phosphate could be affected while that of substrate remained unchanged. Study of the aminotransferase should include a search for cytosol and mitochondrial activators in normal and mutant fibroblasts.

Professor Bremer replied that his patient had a positive DNP test during the neonatal period. Afterwards the DNP test was only periodically positive. Precipitating factors were not detectable. An investigation of the metabolites of the cerebrospinal fluid had not been performed. The increase of the basal lysine levels could not be explained by a reverse direction of the degradative pathway. There had to be other regulative mechanisms influencing lysine uptake or degradation at an earlier stage. In their experience a positive DNP test during the neonatal period should be regarded as a strong indication of congenital metabolic disorders, as there was among these patients a high frequency of metabolic diseases, e.g. maple syrup urine disease, glycogenosis type I, pyruvate dehydrogenase deficiency, glutaric aciduria.

DISCUSSION ON PAPER 21

Dr Schmidt said that in her unit after preliminary classification based on clinical signs, data from sibs and phenylalanine levels on a normal diet, the following parameters were correlated with the initial diagnosis:

(1) a protein load of 180 mg/kg for 3 days
(2) a phenylalanine load of 0·1 g/kg in a single dose superimposed on the (usually restricted) diet
(3) phenylalanine hydroxylase assay
(4) urinary metabolites of phenylalanine
(5) heterozygote tests in parents

The best discrimination between phenylketonuria and hyperphenylalaninaemia was obtained by the protein load, where there was no overlap in phenylalanine values after 72 hours. In the single load test the 24-hour value was most useful, but not conclusive, because of the difficulties in standardising the conditions. Patients with hyperphenylalaninaemia were not treated but kept under observation. They had seen a few patients of the Blaskovics type III variant in whom the biochemical abnormalities produce mental retardation in some and allow normal development in other cases.

Professor Tada presented a family with hyperphenylalaninaemia (serum levels 8–13 mg/100 ml) and the results of load tests, and liver phenylalanine hydroxylase assays. In contrast to PKU, slight enzyme activity was demonstrated. Professor Tada suggested that the persistent form of hyperphenylalaninaemia was a genetic variant of PKU. As the siblings had borderline IQs he advocated treatment, particularly in infancy, if the blood phenylalanine level exceeds 10 mg/100 ml.

Dr Scriver pointed out that some individuals excrete PPA at blood phenylalanine levels as low as 0·75 mM, most at 1 mM (16·5 mg/100 ml) and nearly 100% by 1·75–2 mM indicating individual variation in transaminase activity. Furthermore, transaminase activity is inducible.

Dr Winokur said that there were almost as many classifications as there were writers on the subject. The only constant abnormality was the raised blood phenylalanine. The results of treatment were judged by whether or not subnormality developed. All the IQs quoted here had fallen within the normal range. The IQ could and did fluctuate. The cut-off point between normality and subnormality was 70 and not just any figure below 100.

Dr Woolf wondered if Dr Toothill had used a sufficiently sensitive method for estimating PPA such as the borate–arsenate method or ether extraction and colorimetry. The ferric chloride and dinitrophenylhydrazine (visual) screening tests were insensitive, the latter unreliable at low concentrations because of the solubility of the hydrazone.

Dr Blau had used gas chromatography to measure phenylpyruvic, phenyllactic and *o*-hydroxyphenylacetic acids, all of which appeared at the same blood phenylalanine threshold. There was evidence of two populations with thresholds at 8 and 16 mg/100 ml respectively. Could one speculate that patients with a higher threshold were better protected against the toxic effects of hyperphenylalaninaemia, and that the aromatic acids were incriminated as toxic metabolites.

Dr Buist said that in discussing fasting blood phenylalanine levels the phenylalanine intake should be specified not only for patients on a restricted diet but also for those on a free diet.

Dr Holton suggested that if different thresholds exist this might arise from an altered distribution of phenylalanine between blood and cells rather than from an altered threshold for induction of enzymes.

Dr Watts asked how frequently the author had checked blood phenylalanine levels before arriving at a definite classification. He felt that aromatic acids should be studied by quantitative gas chromatography avoiding extraction into organic solvents. Aromatic acids had high renal clearances. Could renal factors, particularly maturation of renal function, play a part during early life.

Professor Bickel questioned if Dr Toothill's treatment levels had been satisfactory. In case 5, levels of 12–18 mg/100 ml had been mentioned. In his experience such levels were not without danger for the developing brain. Even if the child appeared normal, mild brain damage might not manifest itself as a serious disadvantage until the child was at school.

Dr Blaskovics thought that the methods used by the author, while helpful, were not fully adequate. Some differences in the plasma levels could be related to differences in phenylalanine intake rather than altered enzyme activity. Lack of standardisation in classification between centres and countries had caused confusion regarding prognosis, duration of treatment, etc. In Los Angeles, studies had been initiated in which the response to a standard intake of phenylalanine was used to assess variability in clinically dissimilar groups. All patients received 180 mg/kg/24 h for three days. Patients seemed to divide into five groups, types I–V. Types I and II were true PKU and had to be treated; type III was atypical PKU, and although not necessarily associated with mental retardation, should as a precaution also be treated. Types IV and V correspond to what had been called hyperphenylalaninaemia and, he thought, did not require treatment. When, very rarely, retardation was found, patients were as those described by Professor Clayton and Dr Bartholomé, that is even with early diagnosis and adequate treatment they did not follow the course of PKU. He felt he could not treat 95% of patients unnecessarily for the sake of 5% (probably less) who might be retarded for reasons unrelated to phenylalanine levels. For fuller details, see Blaskovics, *Clin. Endocrinol. Metab.*, **3**, 87, 1974.

DISCUSSION ON PAPER 22

Dr Scriver said that the present assay for phenylalanine hydroxylase was precise but restricted to measurement only of the apoprotein catalysing conversion of phenylalanine to tyrosine. There was unequivocal evidence for genetic heterogeneity at the hydroxylase gene locus. Small residual activity could convert a phenotype requiring treatment to one who did not. The PKU patients with normal hydroxylase activity could have a defect in the enzyme regenerating tetrahydrobiopterin, the cofactor for the hydroxylase. Genetic heterogeneity at two loci might have to be invoked in some patients to explain the phenylketonuria.

Professor Clayton had seen three cases who were originally thought to have classical PKU, but who died after profound neurological degeneration. The youngest of these patients was treated with a satisfactory phenylalanine-low diet, and his liver hydroxylase activity was normal. The enzyme defect in these patients would in due course be classified but even if more was learnt about the enzymic activities in PKU the cause of the brain damage was still unknown.

Dr Buist wondered if use of phenylalanine concentrations higher than 0·2 mM might reveal high K_m variants.

Dr Blau suggested that the clinical course in the patients of Dr Bartholomé and Professor Clayton might be explained by a defect in dihydropteridine reductase, as had been implied. This system also provides reduced biopterin cofactor for tyrosine hydroxylase, the rate-limiting step in catecholamine synthesis, and for tryptophan hydroxylase, rate-limiting for serotonin biosynthesis. Any deficiency in these putative neurotransmitters could be a grave insult to the organism. Dr Watts predicted that we might have to look for the 'K_m mutants' for the cofactors as well as for phenylalanine.

Dr Bartholomé in reply to Dr Buist explained that the reason for using 0·1 mM phenylalanine in the assay was technical. Increasing the amount of labelled phenylalanine increased the background radiation in the thin layer chromatography. On the other hand, an increase in the amount of unlabelled phenylalanine caused a relative decrease in the quantity of labelled tyrosine formed, thereby decreasing the sensitivity.

DISCUSSION ON PAPER 23

Dr Blau offered facilitated phenylalanine transamination with normal phenylalanine hydroxylase as an explanation of Dr Wadman's data. There might be a classical Hardy–Weinberg equilibrium with the transaminase segregating independently of the hydroxylase locus: one could postulate a large population of normal homozygotes with high threshold. The affected PKU patients (and other non-PKU subjects) were heterozygotes with intermediate threshold and Dr Wadman's patient homozygous for the mutant gene with an extremely low threshold.

Professor Bickel wondered if the fact that the patient was mentally normal implied that brain damage is not due to phenylpyruvic, phenyllactic or *o*-hydroxyphenylacetic acid, increased in this patient as well as in true PKU.

Professor Tada thought that the clinical course was evidence that phenylpyruvic acid and the other metabolites are not toxic to the developing brain.

Dr Buist agreed that a low K_m transmaninase might be present. The IQ could be normal because the mutant enzyme was not present in the brain so that no increase in phenylpyruvate was produced there. If the mutant enzyme were present in muscle several amino acid transaminations might be affected. This would not necessarily be obvious *in vivo* as the reaction products might be metabolised.

Dr Wadman replied that as far as he knew phenylalanine transamination is non-specific. One possible explanation of the accumulation of phenylpyruvic acid could be enhanced transamination at low phenylalanine levels due to a transaminase with low K_m for phenylalanine and high or normal K_m for phenylpyruvate. However, it was improbable that a mutation of a non-specific transaminase would affect only its affinity for phenylalanine. They had not seen accumulation of other ketoacids. Another possibility was defective decarboxylation of phenylpyruvic acid but a specific phenylpyruvate decarboxylase had never been demonstrated in man. He thought that the concentration of phenylpyruvic, phenyllactic and *o*-hydroxyphenylacetic acids might be too low to cause damage to the brain or to disturb its normal development.

DISCUSSION ON PAPER 24

Professor Dent asked if after 4-methoxyphenylalanine loading much of the compound appeared in the urine.

Dr Allan was interested in the application of the method to cystic fibrosis. He had used an amino acid hydrolysate as part of an artificial diet for over 5 years. In patients on orthodox therapy plasma amino acid levels were lower than normal with no characteristic pattern. On the diet the pattern reverted to normal. He believed that protein hydrolysates should be used in cystic fibrosis and that their apparent relative failure in absorption was not intrinsic to the hydrolysate but more likely related to contamination with an as yet unknown antigen in the ordinary diet, possibly involved in an immunological reaction at gut level interfering with normal absorptive function.

Dr Scriver pointed out some difficulties in the interpretation of plasma response curves. Up-slope and peak height might largely reflect absorption, but peak height and down-slope also reflected distribution and disposal through various pools in series. The Hartnup data with a steep down-slope, perhaps because of rapid renal loss, seemed clear enough in their message about absorption, however, he remained worried that absorption data obtained with this method might be over interpreted. He still preferred measurement of net disappearance rates to plasma response data, even if the latter were done as well as in this study.

Dr Gompertz asked if anaerobic bacteria as found in the 'stagnant loop' or 'contaminated bowel' syndrome could demethylate the test substance.

Professor Bickel asked if 4-methoxyphenyl-L-alanine absorption had been tested in other diseases, not mentioned so far.

Dr Wadman enquired about the fate of unabsorbed methoxyphenylalanine. Bacterial metabolites might be formed and excreted in the urine.

Dr Brenton wondered how much of the unaltered substance appeared in the urine. Could it interfere with the renal tubular reabsorption of tyrosine or phenylalanine.

Dr Watts wanted to know if *p*-methoxyphenylalanine inhibits phenylalanine hydroxylase, also if animals had been studied at different ages to see if age altered absorption. While not directly relevant to man this would be helpful information in the absence of human controls. Studies with stable isotopes were not always physiological in terms of dose, route of administration, etc. The speaker had not mentioned the use of ^{3}H as a tracer, which had a shorter half life and softer β-emission than ^{14}C.

Dr Seakins replied that *in vivo* studies in rats indicated that renal reabsorption of 4-methoxyphenylalanine was similar to that of tyrosine (Huang, *J. Pharmacol. Exp. Ther.*, **134**, 257, 1961). Urine samples collected from an adult after a loading dose (25 mg/kg) contained only trace amounts (approx. 40 mg 4-methoxyphenylalanine/24 h). The excretion of phenylalanine and tyrosine was not affected.

Deductions from plasma response curves were based not on decay slopes but on maximum values achieved and the time of the maximum.

Dr Seakins anticipated that in common with other aromatic amino acids unabsorbed 4-methoxyphenylalanine would undergo decarboxylation. Some of the product would be absorbed and oxidised in the liver to *p*-methoxyphenylacetic acid. The metabolism of this compound was not fully understood (Oakley and Seakins, *Biochem. J.*, **121**, 17P, 1970).

There was no evidence that 4-methoxyphenylalanine inhibited phenylalanine hydroxylase *in vivo*. Fasting phenylalanine/tyrosine ratios and fasting phenylalanine levels remained constant or fell slightly during tests on now over 60 patients.

DISCUSSION ON PAPER 25

Professor Bickel accepted that 40–50% of histidinaemic patients were liable to suffer brain damage, and advocated, therefore, that every histidinaemic infant should receive dietary treatment. Problems might arise if at a later age histidine ceased to be an essential amino acid. Was there any evidence that this happened in childhood.

Dr Wadman recalled that in a histidinaemic boy aged 11–12 years blood histidine levels could be normalised by dietary restriction.

Professor Clayton had used a low histidine diet in several children in the early days of her interest in this condition. Amongst them was a 12-year-old boy who was presumably approaching the age when histidine may not be essential. With the diet, the blood histidine level was lowered, but there was no clinical change. In co-operation with Dr Brian Neville they were screening about 100 000 infants a year in London for histidinaemia, and had found an incidence of 1 in 14 000 to 1 in 16 000. In all, 19 histidinaemic infants had been followed for up to 3 years. On repeated neurological examination only one infant showed abnormal development and he had a 60% decibel hearing loss. The remainder had a distribution of abilities one might expect to find when any series of young children are examined. So far they had no evidence that biochemical histidinaemia resulted in any clinical condition, and nothing to suggest that their decision not to treat these infants had been wrong.

Dr Scriver contrasted the attitudes to the treatment of phenylketonuria and histidinaemia, and supported the view that with care, special diets need not be harmful. Data from Massachusetts (Levy, Shih and Madigan, *N. Engl. J. Med.*, **291,** 1214, 1974) also suggested that in histidinaemia assessment could be overoptimistic. Here the relevance of animal experiments was important. The experimental results presented were clear cut, but was the model real, because the main metabolic pathway for histidine was flooded whereas, in the disease, it was blocked. Biochemical *and* psychological evaluation was needed and such studies were full of pitfalls. Dr Scriver advocated prospective collaborative studies concerning the need for and possible efficacy of the treatment in histidinaemia.

Dr Gompertz stressed the psychological risks to child and family inherent in the use of semi-synthetic diets which involved isolation of the patient from the rest of the family during meal times. We should not lightly place a group of children on semi-synthetic diets for a biochemical condition which may cause no physical damage.

Dr Holton, in reply, accepted that these animal experiments could not provide a true model for histidinaemia. Nevertheless, the acute studies did show that high levels of histidine in the blood affect the transport of amino acids into the brain. Further work in the immature animal, at a time later than one hour after histidine injection, may give some indication of the effects of a more sustained rise in brain histidine.

DISCUSSION ON PAPER 26

Professor Bickel asked when cataract formation starts in galactokinase deficiency. Were there congenital cataracts as in transferase deficiency, and if so, was prenatal diagnosis indicated so that the mother could perhaps be treated with a galactose-free diet during the second half of her pregnancy.

Dr Carson enquired if early dietary treatment could prevent formation of cataracts in galactokinase deficiency.

Dr Lutz reported that in uridyl transferase deficiency they had always found raised levels of direct reacting (glucuronic acid linked) bilirubin. Was this also the case in galactokinase deficiency?

Dr Scriver thought the yield of homozygote ascertainment in screening for galactokinase deficiency would certainly be low. Heterozygote screening would be of greater interest if technically feasible. It had been reported that maternal heterozygotes gave birth with increased frequency to offspring with congenital cataracts. Heterozygote screening could play a part in cataract prevention if dietary treatment in pregnancy proved effective. Had the authors considered treating heterozygous women in their pedigree during their pregnancies.

Dr Blau suggested that if we were ever to prevent the appearance of homozygous patients with inborn errors of metabolism that have to be treated, detection of heterozygotes would have to be practised on a large scale so that at risk marriages could be ascertained before the birth of affected homozygotes.

Dr Carnevale replied to Professor Bickel and Dr Carson that in their case bilateral cataracts were diagnosed at $5\frac{1}{2}$ months but failing vision was noticed earlier by the parents. Cataract formation was observed as early as 3 weeks of age by Thalhammer *et al.* (1968) and Dahlquist *et al.* (1970). Dietary galactose restriction is effective in preventing cataracts and even regression of lens opacities has been reported when treatment was begun at 4–6 weeks of age (Thalhammer *et al.*, 1968; Linnevah *et al.*, 1970; Dahlquist *et al.*, 1971; Cook *et al.*, 1971). In fact, under dietary control new lens fibres should develop normally and unruptured old ones might clear. Prenatal diagnosis of the disorder while desirable was not technically feasible on a large scale at present. The efficacy of a galactose-free diet in pregnant heterozygotes required further investigation.

As to bilirubin levels, in their case they were only told about a 'severe and protracted jaundice'. High levels of unconjugated bilirubin were, however, reported in the cases of Kerr *et al.* (1971) and Cook *et al.* (1971). He considered that the association of galactokinase deficiency and neonatal jaundice was incidental.

They had been able to examine only two women in their pedigree, the mother and sister of the propositus. Both had low galactokinase levels in their blood but normal visual acuity. However, slit lamp examination revealed slight opacities in the lens of the mother who is currently under dietary treatment.

DISCUSSION ON PAPER 27

Dr Brenton asked if it was the authors' experience that in treating patients with homocystinuria the sequence of events was usually that the homocystine diminished before the mixed disulphide, and that the plasma cystine concentration only rose as homocystine and the mixed disulphide disappeared.

Dr Sardharwalla replied that there was probably no mechanism for removing the homocystine–cystine disulphide once formed in the body except excretion by the kidney. This might explain why the fall in 'mixed disulphide' lagged behind that of homocystine. Their studies showed that so long as homocystine and mixed disulphide were present in the plasma it was difficult to achieve normal plasma cystine levels.

Index